BATES'
Pocket Guide to
Physical Examination
and History Taking

BATES'
Pocket Guide to Physical Examination and History Taking

Seventh Edition

Lynn S. Bickley, MD, FACP
Clinical Professor of Internal Medicine
School of Medicine
University of New Mexico
Albuquerque, New Mexico

Peter G. Szilagyi, MD, MPH
Professor of Pediatrics
Chief, Division of General Pediatrics
University of Rochester School of Medicine and Dentistry
Rochester, New York

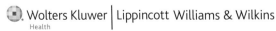

Wolters Kluwer | Lippincott Williams & Wilkins
Health
Philadelphia · Baltimore · New York · London
Buenos Aires · Hong Kong · Sydney · Tokyo

Acquisitions Editor: Elizabeth Nieginski/Susan Rhyner
Product Manager: Annette Ferran
Editorial Assistant: Ashley Fischer
Design Coordinator: Joan Wendt
Art Director, Illustration: Brett MacNaughton
Manufacturing Coordinator: Karin Duffield
Indexer: Angie Allen
Prepress Vendor: Aptara, Inc.

7th Edition

Copyright © 2013 Wolters Kluwer Health | Lippincott Williams & Wilkins.
Copyright © 2009 by Wolters Kluwer Health | Lippincott Williams & Wilkins. Copyright © 2007, 2004, 2000 by Lippincott Williams & Wilkins. Copyright © 1995, 1991 by J. B. Lippincott Company. All rights reserved. This book is protected by copyright. No part of this book may be reproduced or transmitted in any form or by any means, including as photocopies or scanned-in or other electronic copies, or utilized by any information storage and retrieval system without written permission from the copyright owner, except for brief quotations embodied in critical articles and reviews. Materials appearing in this book prepared by individuals as part of their official duties as U.S. government employees are not covered by the above-mentioned copyright. To request permission, please contact Lippincott Williams & Wilkins at Two Commerce Square, 2001 Market Street, Philadelphia PA 19103, via email at permissions@lww.com or via website at lww.com (products and services).

9 8 7 6 5 4 3 2 1

Printed in China

Library of Congress Cataloging-in-Publication Data

Bickley, Lynn S.
 Bates' pocket guide to physical examination and history taking / Lynn S. Bickley, Peter G. Szilagyi. — 7th ed.
   p. ; cm.
 Pocket guide to physical examination and history taking
 Abridgement of: Bates' guide to physical examination and history-taking. 11th ed. / Lynn S. Bickley, Peter G. Szilagyi. c2013.

 Includes bibliographical references and index.
 Summary: "This concise pocket-sized guide presents the classic Bates approach to physical examination and history taking in a quick-reference outline format. It contains all the critical information needed to obtain a clinically meaningful health history and to conduct a thorough physical assessment. Fully revised and updated, the Seventh Edition will help health professionals elicit relevant facts from the patient's history, review examination procedures, highlight common findings, learn special assessment techniques, and sharpen interpretive skills. The book features a vibrant full-color art program and an easy-to-follow two-column format with step-by-step examination techniques on the left and abnormalities with differential diagnoses on the right."—Provided by publisher.

 ISBN 978-1-4511-7322-2 (pbk. : alk. paper)
 I. Bates, Barbara, 1928-2002. II. Szilagyi, Peter G. III. Bickley, Lynn S. Bates' guide to physical examination and history-taking. IV. Title. V. Title: Pocket guide to physical examination and history taking.
 [DNLM: 1. Physical Examination—methods—Handbooks. 2. Medical History Taking—methods—Handbooks. WB 39]
 616.07'51—dc23   2012030529

 Care has been taken to confirm the accuracy of the information presented and to describe generally accepted practices. However, the authors, editors, and publisher are not responsible for errors or omissions or for any consequences from application of the information in this book and make no warranty, expressed or implied, with respect to the currency, completeness, or accuracy of the contents of the publication. Application of this information in a particular situation remains the professional responsibility of the practitioner; the clinical treatments described and recommended may not be considered absolute and universal recommendations.
 The authors, editors, and publisher have exerted every effort to ensure that drug selection and dosage set forth in this text are in accordance with the current recommendations and practice at the time of publication. However, in view of ongoing research, changes in government regulations, and the constant flow of information relating to drug therapy and drug reactions, the reader is urged to check the package insert for each drug for any change in indications and dosage and for added warnings and precautions. This is particularly important when the recommended agent is a new or infrequently employed drug.
 Some drugs and medical devices presented in this publication have Food and Drug Administration (FDA) clearance for limited use in restricted research settings. It is the responsibility of the health care provider to ascertain the FDA status of each drug or device planned for use in his or her clinical practice.

LWW.COM

*To Randolph B. Schiffer, for lifelong care and support,
and to students world-wide committed to clinical excellence.*

Introduction

The *Pocket Guide to Physical Examination and History Taking*, 7th edition is a concise, portable text that:

- Describes how to interview the patient and take the health history.
- Provides an illustrated review of the physical examination.
- Reminds students of common, normal, and abnormal physical findings.
- Describes special techniques of assessment that students may need in specific instances.
- Provides succinct aids to interpretation of selected findings.

There are several ways to use the *Pocket Guide*:

- To review and remember the content of a health history.
- To review and rehearse the techniques of examination. This can be done while learning a single section and again while combining the approaches to several body systems or regions into an integrated examination (see Chap. 1).
- To review common variations of normal and selected abnormalities. Observations are keener and more precise when the examiner knows what to look, listen, and feel for.
- To look up special techniques as the need arises. Maneuvers such as The Timed Get Up and Go test are included in the Special Techniques sections in each chapter.
- To look up additional information about possible findings, including abnormalities and standards of normal.

The *Pocket Guide* is not intended to serve as a primary text for learning the skills of history taking or physical examination. Its detail is too brief for these purposes. It is intended instead as an aid for student review and recall and as a convenient, brief, and portable reference.

Contents

CHAPTER 1 **Overview: Physical Examination and History Taking** 1

CHAPTER 2 **Clinical Reasoning, Assessment, and Recording Your Findings** 15

CHAPTER 3 **Interviewing and the Health History** 31

CHAPTER 4 **Beginning the Physical Examination: General Survey, Vital Signs, and Pain** 49

CHAPTER 5 **Behavior and Mental Status** 67

CHAPTER 6 **The Skin, Hair, and Nails** 83

CHAPTER 7 **The Head and Neck** 99

CHAPTER 8 **The Thorax and Lungs** 127

CHAPTER 9 **The Cardiovascular System** 147

CHAPTER 10 **The Breasts and Axillae** 167

CHAPTER 11 **The Abdomen** 179

CHAPTER 12 **The Peripheral Vascular System** 199

CHAPTER 13 **Male Genitalia and Hernias** 211

CHAPTER 14 **Female Genitalia** 225

CHAPTER 15 **The Anus, Rectum, and Prostate** 241

CHAPTER 16 **The Musculoskeletal System** 251

CHAPTER 17 **The Nervous System** 285

CHAPTER 18 **Assessing Children: Infancy Through Adolescence** 323

CHAPTER 19 **The Pregnant Woman** 359

CHAPTER 20 **The Older Adult** 373

Index 395

CHAPTER 1

Overview: Physical Examination and History Taking

This chapter provides a road map to clinical proficiency in two critical areas: the health history and the physical examination.

For adults, the comprehensive history includes *Identifying Data and Source of the History, Chief Complaint(s), Present Illness, Past History, Family History, Personal and Social History,* and *Review of Systems.* New patients in the office or hospital merit a *comprehensive health history;* however, in many situations, a more flexible *focused,* or *problem-oriented, interview* is appropriate. The components of the comprehensive health history structure the patient's story and the format of your written record, but the order shown below should not dictate the sequence of the interview. The interview is more fluid and should follow the patient's leads and cues, as described in Chapter 3.

Overview: Components of the Adult Health History

Identifying Data	▸ *Identifying data*—such as age, gender, occupation, marital status
	▸ *Source of the history*—usually the patient, but can be a family member or friend, letter of referral, or the medical record
	▸ If appropriate, establish *source of referral* because a written report may be needed
Reliability	▸ Varies according to the patient's memory, trust, and mood
Chief Complaint(s)	▸ The one or more symptoms or concerns causing the patient to seek care

(continued)

Overview: Components of the Adult Health History (continued)

Present Illness	▸ Amplifies the *Chief Complaint*; describes how each symptom developed
	▸ Includes patient's thoughts and feelings about the illness
	▸ Pulls in relevant portions of the *Review of Systems*, called "pertinent positives and negatives" (see p. 3)
	▸ May include *medications*, *allergies*, habits of *smoking* and *alcohol*, which frequently are pertinent to the present illness
Past History	▸ Lists childhood illnesses
	▸ Lists adult illnesses with dates for at least four categories: medical, surgical, obstetric/gynecologic, and psychiatric
	▸ Includes health maintenance practices such as immunizations, screening tests, lifestyle issues, and home safety
Family History	▸ Outlines or diagrams age and health, or age and cause of death, of siblings, parents, and grandparents
	▸ Documents presence or absence of specific illnesses in family, such as hypertension, coronary artery disease, etc.
Personal and Social History	▸ Describes educational level, family of origin, current household, personal interests, and lifestyle
Review of Systems	▸ Documents presence or absence of common symptoms related to each major body system

Be sure to distinguish *subjective* from *objective* data. Decide if your assessment will be comprehensive or focused.

Subjective Data	Objective Data
What the patient tells you	What you detect during the examination
The history, from Chief Complaint through Review of Systems	All physical examination findings

The Comprehensive Adult Health History

As you elicit the adult health history, be sure to include the following: date and time of history; identifying data, which include age, gender, marital status, and occupation; and reliability, which reflects the quality of information the patient provides.

Chapter 1 | Overview: Physical Examination and History Taking

 ## CHIEF COMPLAINT(S)

Quote the patient's own words. "My stomach hurts and I feel awful"; or "I have come for my regular check-up."

 ## PRESENT ILLNESS

This section is a complete, clear, and chronologic account of the problems prompting the patient to seek care. It should include the problem's onset, the setting in which it has developed, its manifestations, and any treatments.

Every principal symptom should be well characterized, with descriptions of the seven features listed below and *pertinent positives* and *negatives* from relevant areas of the Review of Systems that help clarify the *differential diagnosis*.

> **The Seven Attributes of Every Symptom**
>
> - Location
> - Quality
> - Quantity or severity
> - Timing, including onset, duration, and frequency
> - Setting in which it occurs
> - Aggravating and relieving factors
> - Associated manifestations

In addition, list **medications**, including name, dose, route, and frequency of use; **allergies**, including *specific reactions* to each medication; **tobacco** use; and **alcohol** and **drug** use.

 ## HISTORY

List **childhood illnesses**, then list **adult illnesses** in each of four areas:

- *Medical* (e.g., diabetes, hypertension, hepatitis, asthma, HIV), with dates of onset; also information about hospitalizations with dates; number and gender of sexual partners; risky sexual practices

- *Surgical* (dates, indications, and types of operations)

- *Obstetric/gynecologic* (obstetric history, menstrual history, birth control, and sexual function)

- *Psychiatric* (illness and time frame, diagnoses, hospitalizations, and treatments)

Also discuss **Health Maintenance**, including *immunizations,* such as tetanus, pertussis, diphtheria, polio, measles, rubella, mumps, influenza, varicella, hepatitis B, *Haemophilus influenzae* type b, pneumococcal vaccine, and herpes zoster vaccine; and *screening tests,* such as tuberculin tests, Pap smears, mammograms, stool tests, for occult blood colonoscopy, and cholesterol tests, together with the results and the dates they were last performed.

FAMILY HISTORY

Outline or diagram the age and health, or age and cause of death, of each immediate relative, including grandparents, parents, siblings, children, and grandchildren. Record the following conditions as either *present or absent* in the family: hypertension, coronary artery disease, elevated cholesterol levels, stroke, diabetes, thyroid or renal disease, cancer (specify type), arthritis, tuberculosis, asthma or lung disease, headache, seizure disorder, mental illness, suicide, alcohol or drug addiction, and allergies, as well as conditions that the patient reports.

PERSONAL AND SOCIAL HISTORY

Include occupation and the last year of schooling; home situation and significant others; sources of stress, both recent and long term; important life experiences, such as military service; leisure activities; religious affiliation and spiritual beliefs; and activities of daily living (ADLs). Also include lifestyle habits such as *exercise* and *diet, safety measures,* and *alternative health care* practices.

REVIEW OF SYSTEMS (ROS)

These "yes/no" questions go from "head to toe" and conclude the interview. Selected sections can also clarify the Chief Complaint; for example, the respiratory ROS helps characterize the symptom of cough. Start with a fairly general question. This allows you to shift to more specific questions about systems that may be of concern. For example, "How are your ears and hearing?" "How about your lungs and breathing?" "Any trouble with your heart?" "How is your digestion?" The *Review of Systems* questions may uncover problems that the patient overlooked. *Remember to move major health events to the Present Illness or Past History in your write-up.*

Some clinicians do the *Review of Systems* during the physical examination. If the patient has only a few symptoms, this combination can be efficient but may disrupt the flow of both the history and the examination.

General. Usual weight, recent weight change, clothing that fits more tightly or loosely than before; weakness, fatigue, fever.

Skin. Rashes, lumps, sores, itching, dryness, color change; changes in hair or nails; changes in size or color of moles.

Head, Eyes, Ears, Nose, Throat (HEENT). *Head:* Headache, head injury, dizziness, lightheadedness. *Eyes:* Vision, glasses or contact lenses, last examination, pain, redness, excessive tearing, double or blurred vision, spots, specks, flashing lights, glaucoma, cataracts. *Ears:* Hearing, tinnitus, vertigo, earache, infection, discharge. If hearing is decreased, use or nonuse of hearing aid. *Nose and sinuses:* Frequent colds, nasal stuffiness, discharge or itching, hay fever, nosebleeds, sinus trouble. *Throat (or mouth and pharynx):* Condition of teeth and gums; bleeding gums; dentures, if any, and how they fit; last dental examination; sore tongue; dry mouth; frequent sore throats; hoarseness.

Neck. Lumps, "swollen glands," goiter, pain, stiffness.

Breasts. Lumps, pain or discomfort, nipple discharge, self-examination practices.

Respiratory. Cough, sputum (color, quantity), hemoptysis, dyspnea, wheezing, pleurisy, last chest x-ray. You may wish to include asthma, bronchitis, emphysema, pneumonia, and tuberculosis.

Cardiovascular. "Heart trouble," hypertension, rheumatic fever, heart murmurs, chest pain or discomfort, palpitations, dyspnea, orthopnea, paroxysmal nocturnal dyspnea, edema, past electrocardiographic or other cardiovascular tests.

Gastrointestinal. Trouble swallowing, heartburn, appetite, nausea. Bowel movements, color and size of stools, change in bowel habits, rectal bleeding or black or tarry stools, hemorrhoids, constipation, diarrhea. Abdominal pain, food intolerance, excessive belching or passing of gas. Jaundice, liver or gallbladder trouble, hepatitis.

Peripheral Vascular. Intermittent claudication; leg cramps; varicose veins; past clots in veins; swelling in calves, legs, or feet; color change in fingertips or toes during cold weather; swelling with redness or tenderness.

Urinary. Frequency of urination, polyuria, nocturia, urgency, burning or pain on urination, hematuria, urinary infections, kidney stones, incontinence; in males, reduced caliber or force of urinary stream, hesitancy, dribbling.

Genital. *Male:* Hernias, discharge from or sores on penis, testicular pain or masses, history of sexually transmitted infections (STIs) or diseases (STDs) and treatments, testicular self-examination practices. Sexual habits, interest, function, satisfaction, birth control methods, condom use, problems. Concerns about HIV infection. *Female:* Age at menarche; regularity, frequency, and duration of periods; amount of bleeding, bleeding between periods or after intercourse, last menstrual period; dysmenorrhea, premenstrual tension. Age at menopause, menopausal symptoms, postmenopausal bleeding. In patients born before 1971, exposure to diethylstilbestrol (DES) from maternal use during pregnancy. Vaginal discharge, itching, sores, lumps, STIs and treatments. Number of pregnancies, number and type of deliveries, number of abortions (spontaneous and induced), complications of pregnancy, birth control methods. Sexual preference, interest, function, satisfaction, problems (including dyspareunia). Concerns about HIV infection.

Musculoskeletal. Muscle or joint pain, stiffness, arthritis, gout, backache. If present, describe location of affected joints or muscles, any swelling, redness, pain, tenderness, stiffness, weakness, or limitation of motion or activity; include timing of symptoms (e.g., morning or evening), duration, and any history of trauma. Neck or low back pain. Joint pain with systemic features such as fever, chills, rash, anorexia, weight loss, or weakness.

Psychiatric. Nervousness; tension; mood, including depression, memory change, suicide attempts, if relevant.

Neurologic. Changes in mood, attention, or speech; changes in orientation, memory, insight, or judgment; headache, dizziness, vertigo; fainting, blackouts, seizures, weakness, paralysis, numbness or loss of sensation, tingling or "pins and needles," tremors or other involuntary movements, seizures.

Hematologic. Anemia, easy bruising or bleeding, past transfusions, transfusion reactions.

Endocrine. "Thyroid trouble," heat or cold intolerance, excessive sweating, excessive thirst or hunger, polyuria, change in glove or shoe size.

The Physical Examination: Approach and Overview

Conduct a *comprehensive physical examination* on most new patients or patients being admitted to the hospital. For more *problem-oriented*, or *focused, assessments*, the presenting complaints will dictate which segments you elect to perform.

- *The key to a thorough and accurate physical examination is a systematic sequence of examination.* With effort and practice, you will acquire your own routine sequence. This book recommends examining from the patient's *right side*.

- Apply the techniques of inspection, palpation, auscultation, and percussion to each body region, but be sensitive to the whole patient.

- *Minimize the number of times you ask the patient to change position* from supine to sitting, or standing to lying supine.

- For an overview of the physical examination, study the sequence that follows. *Note that clinicians vary in where they place different segments, especially for the musculoskeletal and nervous systems.*

BEGINNING THE EXAMINATION: SETTING THE STAGE

Take the following steps to prepare for the physical examination.

Preparing for the Physical Examination

- Reflect on your approach to the patient.
- Adjust the lighting and the environment.
- Make the patient comfortable.
- Determine the scope of the examination.
- Choose the sequence of the examination.
- Observe the correct examining position (the patient's right side) and handedness.

Think through your approach, your professional demeanor, and how to make the patient comfortable and relaxed. *Always wash your hands in the patient's presence before beginning the examination.*

The Physical Examination: Suggested Sequence and Positioning

- General survey
- Vital signs
- Skin: upper torso, anterior and posterior
- Head and neck, including thyroid and lymph nodes
- *Optional:* Nervous system (mental status, cranial nerves, upper extremity motor strength, bulk, tone, cerebellar function)
- Thorax and lungs
- Breasts
- Musculoskeletal as indicated: upper extremities
- Cardiovascular, including JVP, carotid upstrokes and bruits, PMI, etc.
- Cardiovascular, for S_3 and murmur of mitral stenosis
- Nervous system: lower extremity motor strength, bulk, tone, sensation; reflexes; Babinskis
- Musculoskeletal, as indicated
- *Optional:* Skin, anterior and posterior
- *Optional:* Nervous system, including gait
- *Optional:* Musculoskeletal, comprehensive
- *Women:* Pelvic and rectal examination
- *Men:* Prostate and rectal examination
- Cardiovascular, for murmur of aortic insufficiency
- *Optional:* Thorax and lungs—anterior
- Breasts and axillae
- Abdomen
- Peripheral vascular; *Optional:* Skin—lower torso and extremities

Key to the Symbols for the Patient's Position

- Sitting
- Lying supine, with head of bed raised 30 degrees
- Same, turned partly to left side
- Standing
- Lying supine, with hips flexed, abducted, and externally rotated, and knees flexed (lithotomy position)
- Lying on the left side (left lateral decubitus)
- Sitting, leaning forward
- Lying supine

Each symbol pertains until a new one appears. Two symbols separated by a slash indicate either or both positions.

Reflect on Your Approach to the Patient. Identify yourself as a student. Try to appear calm, organized, and competent, even if you feel differently. If you forget to do part of the examination, this is not uncommon, especially at first! Simply examine that area out of sequence, but smoothly.

Adjust Lighting and the Environment. Adjust the bed to a convenient height (be sure to lower it when finished!). Ask the patient to move toward you if this makes it easier to do your physical examination. Good lighting and a quiet environment are important. *Tangential lighting* is optimal for structures such as the jugular venous pulse, the thyroid gland, and the apical impulse of the heart. It throws contours, elevations, and depressions, whether moving or stationary, into sharper relief.

Make the Patient Comfortable. Show concern for privacy and modesty.

- Close nearby doors and draw curtains before beginning.

- Acquire the art of *draping the patient* with the gown or draw sheet as you learn each examination segment in future chapters. *Your goal is to visualize one body area at a time.*

- As you proceed, keep the patient informed, especially when you anticipate embarrassment or discomfort, as when checking for the femoral pulse. Also try to gauge how much the patient wants to know.

- Make sure your instructions to the patient at each step are courteous and clear.

- Watch the patient's facial expression and even ask "Is it okay?" as you move through the examination.

When you have finished, tell the patient your general impressions and what to expect next. Lower the bed to avoid risk of falls and raise the bedrails if needed. As you leave, clean your equipment, dispose of waste materials, and wash your hands.

Determine the Scope of the Examination. *Comprehensive or Focused?* Choose whether to do a *comprehensive* or *focused examination*.

Choose the Sequence of the Examination.   The sequence of the examination should

- maximize the patient's comfort
- avoid unnecessary changes in position, and
- enhance the clinician's efficiency.

In general, move from "head to toe." An important goal as a student is to develop your own sequence with these principles in mind. See Chapter 1 of the textbook for a suggested examination sequence.

Observe the Correct Examining Position and Handedness.   Examine the patient from the patient's *right side*. Note that it is more reliable to estimate jugular venous pressure from the right, the palpating hand rests more comfortably on the apical impulse, the right kidney is more frequently palpable than the left, and examining tables are frequently positioned to accommodate a right-handed approach. To examine the *supine patient,* you can examine the head, neck, and anterior chest. Then roll the patient onto each side to listen to the lungs, examine the back, and inspect the skin. Roll the patient back and finish the rest of the examination with the patient again supine.

The Comprehensive Adult Physical Examination

General Survey.   Continue this survey throughout the patient visit. Observe general state of health, height, build, and sexual development. Note posture, motor activity, and gait; dress, grooming, and personal hygiene; and any odors of the body or breath. Watch facial expressions and note manner, affect, and reactions to persons and things in the environment. Listen to the patient's manner of speaking and note the state of awareness or level of consciousness.

Vital Signs.   Ask the patient **to sit** on the edge of the bed or examining table, unless this position is contraindicated. Stand in front of the patient, moving to either side as needed. Measure the blood pressure. Count pulse and respiratory rate. If indicated, measure body temperature.

Skin.   Observe the face. Identify any lesions, noting their location, distribution, arrangement, type, and color. Inspect and palpate the hair and nails. Study the patient's hands. Continue to assess the skin as you examine the other body regions.

HEENT.   Darken the room to promote pupillary dilation and visibility of the fundi. ***Head:*** Examine the hair, scalp, skull, and face. ***Eyes:*** Check visual acuity and screen the visual fields. Note position and alignment of the eyes. Observe the eyelids. Inspect the sclera and conjunctiva of each eye. With oblique lighting, inspect each cornea, iris, and lens. Compare the pupils, and test their reactions to light. Assess extraocular movements. With an ophthalmoscope, inspect the ocular fundi. ***Ears:*** Inspect the auricles, canals, and drums. Check auditory acuity. If acuity is diminished, check lateralization (Weber test) and compare air and bone conduction (Rinne test). ***Nose and sinuses:*** Examine the external nose; using a light and nasal speculum, inspect nasal mucosa, septum, and turbinates. Palpate for tenderness of the frontal and maxillary sinuses. ***Throat (or mouth and pharynx):*** Inspect the lips, oral mucosa, gums, teeth, tongue, palate, tonsils, and pharynx. *(You may wish to assess the Cranial Nerves at this point in the examination.)*

Neck.   Move behind the sitting patient to feel the thyroid gland and to examine the back, posterior thorax, and lungs. Inspect and palpate the cervical lymph nodes. Note any masses or unusual pulsations in the neck. Feel for any deviation of the trachea. Observe sound and effort of the patient's breathing. Inspect and palpate the thyroid gland.

Back.   Inspect and palpate the spine and muscles.

Posterior Thorax and Lungs.   Inspect and palpate the spine and muscles of the *upper* back. Inspect, palpate, and percuss the chest. Identify the level of diaphragmatic dullness on each side. Listen to the breath sounds; identify any adventitious (or added) sounds, and, if indicated, listen to transmitted voice sounds (see p. 133).

Breasts, Axillae, and Epitrochlear Nodes.   The patient is **still sitting**. Move to the front again. ***In a woman***, inspect the breasts with patient's arms relaxed, then elevated, and then with her hands pressed on her hips. ***In either sex***, inspect the axillae and feel for the axillary nodes; feel for the epitrochlear nodes.

A Note on the Musculoskeletal System. By now, you have made preliminary observations of the musculoskeletal system, including the hands, the upper back, and, in women, the shoulders' range of motion (ROM). Use these observations to decide whether a full musculoskeletal examination is warranted: *With the patient still sitting,* examine the hands, arms, shoulders, neck, and temporomandibular joints. Inspect and palpate the joints and check their ROM.

(You may choose to examine upper extremity muscle bulk, tone, strength, and reflexes at this time, or you may decide to wait until later.)

Palpate the breasts, while continuing your inspection.

Anterior Thorax and Lungs. The patient position is supine. Ask the patient to lie down. Stand at the *right side* of the patient's bed. Inspect, palpate, and percuss the chest. Listen to the breath sounds, any adventitious sounds, and, if indicated, transmitted voice sounds.

Cardiovascular System. Elevate head of bed to about 30 degrees, adjusting as necessary to see the jugular venous pulsations. Observe the jugular venous pulsations, and measure the jugular venous pressure in relation to the sternal angle. Inspect and palpate the carotid pulsations. Listen for carotid bruits.

Ask the patient to roll partly onto the left side while you listen at the apex. Then have the patient roll back to supine while you listen to the rest of the heart. Ask the patient to sit, lean forward, and exhale while you listen for the murmur of aortic regurgitation. Inspect and palpate the precordium. Note the location, diameter, amplitude, and duration of the apical impulse. Listen at the apex and the lower sternal border with the bell of a stethoscope. Listen at each auscultatory area with the diaphragm. Listen for S_1 and S_2 and for physiologic splitting of S_2. Listen for any abnormal heart sounds or murmurs.

Abdomen. Lower the head of the bed to the flat position. **The patient should be supine.** Inspect, auscultate, and percuss. Palpate lightly, then deeply. Assess the liver and spleen by percussion and then palpation. Try to feel the kidneys; palpate the aorta and its pulsations. If you suspect kidney infection, percuss posteriorly over the costovertebral angles.

Peripheral Vascular System. With the patient supine, palpate the femoral pulses and, if indicated, popliteal pulses. Palpate the inguinal lymph nodes. Inspect for edema, discoloration, or ulcers in the lower extremities. Palpate for pitting edema. **With the patient standing,** inspect for varicose veins.

Lower Extremities. Examine the legs, assessing the three systems (see next page) while the patient is still supine. Each of these systems can be further assessed when the patient stands.

Nervous System. The patient is sitting or supine. The examination of the nervous system can also be divided into the upper extremity examination (when the patient is still sitting) and the lower extremity examination (when the patient is supine) after examination of the peripheral nervous system.

Mental Status. If indicated and not done during the interview, assess orientation, mood, thought process, thought content, abnormal perceptions, insight and judgment, memory and attention, information and vocabulary, calculating abilities, abstract thinking, and constructional ability.

Cranial Nerves. If not already examined, check sense of smell, funduscopic examination, strength of the temporal and masseter muscles, corneal reflexes, facial movements, gag reflex, strength of the trapezia and sternomastoid muscles, and protrusion of tongue.

Motor System. Muscle bulk, tone, and strength of major muscle groups. *Cerebellar function:* rapid alternating movements (RAMs), point-to-point movements such as finger to nose (F → N) and heel to shin (H → S); gait. Observe patient's gait and ability to walk heel to toe, on toes, and on heels; to hop in place; and to do shallow knee bends. Do a Romberg test; check for pronator drift.

Sensory System. Pain, temperature, light touch, vibrations, and discrimination. Compare right and left sides and distal with proximal areas on the limbs.

Reflexes. Include biceps, triceps, brachioradialis, patellar, Achilles deep tendon reflexes; also plantar reflexes or Babinski reflex (see pp. 301–303).

Additional Examinations. The *rectal* and *genital* examinations are often performed at the end of the physical examination.

Male Genitalia and Hernias. Examine the penis and scrotal contents. Check for hernias.

Rectal Examination in Men. The patient is **lying on his left side** for the rectal examination. Inspect the sacrococcygeal and perianal areas. Palpate the anal canal, rectum, and prostate. (If the patient cannot stand, examine the genitalia before doing the rectal examination.)

Genital and Rectal Examination in Women. The patient is **supine in the lithotomy position.** Sit during the examination with the speculum, then stand during bimanual examination of uterus, adnexa, and rectum. Examine the external genitalia, vagina, and cervix. Obtain a Pap smear. Palpate the uterus and adnexa. Do a bimanual and rectal examination.

Standard and Universal Precautions

The Centers for Disease Control and Prevention (CDC) have issued several guidelines to protect patients and examiners from the spread of infectious disease. All clinicians examining patients are well advised to study and observe these precautions at the CDC Web sites. Advisories for standard and methicillin-resistant *Staphylococcus aureus* (*MRSA*) precautions and for universal precautions are briefly summarized below.

- *Standard and MRSA precautions:* Standard precautions are based on the principle that all blood, body fluids, secretions, excretions except sweat, nonintact skin, and mucous membranes may contain transmissible infectious agents. These practices apply to all patients in any setting. They include hand hygiene; when to use gloves, gowns, and mouth, nose, and eye protection; respiratory hygiene and cough etiquette; patient isolation criteria; precautions relating to equipment, toys and solid surfaces, and handling of laundry; and safe needle-injection practices.

    Be sure to wash your hands before and after examining the patient. This will show your concern for the patient's welfare and display your awareness of a critical component of patient safety. Antimicrobial fast-drying soaps are often within easy reach. *Change your white coat frequently*, because cuffs can become damp and smudged and transmit bacteria.

- *Universal precautions:* Universal precautions are a set of precautions designed to prevent transmission of HIV, hepatitis B virus (HBV), and other blood-borne pathogens when providing first aid or health care. The following fluids are considered potentially infectious: all blood and other body fluids containing visible blood, semen, and vaginal secretions; and cerebrospinal, synovial, pleural, peritoneal, pericardial, and amniotic fluids. Protective barriers include gloves, gowns, aprons, masks, and protective eyewear. All health care workers should *observe the important precautions for safe injections and prevention of injury from needlesticks, scalpels, and other sharp instruments and devices.* Report to your health service immediately if such injury occurs.

CHAPTER 2

Clinical Reasoning, Assessment, and Recording Your Findings

Assessment and Plan: the Process of Clinical Reasoning

Because assessment takes place in the clinician's mind, the process of clinical reasoning often seems inaccessible to beginning students. As an active learner, ask your teachers and clinicians to elaborate on the fine points of their clinical reasoning and decision making.

As you gain experience, your clinical reasoning will begin at the outset of the patient encounter, not at the end. Listed below are principles underlying the process of clinical reasoning and certain explicit steps to help guide your thinking.

Identifying Problems and Making Diagnoses: Steps in Clinical Reasoning

- **Identify abnormal findings.** Make a list of the patient's *symptoms*, the *signs* you observed during the physical examination, and available laboratory reports.
- **Localize these findings anatomically.** The symptom of a scratchy throat and the sign of an erythematous inflamed pharynx, for example, clearly localize the problem to the pharynx. Some symptoms and signs, such as fatigue or fever, cannot be localized but are useful in the next steps.
- **Interpret the findings in terms of the probable process.** There are a number of *pathologic* processes, including congenital, inflammatory or infectious, immunologic, neoplastic, metabolic, nutritional, degenerative, vascular, traumatic, and toxic. Other problems are *pathophysiologic*, reflecting derangements of biologic functions, such as heart failure. Still other problems are *psychopathologic*, such as headache as an expression of a somatization disorder.

(continued)

Identifying Problems and Making Diagnoses: Steps in Clinical Reasoning (continued)

- **Make hypotheses about the nature of the patient's problems.** Draw on your knowledge, experience, and reading about patterns of abnormalities and diseases. By consulting the clinical literature, you embark on the lifelong goal of *evidence-based decision making*. The following steps should help:
  1. Select the most specific and critical findings to support your hypothesis.
  2. Match your findings against all the conditions you know that can produce them.
  3. Eliminate the diagnostic possibilities that fail to explain the findings.
  4. Weigh the competing possibilities and select the most likely diagnosis.
  5. Give special attention to potentially life-threatening and treatable conditions. One rule of thumb is *always to include "the worst-case scenario"* in your list of differential diagnoses and make sure you have ruled out that possibility based on your findings and patient assessment.
- **Test your hypotheses.** You may need further history, additional maneuvers on physical examination, or laboratory studies or x-rays to confirm or to rule out your tentative diagnosis or to clarify which possible diagnosis is most likely.
- **Establish a working diagnosis.** Make this at the highest level of explicitness and certainty that the data allow. You may be limited to a symptom, such as "tension headache, cause unknown." At other times, you can define a problem explicitly in terms of its structure, process, and cause, such as "bacterial meningitis, pneumococcal." Routinely listing *Health Maintenance* helps you track several important health concerns more effectively: immunizations, screening measures (e.g., mammograms, prostate examinations), instructions regarding nutrition and breast or testicular self-examinations, recommendations about exercise or use of seat belts, and responses to important life events.
- **Develop a plan agreeable to the patient.** Identify and record a *Plan* for each patient problem, ranging from tests to confirm or further evaluate a diagnosis; to consultations for subspecialty evaluation; to additions, deletions, or changes in medication; or to arranging a family meeting.

The Case of Mrs. N

Now study the case of Mrs. N. Scrutinize the findings recorded, apply your clinical reasoning, and analyze the assessment and plan.

Health History

8/25/12 11:00 AM

Mrs. N is a pleasant, 54-year-old widowed saleswoman residing in Espanola, New Mexico.

Referral. None

Source and Reliability. Self-referred; seems reliable.

Chief Complaint: "My head aches."

Present Illness: For about 3 months, Mrs. N has had increasing problems with frontal headaches. These are usually bifrontal, throbbing, and mild to moderately severe. She has missed work on several occasions because of associated nausea and vomiting. Headaches now average once a week, usually are related to stress, and last 4 to 6 hours. They are relieved by sleep and putting a damp towel over the forehead. There is little relief from aspirin. No associated visual changes, motor-sensory deficits, or paresthesias.

"Sick headaches" with nausea and vomiting began at age 15, recurred throughout her mid-20s, then decreased to one every 2 or 3 months and almost disappeared.

The patient reports increased pressure at work from a new and demanding boss; she is also worried about her daughter (see *Personal and Social History*). She thinks her headaches may be like those in the past but wants to be sure, because her mother died following a stroke. She is concerned that they interfere with her work and make her irritable with her family. She eats three meals a day and drinks three cups of coffee a day and tea at night.

Medications. Aspirin, 1 to 2 tablets every 4 to 6 hours as needed. "Water pill" in the past for ankle swelling, none recently.

*Allergies. Ampicillin causes rash.

Tobacco. About 1 pack of cigarettes per day since age 18 (36 pack-years).

Alcohol/drugs. Wine on rare occasions. No illicit drugs.

Past History

Childhood Illnesses. Measles, chickenpox. No scarlet fever or rheumatic fever.
Adult Illnesses. Medical: Pyelonephritis, 1998, with fever and right flank pain; treated with ampicillin; developed generalized rash with itching several days later. Reports x-rays were normal; no recurrence of infection. ***Surgical:*** Tonsillectomy, age 6; appendectomy, age 13. Sutures for laceration, 2001, after stepping on glass. ***Ob/Gyn:*** 3-3-0-3, with normal vaginal deliveries. Three living children. Menarche age 12. Last menses 6 months ago. Little interest in sex, and not sexually active. No concerns about HIV infection.
Psychiatric: None.
Health Maintenance. Immunizations: Oral polio vaccine, year uncertain; tetanus shots × 2, 1991, followed with booster 1 year later; flu vaccine, 2000, no reaction. ***Screening tests:*** Last Pap smear, 2008, normal. No mammograms to date.

---

*You may wish to add an asterisk or underline important points.

(continued)

Family History

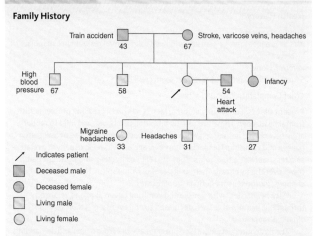

OR

Father died at age 43 in train accident. Mother died at age 67 from stroke; had varicose veins, headaches.

One brother, 61, with hypertension, otherwise well; second brother, 58, well except for mild arthritis; one sister, died in infancy of unknown cause.

Husband died at age 54 of heart attack.

Daughter, 33, with migraine headaches, otherwise well; son, 31, with headaches; son, 27, well.

No family history of diabetes, tuberculosis, heart or kidney disease, cancer, anemia, epilepsy, or mental illness.

Personal and Social History: Born and raised in Las Cruces, finished high school, married at age 19. Worked as sales clerk for 2 years, then moved with husband to Amarillo, had 3 children. Returned to work 15 years ago because of financial pressures. Children all married. Four years ago, Mr. N died suddenly of a heart attack, leaving little savings. Mrs. N has moved to small apartment to be near her daughter, Isabel. Isabel's husband, John, has an alcohol problem. Mrs. N's apartment now a haven for Isabel and her 2 children, Kevin, 6 years, and Lucia, 3 years. Mrs. N feels responsible for helping them; feels tense and nervous but denies depression. She has friends but rarely discusses family problems: "I'd rather keep them to myself. I don't like gossip." No church or other organizational support. She is typically up at 7:00 A.M., works 9:00 to 5:30, eats dinner alone.

Exercise and diet. Gets little exercise. Diet high in carbohydrates.

Safety measures. Uses seat belt regularly. Uses sunblock. Medications kept in an unlocked medicine cabinet. Cleaning solutions in unlocked cabinet below sink. Mr. N's shotgun and box of shells in unlocked closet upstairs.

(continued)

Review of Systems

General. *Has gained about 10 lbs in the past 4 years.
Skin. No rashes or other changes.
Head, Eyes, Ears, Nose, Throat (HEENT). See *Present Illness*. No history of head injury. *Eyes:* Reading glasses for 5 years, last checked 1 year ago. No symptoms. *Ears:* Hearing good. No tinnitus, vertigo, infections. *Nose, sinuses:* Occasional mild cold. No hay fever, sinus trouble. *Throat (or mouth and pharynx):* Some bleeding of gums recently. Last dental visit 2 years ago. Occasional canker sore.
Neck. No lumps, goiter, pain. No swollen glands.
Breasts. No lumps, pain, discharge. Does breast self-exam sporadically.
Respiratory. No cough, wheezing, shortness of breath. Last chest x-ray, 1986, St. Vincent's Hospital; unremarkable.
Cardiovascular. No known heart disease or high blood pressure; last blood pressure taken in 2006. No dyspnea, orthopnea, chest pain, palpitations. Has never had an electrocardiogram (ECG).
Gastrointestinal. Appetite good; no nausea, vomiting, indigestion. Bowel movement about once daily, *though sometimes has hard stools for 2 to 3 days when especially tense; no diarrhea or bleeding. No pain, jaundice, gallbladder or liver problems.
Urinary. No frequency, dysuria, hematuria, or recent flank pain; nocturia × 1, large volume. *Occasionally loses some urine when coughs hard.
Genital. No vaginal or pelvic infections. No dyspareunia.
Peripheral Vascular. Varicose veins appeared in both legs during first pregnancy. For 10 years, has had swollen ankles after prolonged standing; wears light elastic pantyhose; tried "water pill" 5 months ago, but it didn't help much; no history of phlebitis or leg pain.
Musculoskeletal. Mild, aching, low back pain, often after a long day's work; no radiation down the legs; used to do back exercises but not now. No other joint pain.
Psychiatric. No history of depression or treatment for psychiatric disorders. See also *Present Illness* and *Personal and Social History*.
Neurologic. No fainting, seizures, motor or sensory loss. Memory good.
Hematologic. Except for bleeding gums, no easy bleeding. No anemia.
Endocrine. No known thyroid trouble, temperature intolerance. Sweating average. No symptoms or history of diabetes.

Physical Examination

Mrs. N is a short, overweight, middle-aged woman, who is animated and responds quickly to questions. She is somewhat tense, with moist, cold hands. Her hair is well-groomed. Her color is good, and she lies flat without discomfort.
Vital Signs. Ht (without shoes) 157 cm (5'2"). Wt (dressed) 65 kg (143 lb). BMI 26. BP 164/98 right arm, supine; 160/96 left arm, supine; 152/88 right arm, supine with wide cuff. Heart rate (HR) 88 and regular. Respiratory rate (RR) 18. Temperature (oral) 98.6°F.

(continued)

Skin. Palms cold and moist, but color good. Scattered cherry angiomas over upper trunk. Nails without clubbing, cyanosis.

Head, Eyes, Ears, Nose, Throat (HEENT). ***Head:*** Hair of average texture. Scalp without lesions, normocephalic/atraumatic (NC/AT). ***Eyes:*** Vision 20/30 in each eye. Visual fields full by confrontation. Conjunctiva pink; sclera white. Pupils 4 mm constricting to 2 mm, round, regular, equally reactive to light. Extraocular movements intact. Disc margins sharp, without hemorrhages, exudates. No arteriolar narrowing or A-V nicking. ***Ears:*** Wax partially obscures right tympanic membrane (TM); left canal clear, TM with good cone of light. Acuity good to whispered voice. Weber midline. AC > BC. ***Nose:*** Mucosa pink, septum midline. No sinus tenderness. ***Mouth:*** Oral mucosa pink. Several interdental papillae red, slightly swollen. Dentition good. Tongue midline, with 3 × 4 mm shallow white ulcer on red base on undersurface near tip; tender but not indurated. Tonsils absent. Pharynx without exudates.

Neck. Neck supple. Trachea midline. Thyroid isthmus barely palpable, lobes not felt.

Lymph Nodes. Small (<1 cm), soft, nontender, and mobile tonsillar and posterior cervical nodes bilaterally. No axillary or epitrochlear nodes. Several small inguinal nodes bilaterally, soft and nontender.

Thorax and Lungs. Thorax symmetric with good excursion. Lungs resonant. Breath sounds vesicular with no added sounds. Diaphragms descend 4 cm bilaterally.

Cardiovascular. Jugular venous pressure 1 cm above the sternal angle, with head of examining table raised to 30°. Carotid upstrokes brisk, without bruits. Apical impulse discrete and tapping, barely palpable in the 5th left interspace, 8 cm lateral to the midsternal line. Good S_1, S_2; no S_3 or S_4. A II/VI medium-pitched midsystolic murmur at the 2nd right interspace; does not radiate to the neck. No diastolic murmurs.

Breasts. Pendulous, symmetric. No masses; nipples without discharge.

Abdomen. Protuberant. Well-healed scar, right lower quadrant. Bowel sounds active. No tenderness or masses. Liver span 7 cm in right midclavicular line; edge smooth, palpable 1 cm below right costal margin (RCM). Spleen and kidneys not felt. No costovertebral angle tenderness (CVAT).

Genitalia. External genitalia without lesions. Mild cystocele at introitus on straining. Vaginal mucosa pink. Cervix pink, parous, and without discharge. Uterus anterior, midline, smooth, not enlarged. Adnexa not palpated due to obesity and poor relaxation. No cervical or adnexal tenderness. Pap smear taken. Rectovaginal wall intact.

Rectal. Rectal vault without masses. Stool brown, negative for occult blood.

Extremities. Warm and without edema. Calves supple, nontender.

Peripheral Vascular. Trace edema at both ankles. Moderate varicosities of saphenous veins in both lower extremities. No stasis pigmentation or ulcers. Pulses (2+ = brisk, or normal):

	Radial	**Femoral**	**Popliteal**	**Dorsalis Pedis**	**Posterior Tibial**
RT	2+	2+	2+	2+	2+
LT	2+	2+	2+	2+	2+

(continued)

Musculoskeletal. No joint deformities. Good range of motion in hands, wrists, elbows, shoulders, spine, hips, knees, ankles.

Neurologic. **Mental Status:** Tense but alert and cooperative. Thought coherent. Oriented to person, place, and time. ***Cranial Nerves:*** II–XII intact. ***Motor:*** Good muscle bulk and tone. Strength 5/5 throughout (see p. 295 for grading system). ***Cerebellar:*** Rapid alternating movements (RAMs), point-to-point movements intact. Gait stable, fluid. ***Sensory:*** Pinprick, light touch, position sense, vibration, and stereognosis intact. Romberg negative.
Reflexes:

	Biceps	Triceps	Brachioradialis	Patellar	Achilles	Plantar
RT	2+	2+	2+	2+	1+	↓
LT	2+	2+	2+	2+/2+	1+	↓

Laboratory Data

None Currently. See Plan.

Assessment and Plan

1. **Migraine headaches.** A 54-year-old woman with migraine headaches since childhood, with a throbbing vascular pattern and frequent nausea and vomiting. Headaches are associated with stress and relieved by sleep and cold compresses. There is no papilledema, and there are no motor or sensory deficits on the neurologic examination. The differential diagnosis includes tension headache, also associated with stress, but there is no relief with massage, and the pain is more throbbing than aching. There are no fever, stiff neck, or focal findings to suggest meningitis, and the lifelong recurrent pattern makes subarachnoid hemorrhage unlikely (usually described as "the worst headache of my life").

(continued)

Assessment and Plan (continued)

   Plan:
   - Discuss features of migraine vs. tension headaches.
   - Discuss biofeedback and stress management.
   - Advise patient to avoid caffeine, including coffee, colas, and other caffeinated beverages.
   - Start NSAIDs for headache, as needed.
   - If needed next visit, begin prophylactic medication, because patient is having more than three migraines per month.

2. **Elevated blood pressure.** Systolic hypertension is present. May be related to anxiety from first visit. No evidence of end-organ damage to retina or heart.
   Plan:
   - Discuss standards for assessing blood pressure.
   - Recheck blood pressure in 1 month.
   - Check basic metabolic panel; review urinalysis.
   - Introduce weight reduction and/or exercise programs (see #4).
   - Reduce salt intake.

3. **Cystocele with occasional stress incontinence.** Cystocele on pelvic examination, probably related to bladder relaxation. Patient is perimenopausal. Incontinence reported with coughing, suggesting alteration in bladder neck anatomy. No dysuria, fever, flank pain. Not taking any contributing medications. Usually involves small amounts of urine, no dribbling, so doubt urge or overflow incontinence.
   Plan:
   - Explain cause of stress incontinence.
   - Review urinalysis.
   - Recommend Kegel exercises.
   - Consider topical estrogen cream to vagina next visit if no improvement.

4. Overweight. Patient 5'2", weighs 143 lb. BMI is ~26.
   Plan:
   - Explore diet history; ask patient to keep food intake diary.
   - Explore motivation to lose weight; set target for weight loss by next visit.
   - Schedule visit with dietitian.
   - Discuss exercise program, specifically, walking 30 minutes most days each week.

5. **Family stress.** Son-in-law with alcohol problem; daughter and grandchildren seeking refuge in patient's apartment, leading to tensions in these relationships. Patient also has financial constraints. Stress currently situational. No evidence of major depression at present.
   Plan:
   - Explore patient's views on strategies to cope with stress.
   - Explore sources of support, including Al-Anon for daughter and financial counseling for patient.
   - Continue to monitor for depression.

(continued)

Assessment and Plan (continued)

6. **Occasional musculoskeletal low back pain.** Usually with prolonged standing. No history of trauma or motor vehicle accident. Pain does not radiate; no tenderness or motor-sensory deficits on examination. Doubt disc or nerve root compression, trochanteric bursitis, sacroiliitis.
   Plan:
   - Review benefits of weight loss and exercises to strengthen low back muscles.
7. **Tobacco abuse.** 1 pack per day for 36 years.
   Plan:
   - Check peak flow or FEV_1/FVC on office spirometry.
   - Give strong warning to stop smoking.
   - Offer referral to tobacco cessation program.
   - Offer patch, current treatment to enhance abstinence.
8. **Varicose veins, lower extremities.** No complaints currently.
9. **History of right pyelonephritis, 1998.**
10. **Ampicillin allergy.** Developed rash but no other allergic reaction.
11. **Health maintenance.** Last Pap smear 2004; has never had a mammogram.
    Plan:
    - Teach patient breast self-examination; schedule mammogram.
    - Schedule Pap smear next visit.
    - Provide three stool guaiac cards; next visit discuss screening colonoscopy.
    - Suggest dental care for mild gingivitis.
    - Advise patient to move medications, caustic cleaning agents, gun and ammunition to locked cabinet—if possible, above shoulder height.

Approaching the Challenges of Clinical Data

As you can see from the case of Mrs. N, organizing the patient's clinical data poses several challenges. The following guidelines will help you address these challenges.

- **Clustering data into single vs. multiple problems.** The patient's *age* may help. Young people are more likely to have a single disease, while older people tend to have multiple diseases. The *timing* of symptoms is often useful. For example, an episode of pharyngitis 6 weeks ago probably is unrelated to fever, chills, pleuritic chest pain, and cough that prompt an office visit today.

  If symptoms and signs are in a single system, one disease may explain them. Problems in different, apparently unrelated systems often require more than one explanation. Again, knowledge of disease patterns is necessary.

Some diseases involve *multisystem conditions*. To explain cough, hemoptysis, and weight loss in a 60-year-old plumber who has smoked cigarettes for 40 years, you probably even now would rank lung cancer high in your list of differential diagnoses.

- **Sifting through an extensive array of data.** Try to *tease out separate clusters of observations and analyze one cluster at a time*. You also can *ask a series of key questions* that may steer your thinking in one direction. For example, you may ask what produces and relieves the patient's chest pain. If the answer is exercise and rest, you can focus on the cardiovascular and musculoskeletal systems and set the gastrointestinal system aside.

- **Assessing the quality of the data.** To avoid errors in interpreting clinical information, acquire the habits of skilled clinicians, summarized below.

Tips for Ensuring the Quality of Patient Data

- Ask open-ended questions and listen carefully and patiently to the patient's story.
- Craft a thorough and systematic sequence to history taking and physical examination.
- Keep an open mind toward the patient and the data.
- Always include "the worst-case scenario" in your list of possible explanations of the patient's problem, and make sure it can be safely eliminated.
- Analyze any mistakes in data collection or interpretation.
- Confer with colleagues and review the pertinent medical literature to clarify uncertainties.
- Apply principles of data analysis to patient information and testing.

- **Improving your assessment of clinical data and laboratory tests.** Apply several key principles for selecting and using clinical data and tests: *reliability, validity, sensitivity, specificity,* and *predictive value*. Learn to apply these principles to your clinical findings and the tests you order.

- **Displaying clinical data.** To use these principles, it is important to display the data in the 2 × 2 format diagrammed on page 32. Always using this format will ensure the accuracy of your calculations of sensitivity, specificity, and predictive value.

Principles of Test Selection and Use

Reliability: The reproducibility of a measurement. It indicates how well repeated measurements of the same relatively stable phenomenon will give the same result, also known as precision. Reliability may be measured for one observer or more observers.

Example. If on several occasions one clinician consistently percusses the same span of a patient's liver dullness, *intraobserver reliability* is good. If, on the other hand, several observers find quite different spans of liver dullness on the same patient, *interobserver reliability* is poor.

Validity: The closeness with which a measurement reflects the true value of an object. It indicates how closely a given observation agrees with "the true state of affairs," or the best possible measure of reality.

Example. Blood pressure measurements by mercury-based sphygmomanometers are less valid than intra-arterial pressure tracings.

Sensitivity: Identifies the proportion of people who test positive in a group of people known to have the disease or condition, or the proportion of people who are *true positives* compared with the total number of people who actually have the disease. When the observation or test is negative in people who have the disease, the result is termed *false negative*. Good observations or tests have a sensitivity of more than 90% and when negative help "rule out" disease because false negatives are few. Such observations or tests are especially useful for screening.

Example. The sensitivity of Homan's sign in the diagnosis of deep venous thrombosis (DVT) of the calf is 50%. In other words, compared with a group of patients with DVT confirmed by venous ultrasound, a much better test, only 50% will have a positive Homan's sign, so this sign, if absent, is not helpful, because 50% of patients may have DVT.

Specificity: Identifies the proportion of people who test negative in a group known to be *without* a given disease or condition, or the proportion of people who are *true negatives* compared with the total number of people without the disease. When the observation or test is positive in people without the disease, the result is termed *false positive*. Good observations or tests have a specificity of more than 90% and help "rule in" disease, because the test is rarely positive when disease is absent, and false positives are few.

Example: The specificity of serum amylase in patients with possible acute pancreatitis is 70%. In other words, of 100 patients without pancreatitis, 70% will have a normal serum amylase; in 30%, the serum amylase will be falsely elevated.

Predictive value: Indicates how well a given symptom, sign, or test result— either positive or negative—predicts the presence or absence of disease. *Positive predictive value* is the probability of disease in a patient with a positive (abnormal) test, or the proportion of "true positives" out of the total population with the disease. *Negative predictive value* is the probability of not having the condition or disease when the test is negative (normal), or

(continued)

Principles of Test Selection and Use (continued)

the proportion of "true negatives" out of the total population without the disease.

Examples. In a group of women with palpable breast nodules in a cancer screening program, the proportion with confirmed breast cancer would constitute the *positive predictive value* of palpable breast nodules for diagnosing breast cancer. In a group of women without palpable breast nodules in a cancer screening program, the proportion without confirmed breast cancer constitutes the *negative predictive value* of absence of breast nodules.

Sensitivity, specificity, and *predictive values* are illustrated in a 2 × 2 table, as shown below in an example of 200 people, half of whom have the disease in question. In this example, the disease prevalence of 50% is much higher than in most clinical situations. Because the positive predictive value increases with prevalence, its calculated value here is unusually high.

	Disease Present	Disease Absent	
Observation +	95 true-positive observations (a)	95 false-positive observations (b)	105 total positive observations
Observation −	5 false-negative observations (c)	90 true-negative observations (d)	95 total negative observations
	100 total persons with the disease	100 total persons without the disease	200 total persons

$$\text{Sensitivity} = \frac{a}{a+c} = \frac{95}{95+5} \times 100 = 95\%$$

$$\text{Specificity} = \frac{d}{b+d} = \frac{90}{90+10} \times 100 = 90\%$$

$$\text{Positive predictive value} = \frac{a}{a+b} = \frac{95}{95+10} \times 100 = 90.5\%$$

$$\text{Negative predictive value} = \frac{d}{c+d} = \frac{90}{90+5} \times 100 = 94.7\%$$

Likelihood ratio (LR): Conveys the odds that a finding occurs in a patient with the condition compared with a patient without the condition. When the LR is >1.0, the probability of the condition goes up; when the LR is < 1.0, the probability of the condition goes down.

(continued)

Principles of Test Selection and Use (continued)

- A positive LR = $\dfrac{sensitivity}{(1 - specificity)}$
- A negative LR = $\dfrac{(1 - sensitivity)}{specificity}$

Example. The LR of a subarachnoid hemorrhage (SAH) is 10 if neck stiffness is present and 0.4 if neck stiffness is absent. The odds of SAH are 10 times higher if neck stiffness is present compared with patients without SAH. When neck stiffness is absent, the odds the patient has SAH are reduced by a factor of 0.4.

For example, suppose the pre-test probability of SAH in the patient is 25% or a pre-test odds of 1:3. If the patient has neck stiffness, the post-test probability is revised upward by the LR to 77% (post-test odds of 10.3). If there is no neck stiffness, the post-test probability is revised downward by the negative LR to 12% (post-test odds of 4:30).

Organizing the Patient Record

A clear, well-organized clinical record is one of the most important adjuncts to your patient care. Think about the *order and readability* of the record and the *amount of detail* needed. Use the following checklist to make sure your record is clear, informative, and easy to follow.

Checklist for a Clear Patient Record

Is the order clear?

Order is imperative. Make sure that future readers, including you, can find specific points of information easily. Keep the *subjective* items of the history, for example, in the history; do not let them stray into the physical examination. Did you . . .

- Make the headings clear?
- Accent your organization with indentations and spacing?
- Arrange the *Present Illness* in chronologic order, starting with the current episode, then filling in relevant background information?

Do the data included contribute directly to the assessment?

Spell out the supporting data—both positive and negative—for every problem or diagnosis that you identify.

(continued)

Checklist for a Clear Patient Record (continued)

Are pertinent negatives specifically described?

Often portions of the history or examination suggest a potential or actual abnormality.

Examples. For the patient with notable bruises, record the "pertinent negatives," such as the absence of injury or violence, familial bleeding disorders, or medications or nutritional deficits that might lead to bruising.

For the patient who is depressed but not suicidal, record both facts. In the patient with a transient mood swing, on the other hand, a comment on suicide is unnecessary.

Are there overgeneralizations or omissions of important data?

Remember that data not recorded are data lost. No matter how vividly you can recall selected details today, you probably will not remember them in a few months. The phrase "neurologic exam negative," even in your own handwriting, may leave you wondering in a few months' time, "Did I really do the sensory exam?"

Is there too much detail?

Avoid burying important information in a mass of excessive detail, to be discovered by only the most persistent reader. *Omit most negative findings* unless they relate directly to the patient's complaints or to specific exclusions in your diagnostic assessment. *Do not list abnormalities that you did not observe. Instead, concentrate on a few major ones,* such as "no heart murmurs," and try to describe structures concisely and positively.

Examples. "Cervix pink and smooth" indicates you saw no redness, ulcers, nodules, masses, cysts, or other suspicious lesions, but the description is shorter and much more readable.

You can omit certain body structures even though you examined them, such as normal eyebrows and eyelashes.

Are phrases and short words used appropriately? Is there unnecessary repetition of data?

Omit unnecessary words, such as those in parentheses in the examples below. This saves valuable time and space.

Examples. "Cervix is pink (in color)." "Lungs are resonant (to percussion)." "Liver is tender (to palpation)." "Both (right and left) ears with cerumen." "II/VI systolic ejection murmur (audible)." "Thorax symmetric (bilaterally)."

Omit repetitive introductory phrases such as "The patient reports no . . . ," because readers assume the patient is the source of the history unless otherwise specified.

Use short words instead of longer, fancier ones when they mean the same thing, such as "felt" for "palpated" or "heard" for "auscultated."

Describe what you observed, not what you did. "Optic discs seen" is less informative than "disc margins sharp," even if it marks your first glimpse as an examiner!

(continued)

Checklist for a Clear Patient Record (continued)

Is the written style succinct? Is there excessive use of abbreviations?

Records are scientific and legal documents, so they should be clear and understandable. Using words and brief phrases instead of whole sentences is common, but abbreviations and symbols should be used only if they are readily understood. Likewise, an overly elegant style is less appealing than a concise summary.

Be sure your record is legible; otherwise, all that you have recorded is worthless to your readers.

Are diagrams and precise measurements included where appropriate?

Diagrams add greatly to the clarity of the record.

Examples. Study the examples below:

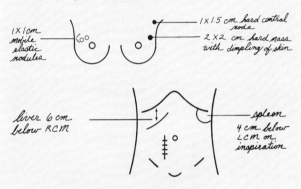

To ensure accurate evaluations and future comparisons, make measurements in centimeters, not in fruits, nuts, or vegetables.

Example. "1 × 1 cm lymph node" vs. "a pea-sized lymph node . . ." Or "2 × 2 cm mass on the left lobe of the prostate" vs. "a walnut-sized prostate mass."

Is the tone of the write-up neutral and professional?

It is important to be objective. Hostile, moralizing, or disapproving comments have no place in the patient's record. Never use words, penmanship, or punctuation that are inflammatory or demeaning.

Example. Comments such as "Patient DRUNK and LATE TO CLINIC AGAIN!!" are unprofessional and set a bad example for other providers reading the chart. They also might prove difficult to defend in a legal setting.

After you have completed your assessment and written record, you will find it helpful to generate a *Problem List* that summarizes the patient's problems for the front of the office or hospital chart. A sample *Problem List* for Mrs. N is provided below.

Sample Problem List

Date Entered	Problem No.	Problem
8/30/12	1	Migraine headaches
	2	Elevated blood pressure
	3	Cystocele with occasional stress incontinence
	4	Overweight
	5	Family stress
	6	Low back pain
	7	Tobacco abuse
	8	Varicose veins
	9	History of right pyelonephritis
	10	Allergy to ampicillin
	11	Health maintenance

CHAPTER 3

Interviewing and the Health History

The health history is a conversation with a purpose. In social conversation, you express your own needs and interests with responsibility only for yourself. The primary goal of the clinician–patient interview is to *listen* and improve the well-being of the patient through a trusting and supportive relationship. The interviewing process differs significantly from the format for the health history presented in Chapter 1. Both are fundamental to your work with patients but serve different purposes.

- The *interviewing process* that generates the patient's story is fluid and requires empathy, effective communication, and the relational skills to respond to patient cues, feelings, and concerns. It is "open-ended," drawing on a range of techniques that affirm and empower the patient—active listening, guided questioning, nonverbal affirmation, empathic responses, validation, reassurance, and partnering. These techniques are especially pertinent to eliciting the patient's chief concerns and the History of the Present Illness.

- The *health history format* is a structured framework for organizing patient information into written or verbal form. This format focuses your attention on the specific kinds of information you need to obtain, facilitates clinical reasoning, and clarifies communication of patient concerns, diagnoses, and plans to other health care providers involved in the patient's care. More "clinician-centered" closed-ended yes/no questions are more pertinent to the Medical History, the Family History, the Personal and Social History, and, most closed-ended of all, the Review of Systems.

For new patients in the office, hospital, or long-term care setting, you will do a *comprehensive health history*, described for adults in Chapter 1. For patients who seek care for a specific complaint, such as painful urination, a more limited interview, tailored to that specific problem—sometimes called a *focused* or *problem-oriented history*—may be indicated.

The Fundamentals of Skilled Interviewing

Skilled interviewing requires the use of specific learnable techniques perfected over a lifetime. Practice these techniques and find ways to be observed or recorded so that you can receive feedback on your progress.

Active Listening. This requires listening closely to what the patient is communicating, being aware of the patient's emotional state, and using verbal and nonverbal skills to encourage the patient to continue and expand both concerns and fears.

Empathic Responses. Patients may express—with or without words—feelings they have not consciously acknowledged. Emphatic responses are vital to patient rapport and healing and convey that you experience some of the patient's suffering. *To express empathy, you must first recognize the patient's feelings.* Elicit these feelings rather than assume how the patient feels.

Respond with understanding and acceptance. Responses may be as simple as "I understand," "That sounds upsetting," or "You seem sad." Empathy also may be nonverbal—for example, placing your hand on the patient's arm if the patient is crying.

Guided Questioning. It is important to adapt your questioning to the patient's verbal and nonverbal cues.

Types of Guided Questioning

- Moving from open-ended to focused questions
- Using questioning that elicits a graded response
- Asking a series of questions, one at a time
- Offering multiple choices for answers
- Clarifying what the patient means
- Encouraging with continuers
- Using echoing

Proceed from the general to the specific. Directed questions should not be leading questions that call for a "yes" or "no" answer: not "Did your stools look like tar?" but "Please describe your stools."

Ask questions that require *a graded response* rather than a single answer. "What physical activity do you do that makes you short of breath?" is better than "Do you get short of breath climbing stairs?" Be sure to *ask one question at a time.* Try "Do you have any of the following problems?" Be sure to pause and establish eye contact as you list each problem.

Sometimes patients seem unable to describe symptoms. *Offer multiple-choice answers.*

For patients using words that are ambiguous, *request clarification,* as in "Tell me exactly what you meant by 'the flu.'"

Posture, actions, or words encourage the patient to say more but do not specify the topic. Nod your head or remain silent. Lean forward, make eye contact, and use **continuers** like "Mm-hmm," "Go on," or "I'm listening."

Repetition and **echoing** of the patient's words encourage the patient to express both factual details and feelings.

Nonverbal Communication. Being sensitive to nonverbal messages allows you to both "read the patient" more effectively and send messages of your own. Pay close attention to eye contact, facial expression, posture, head position and movement such as shaking or nodding, interpersonal distance, and placement of the arms or legs, such as crossed, neutral, or open. Physical contact (like placing your hand on the patient's arm) can convey empathy or help the patient gain control of feelings. You also can mirror the patient's *paralanguage,* or qualities of speech such as pacing, tone, and volume, to increase rapport. Be sensitive to cultural variations in uses and meanings of nonverbal behaviors.

Validation. An important way to make a patient feel accepted is to provide verbal support that legitimizes or validates the patient's emotional experience.

Reassurance. Avoid premature or false reassurance. Such reassurance may block further disclosures, especially if the patient feels that exposing anxiety is a weakness. *The first step to effective reassurance is identifying and accepting the patient's feelings without offering reassurance at that moment.*

Partnering. Express your desire to work with patients in an ongoing way. Reassure patients that regardless of what happens with their disease, as their provider, you are committed to a continuing partnership. Even in your role as a student, such support can make a big difference.

Summarization. Giving a capsule summary lets the patient know that you have been listening carefully. It also clarifies what you know and what you don't know. Summarization allows you to organize your clinical reasoning and to convey your thinking to the patient, which makes the relationship more collaborative.

Transitions. Tell patients when you are changing directions during the interview. This gives patients a greater sense of control.

Empowering the Patient. The clinician–patient relationship is inherently unequal. Patients have many reasons to feel vulnerable: pain, worry, feeling overwhelmed with the health care system, lack of familiarity with the clinical evaluation process. Differences of gender, ethnicity, race, or class may also create power differentials. Ultimately, patients must be empowered to take care of themselves and feel confident about following through on your advice. Review the principles below.

> **Empowering the Patient: Principles of Sharing Power**
>
> - Evoke the patient's perspective.
> - Convey interest in the person, not just the problem.
> - Follow the patient's lead.
> - Elicit and validate emotional content.
> - Share information with the patient, especially at transition points during the visit.
> - Make your clinical reasoning transparent to the patient.
> - Reveal the limits of your knowledge.

The Sequence and Context of the Interview

PREPARATION

Interviewing patients to elicit their health history requires planning.

- **Review the medical record.** Before seeing the patient, review the medical record or chart. It often provides valuable information about past diagnoses and treatments; however, data may be incomplete or even disagree with what you learn from the patient, so be open to developing new approaches or ideas.

- **Set goals for the interview.** Clarify your goals for the interview. A clinician must balance **provider-centered goals** with **patient-centered goals.** The clinician's task is to balance these multiple agendas.

- **Review your clinical behavior and appearance.** Consciously or not, you send messages through your behavior. Posture, gestures, eye contact, and tone of voice all can express interest, attention, acceptance, and understanding. The skilled interviewer is calm and unhurried, even when time is limited. Reactions that betray disapproval, embarrassment, impatience, or boredom block communication. Patients find cleanliness, neatness, conservative dress, and a name tag reassuring.

- **Adjust the environment.** Always consider the patient's privacy. Pull shut any bedside curtains. Suggest moving to an empty room rather than having a conversation that can be overheard.

THE SEQUENCE OF THE INTERVIEW

In general, an interview moves through several stages. *Throughout this sequence, as the clinician, you must always stay attuned to the patient's feelings, help the patient express them, respond to their content, and validate their significance.*

- **Greet the patient and establish rapport.** *Greet the patient* by name and introduce yourself, giving your name. If possible, shake hands. If this is the first contact, explain your role, including your status as a student and how you will be involved in the patient's care. Using a title to address the patient (e.g., Mr. O'Neil, Ms. Wu) is always best. **Avoid first names** unless you have specific permission from the patient.

  Whenever visitors are present, *maintain confidentiality.* Let the **patient** decide if visitors or family members should remain in the room, and ask for the patient's permission before conducting the interview in front of them.

  Attend to the patient's comfort. Ask how he or she is feeling and if you are coming at a convenient time. Look for signs of discomfort, such as frequent changes of position or facial expressions that show pain or anxiety. Arranging the bed may make the patient more comfortable.

Consider the best way to *arrange the room*. Choose a distance that facilitates conversation and good eye contact. Try to sit at eye level with the patient. Move any physical barriers between you and the patient, such as desks or bedside tables, out of the way.

Give the patient your undivided attention. Spend enough time on small talk to put the patient at ease. If necessary, jot down short phrases, specific dates, or words rather than trying to put them into a final format. Maintain good eye contact, and whenever the patient is talking about sensitive or disturbing material, put down your pen.

- **Establish an agenda.** It is important to identify both your own and the patient's issues at the beginning of the encounter. Often, you may need to focus the interview by asking the patient which problem is most pressing. For example, "Do you have some special concerns today? Which one are you most concerned about?" Some patients may not have a specific complaint or problem. *It is still important to start with the patient's story.*

- **Invite the patient's story.** As you probe the patient's concern, begin with **open-ended questions** that allow full freedom of response: "Tell me more about…." Avoid questions that restrict the patient to a minimally informative "yes" or "no" answer. *Listen to the patient's answers without interrupting.*

  Train yourself to *follow the patient's leads*. Use verbal and nonverbal cues that prompt patients to recount their stories spontaneously. Use *continuers,* especially at the outset, such as nodding your head and using phrases such as "Uh huh," "Go on," and "I see."

- **Explore the patient's perspective.** The *disease/illness model* helps you understand the difference between your perspective and the patient's perspective. In this model, *disease* is the explanation that the *clinician* brings to the symptoms. It is the way that the clinician organizes what he or she learns from the patient into a coherent picture that leads to a clinical diagnosis and treatment plan. **Illness** can be defined as how the *patient* experiences symptoms. *The health history interview needs to include both of these views of reality.*

  Learning how patients perceive illness means asking patient-centered questions in the four domains listed below, which follow the mnemonic "FIFE"—Feelings, Ideas, effect on Function, and Expectations. This is crucial to patient satisfaction, effective health care, and patient follow-through.

Exploring the Patient's Perspective (F-I-F-E)

- The patient's **F**eelings, including fears or concerns, about the problem
- The patient's **I**deas about the nature and the cause of the problem
- The effect of the problem on the patient's life and **F**unction
- The patient's **E**xpectations of the disease, of the clinician, or of health care, often based on prior personal or family experiences

- **Identify and respond to the patient's emotional cues.** Patients offer various clues to their concerns that may be direct or indirect, verbal or nonverbal; they may express them as ideas or emotions. Acknowledging and responding to these clues help build rapport, expand the clinician's understanding of the illness, and improve patient satisfaction. Clues to the patient's perspective on illness are provided in the box below.

Clues to the Patient's Perspective on Illness

- Direct statement(s) by the patient of explanations, emotions, expectations, and effects of the illness
- Expression of feelings about the illness without naming the illness
- Attempts to explain or understand symptoms
- Speech clues (e.g., repetition, prolonged reflective pauses)
- Sharing a personal story
- Behavioral clues indicative of unidentified concerns, dissatisfaction, or unmet needs such as reluctance to accept recommendations, seeking a second opinion, or early appointment

Source: Lang F, Floyd MR, Beine KL. Clues to patients' explanations and concerns about their illnesses: a call for active listening. Arch Fam Med 2000;9(3):222–227.

- **Expand and clarify the patient's story.** Each symptom has attributes that must be clarified, including context, associations, and chronology, especially for pain. It is critical to understand fully every symptom's essential characteristics. *Always elicit the seven features of every symptom.*

The Seven Attributes of a Symptom

1. ***Location.*** Where is it? Does it radiate?
2. ***Quality.*** What is it like?
3. ***Quantity or severity.*** How bad is it? (For pain, ask for a rating on a scale of 1 to 10.)
4. ***Timing.*** When did (does) it start? How long did (does) it last? How often did (does) it occur?
5. ***Setting in which it occurs.*** Include environmental factors, personal activities, emotional reactions, or other circumstances that may have contributed to the illness.
6. ***Remitting or exacerbating factors.*** Does anything make it better or worse?
7. ***Associated manifestations.*** Have you noticed anything else that accompanies it?

To pursue the seven attributes, two mnemonics may help:

- **OLD CARTS,** or **O**nset, **L**ocation, **D**uration, **C**haracter, **A**ggravating/**A**lleviating Factors, **R**adiation, and **T**iming; and

- **OPQRST,** or **O**nset, **P**alliating/**P**rovoking Factors, **Q**uality, **R**adiation, **S**ite, and **T**iming

Use language that is understandable and appropriate to the patient. Technical language confuses patients and blocks communication. Whenever possible, *use the patient's words, making sure you clarify their meaning.*

Facilitate the patient's story by using different types of questions and the techniques of skilled interviewing on pp. 32–34. Often you will need to *use directed questions* (see p. 32) that ask for specific information the patient has not already offered. *In general, the patient interview moves back and forth from an open-ended question to a directed question and then on to another open-ended question.*

Establishing the sequence and time course of the patient's symptoms is important. You can encourage a chronologic account by asking such questions as "What then?" or "What happened next?"

Some students visualize the process of evoking a full description of the symptom as "the cone", as shown on the following page.

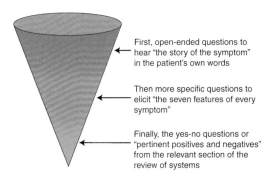

- First, open-ended questions to hear "the story of the symptom" in the patient's own words
- Then more specific questions to elicit "the seven features of every symptom"
- Finally, the yes-no questions or "pertinent positives and negatives" from the relevant section of the review of systems

Each symptom has its own "cone," which becomes a paragraph in the History of Present Illness in the written record.

- **Generate and test diagnostic hypotheses.** As you listen to the patient's concerns, you will begin to *generate hypotheses* about what disease process might be the cause. Identifying the various attributes of the patient's symptoms and pursuing specific details are fundamental to recognizing patterns of disease and differentiating one disease from another.

- **Share the treatment plan.** Learning about the disease and conceptualizing the illness give you and the patient the basis for planning further evaluation (physical examination, laboratory tests, consultations, etc.). Motivational interviewing techniques may help the patient achieve desired behavior changes.

- **Close the interview.** Make sure the patient fully understands the plans you have developed together. You can say, "We need to stop now. Do you have any questions about what we've covered?" Review future evaluation, treatments, and follow-up. Give the patient a chance to ask any final questions. Ask the patient to repeat the plan back to you.

- **Take time for self-reflection.** As clinicians, we encounter a wide variety of people, each one unique. Because we bring our own values, assumptions, and biases to every encounter, we must look inward to clarify how our expectations and reactions may affect what we hear and how we behave. *Self-reflection brings a deepening personal awareness to our work with patients and is one of the most rewarding aspects of providing patient care.*

THE CULTURAL CONTEXT OF THE INTERVIEW

Cultural Humility—A Changing Paradigm. As you provide care for an ever-expanding and diverse group of patients, it is important to understand how culture shapes not just the patient's beliefs, but your own. *Culture* is a system of shared ideas, rules, and meanings that influences how we view the world, experience it emotionally, and behave in relation to other people. This definition of culture is broader than the term *ethnicity*. The influence of culture is not limited to minority groups—it is relevant to everyone, including the culture of clinicians and their training. *Cultural competence* commonly is viewed as "a set of attitudes, skills, behaviors, and policies that enable organizations and staff to work effectively in cross-cultural situations. It reflects the ability to acquire and use knowledge of the health-related benefits, attitudes, practices, and communication patterns of clients and their families to improve services, strengthen programs, increase community participation, and close the gaps in health status among diverse population groups."

Clinicians are increasingly challenged to adopt *cultural humility*, a "process that requires humility as individuals continually engage in self-reflection and self-critique as lifelong learners and reflective practitioners." This process includes "the difficult work of examining cultural beliefs and cultural systems of both patients and providers to locate the points of cultural dissonance or synergy that contribute to patients' health outcomes." It calls for clinicians to "bring into check the power imbalances that exist in the dynamics of (clinician)–patient communication" and maintain mutually respectful and dynamic partnerships with patients and communities. The following three-point framework will help you.

- **Self-awareness.** As clinicians, we face the task of bringing our own values and biases to a conscious level. *Values* are the standards we use to measure our own and others' beliefs and behaviors. *Biases* are the attitudes or feelings that we attach to perceived differences, for example, the way an individual relates to time, which can be a culturally determined phenomenon. Are you always on time—a positive value in the dominant Western culture? Or do you tend to run a little late? How do you feel about people whose habits are opposite to yours? Think about the role of physical appearance. Do you consider yourself thin, midsize, or heavy? How do you feel about people who have different weights?

- **Respectful Communication.** Maintain an open, respectful, and inquiring attitude. "What did you hope to get from this visit?" If you have established rapport and trust, patients will be willing to teach you. Be ready to acknowledge your ignorance or bias. "I mistakenly made assumptions about you that are not right. I apologize. Would you be willing to tell me more about yourself and your future goals?"

Learn about different cultures: do pertinent reading; go to movies that are made in different countries; learn about different consumer health agendas.

- **Collaborative Partnerships.** Communication based on trust, respect, and a willingness to re-examine assumptions helps allow patients to express concerns that run counter to the dominant culture. You, the clinician, must be willing to listen to and validate these emotions, and not let your own feelings prevent you from exploring painful areas. You also must be willing to re-examine your beliefs.

Advanced Interviewing

CHALLENGING PATIENTS

Always remember the importance of listening to the patient and clarifying the patient's agenda.

Silent Patient. Silence has many meanings and purposes. Watch closely for nonverbal cues such as difficulty controlling emotions. You may need to shift your inquiry to symptoms of depression or begin an exploratory mental status examination. Silence may be the patient's response to how you are asking questions. Are you asking too many direct questions? Have you offended the patient?

Confusing Patient. Some patients have *multiple symptoms* or a somatization disorder. Focus on the context of the symptoms and guide the interview into a psychosocial assessment. At other times, you may be baffled, frustrated, or confused. The history is vague and difficult to understand, and patients may describe symptoms in bizarre terms. Try to learn more about the unusual symptoms. Watch for delirium in acutely ill or intoxicated patients and for dementia in the elderly. When you suspect a psychiatric or neurologic disorder, shift to a mental status examination, focusing on level of consciousness, orientation, and memory.

Patient With Altered Capacity. Some patients cannot provide their own histories because of delirium, dementia, or other conditions. Others cannot relate certain parts of the history. In such cases, determine whether the patient has *decision-making capacity*, or the ability to understand information related to health, to make medical choices based on reason and a consistent set of values, and to declare preferences about treatments. Many patients with psychiatric or cognitive deficits still retain the ability to make decisions.

For patients with capacity, obtain their consent before talking about their health with others. Maintain confidentiality and clarify what you can discuss with others. They may offer surprising and important information. Consider dividing the interview into two segments—one with the patient and the other with both the patient and a second informant. Also learn the tenets of the *Health Insurance Portability and Accountability Act (HIPAA)* passed by Congress in 1996, which sets strict standards for disclosure for both institutions and providers when sharing patient information. These can be found at www.hhs.gov/ocr/hipaa/.

For patients with impaired capacity, find a *surrogate informant* or *decision maker* to assist with the history. Check whether the patient has a *durable power of attorney for health care* or a *health care proxy*. If not, in many cases, a spouse or family member can represent the patient's wishes.

Talkative Patient. Several techniques are helpful. For the first 5 or 10 minutes, listen closely. Does the patient seem obsessively detailed or unduly anxious? Is there a flight of ideas or disorganized thought process? Try to focus on what seems most important to the patient. "You've described many concerns. Let's focus on the hip pain first. Can you tell me what it feels like?" Or you can ask, "What is your #1 concern today?"

Crying Patient. Usually crying is therapeutic, as is quiet acceptance of the patient's distress. Make a facilitating or supportive remark like "I'm glad that you were able to express your feelings."

Angry or Disruptive Patient. Many patients have reasons to be angry: they are ill, they have suffered a loss, they lack accustomed control over their own lives, and they feel relatively powerless. They may direct this anger toward you. *Accept angry feelings from patients and allow them to express such emotions without getting angry in return*. Validate their feelings without agreeing with their reasons. "I understand that you felt very frustrated by the long wait and answering the same questions over and over." Some angry patients become hostile and disruptive. Before approaching them, alert security. It is important to stay calm, appear accepting, and avoid being challenging. Keep your posture relaxed and nonthreatening. Once you have established rapport, gently suggest moving to a different location.

Patient With a Language Barrier. The ideal interpreter is a neutral, objective person trained in both languages and cultures. Avoid using family members or friends as interpreters: confidentiality may be violated. As you begin working with the interpreter, *make questions clear, short, and simple*. Speak directly to the patient. Bilingual written questionnaires are valuable.

Guidelines for Working With an Interpreter: "INTERPRET"

I	Introductions: Make sure to introduce all the individuals in the room. During the introduction, include information as to the roles individuals will play.
N	Note Goals: Note the goals of the interview. What is the diagnosis? What will the treatment entail? Will there be any follow-up?
T	Transparency: Let the patient know that everything said will be interpreted throughout the session.
E	Ethics: Use qualified interpreters (not family members or children) when conducting an interview. Qualified interpreters allow the patient to maintain autonomy and make informed decisions about his or her care.
R	Respect Beliefs: Limited English Proficient (LEP) patients may have cultural beliefs that need to be taken into account as well. The interpreter may be able to serve as a cultural broker and help explain any cultural beliefs that may exist.
P	Patient Focus: The patient should remain the focus of the encounter. Providers should interact with the patient and not the interpreter. Make sure to ask and address any questions the patient may have prior to ending the encounter. If you don't have trained interpreters on staff, the patient may not be able to call in with questions.
R	Retain Control: It is important as the provider that you remain in control of the interaction and not let the patient or the interpreter take over the conversation.
E	Explain: Use simple language and short sentences when working with an interpreter. This will ensure that comparable words can be found in the second language and that all the information can be conveyed clearly.
T	Thanks: Thank the interpreter and the patient for their time. On the chart, note that the patient needs an interpreter and who served as an interpreter this time.

Source: U.S. Department of Health and Human Services. Interpret Tool: working with interpreters in cultural settings. Available at https://www.thinkculturalhealth.hhs.gov/pdfs/InterpretTool.pdf. Accessed June 6, 2012.

Patient With Low Literacy or Low Health Literacy. Assess the ability to read. Some patients may try to hide their reading problems. Ask the patient to read whatever instructions you have written. Simply handing the patient written material upside-down to see if the patient turns it around may settle the question. Assess *health literacy,* or the skills to function effectively in the health care system: interpreting documents, reading labels and medication instructions, and speaking and listening effectively.

Patient With Hearing Loss. Find out the patient's preferred method of communicating. Patients may use American Sign Language, a unique language with its own syntax, or various other communication forms combining signs and speech. Determine whether the patient identifies with the Deaf or Hearing culture. Handwritten questions and answers may be the best solution. When patients have *partial hearing impairment* or can *read lips,* face them directly, in good light. If the patient has a *unilateral hearing loss,* sit on the hearing side. If the patient has a *hearing aid,* make sure it is working. Eliminate background noise such as television.

Patient With Impaired Vision. Shake hands to establish contact and explain who you are and why you are there. If the room is unfamiliar, orient the patient to the surroundings.

Patient With Limited Intelligence. Patients of moderately limited intelligence usually can give adequate histories. Pay special attention to the patient's schooling and ability to function independently. How far has the patient gone in school? If he or she didn't finish, why not? Assess simple calculations, vocabulary, memory, and abstract thinking. For patients with severe mental retardation, obtain the history from the family or caregivers. Avoid "talking down" or using condescending behavior. The sexual history is equally important and often overlooked.

Patient With Personal Problems. Patients may ask you for advice about personal problems outside the range of health. Letting the patient talk through the problem is usually more valuable and therapeutic than any answer you could give.

Seductive Patient. The emotional and physical intimacy of the clinician–patient relationship may lead to sexual feelings. If you become aware of such feelings, accept them as a normal human response, and bring them to the conscious level so they will not affect your behavior. Denying these feelings makes it more likely that you will act inappropriately. *Any* sexual contact or romantic relationship with patients is *unethical;* keep your relationship with the patient within professional bounds and seek help if you need it.

SENSITIVE TOPICS

The Sexual History. You can introduce questions about sexual function and practices at multiple points in a patient's history. An orienting sentence or two is often helpful. "Now I'd like to ask you some questions about your sexual health and practices" or "I routinely ask all patients about their sexual function."

- "When was the last time you had intimate physical contact with someone?" "Did that contact include sexual intercourse?"

- "Do you have sex with men, women, or both?" The health implications of heterosexual, homosexual, or bisexual experiences are significant.

- "How many sexual partners have you had in the last 6 months?" "In the last 5 years?" "In your lifetime?"

- Because no explicit risk factors may be present, it is important to ask all patients "Do you have any concerns about HIV or AIDS?" Also ask about routine use of condoms.

Mental Health History. Cultural constructs of mental illness vary widely, causing marked differences in acceptance and attitudes. Ask open-ended questions initially: "Have you ever had any problem with emotional or mental illnesses?" Then move to more specific questions: "Have you ever visited a counselor or psychotherapist?" "Have you taken medication for emotional issues?" "Have you or a family member ever been hospitalized for a mental health problem?"

Be sensitive to reports of mood changes or symptoms such as fatigue, tearfulness, appetite or weight changes, insomnia, and vague somatic complaints. Two opening screening questions are: "Over the past 2 weeks, have you felt down, depressed, or hopeless?" and "Over the past 2 weeks, have you felt little interest or pleasure in doing things?" Ask about thoughts of suicide: "Have you ever thought about hurting yourself or ending your life?" Evaluate severity.

Many patients with schizophrenia or other psychotic disorders can function in the community and tell you about their diagnoses, symptoms, hospitalizations, and medications. Investigate their symptoms and assess any effects on mood or daily activities.

Alcohol and Prescription and Illicit Drugs. Clinicians should routinely ask about current and past use of alcohol or drugs, patterns of use, and family history. Be familiar with the definitions below:

- **Tolerance:** A state of adaptation in which exposure to a drug induces changes that result in a diminution of one or more of the drug's effects over time.

- **Physical Dependence:** A state of adaptation that is manifested by a drug class–specific withdrawal syndrome that can be produced by abrupt cessation, rapid dose reduction, decreasing blood level of the drug, and/or administration of an antagonist.

- **Addiction:** A primary, chronic, neurobiologic disease with genetic, psychosocial, and environmental factors influencing its development and manifestations. It is characterized by behaviors that include one or more of the following: impaired control over drug use, compulsive use, continued use despite harm, and craving.

For assessing alcohol intake, "What do you like to drink?" or "Tell me about your use of alcohol" are good opening questions that avoid the easy yes or no response. The most widely used screening questions are the *CAGE* questions about *C*utting down, *A*nnoyance when criticized, *G*uilty feelings, and *E*ye-openers. Two or more affirmative answers to the CAGE questions suggest alcoholism. The CAGE Questionnaire is readily available online.

Also ask about blackouts (loss of memory for events during drinking), seizures, accidents or injuries while drinking, job loss, marital conflict, or legal problems. Ask specifically about drinking while driving or operating machinery.

Questions about drugs are similar. "How much marijuana do you use? Cocaine? Heroin? Amphetamines?" (Ask about each one by name.) "How about prescription drugs such as sleeping pills?" "Diet pills?" "Painkillers?" Use the CAGE questions but relate them to drug use. With adolescents, it may be helpful to ask about substance use by friends or family members first. "A lot of young people are using drugs these days. How about at your school? Your friends?"

Intimate Partner Violence and Domestic Violence. Many authorities recommend routine screening of all female and older adult patients for domestic violence. Start with general "normalizing" questions: "Because abuse is common in many women's lives, I've begun to ask about it routinely." "Are there times in your relationships that you feel unsafe or afraid?" "Have you ever been hit, kicked, punched, or hurt by someone you know?"

Clues to Physical and Sexual Abuse

- Injuries that are unexplained, seem inconsistent with the patient's story, are concealed by the patient, or cause embarrassment
- Delay in getting treatment for trauma
- History of repeated injuries or "accidents"
- If the patient or a person close to the patient has a history of alcohol or drug abuse
- Partner tries to dominate the visit, will not leave the room, or seems unusually anxious or solicitous
- Pregnancy at a young age; multiple partners
- Repeated STIs; vaginal lacerations or bruises
- Fear of the pelvic examination or leaving the examination room

Death and the Dying Patient. Work through your own feelings with the help of reading and discussion. Kübler-Ross has described five stages in our response to loss or the anticipatory grief of impending death: denial and isolation, anger, bargaining, depression or sadness, and acceptance. These stages may occur sequentially or overlap in different combinations. Dying patients rarely want to talk about their illnesses all the time, nor do they wish to confide in everyone they meet. Give them opportunities to talk and then listen receptively, but be supportive if they prefer to stay at a social level.

Understanding the patient's wishes about treatment at the end of life is an important clinician responsibility. Even if discussions of death and dying are difficult, you must learn to ask specific questions. Ask about Do Not Resuscitate (DNR) status. Find out about the patient's frame of reference. "What experiences have you had with the death of a close friend or relative?" "What do you know about cardiopulmonary resuscitation (CPR)?" Assure patients that relieving pain and taking care of their other spiritual and physical needs will be a priority. Encourage any adult, but especially the elderly or chronically ill, to establish a *health care proxy*, an individual who can act for the patient in life-threatening situations.

Ethics and Professionalism

Medical ethics come into play in almost every patient interaction. Fundamental maxims are as follows:

- ***Nonmaleficence*** or ***primum non nocere,*** commonly stated as "First, do no harm"

- ***Beneficence,*** or the dictum that the clinician needs to "do good" for the patient. As clinicians, our actions need to be motivated by what is in the patient's best interest.

- ***Autonomy,*** whereby patients have the right to determine what is in their own best interest

- ***Confidentiality,*** meaning that we are obligated not to tell others what we learn from our patients

The Tavistock Principles guide behavior in health care for both individuals and institutions.

The Tavistock Principles

Rights: People have a right to health and health care.
Balance: Care of individual patients is central, but the health of populations is also our concern.
Comprehensiveness: In addition to treating illness, we have an obligation to ease suffering, minimize disability, prevent disease, and promote health.
Cooperation: Health care succeeds only if we cooperate with those we serve, each other, and those in other sectors.
Improvement: Improving health care is a serious and continuing responsibility.
Safety: Do no harm.
Openness: Being open, honest, and trustworthy is vital in health care.

CHAPTER 4

Beginning the Physical Examination: General Survey, Vital Signs, and Pain

The Health History

Common or Concerning Symptoms

- Fatigue and weakness
- Fever, chills, night sweats
- Changes in weight
- Pain

Fatigue and Weakness. *Fatigue* is a nonspecific symptom with many causes. Use open-ended questions to explore the attributes of the patient's fatigue, and encourage the patient to fully describe what he or she is experiencing.

Weakness differs from fatigue. It denotes a demonstrable loss of muscle power and will be discussed later with other neurologic symptoms.

Fever, Chills, and Night Sweats. Ask about fever if the patient has an acute or chronic illness. Find out whether the patient has used a thermometer to measure the temperature. Distinguish between subjective *chilliness* and a *shaking chill*, with shivering throughout the body and chattering of teeth. *Night sweats* raise concerns about tuberculosis or malignancy.

Focus your questions on the timing of the illness and its associated symptoms. Become familiar with patterns of infectious diseases that may affect your patient. Inquire about travel, contact with sick people, or other unusual exposures. Be sure to inquire about medications, as they may cause fever. In contrast, recent ingestion of aspirin, acetaminophen, corticosteroids, and nonsteroidal anti-inflammatory drugs may mask it.

Weight Changes. Good opening questions include "How often do you check your weight?" and "How is it compared to a year ago?"

- *Weight gain* occurs when caloric intake exceeds caloric expenditure over time. It also may reflect abnormal accumulation of body fluids.

- *Weight loss* has many causes: decreased food intake, dysphagia, vomiting, and insufficient supplies of food; defective absorption of nutrients; increased metabolic requirements; and loss of nutrients through the urine, feces, or injured skin. Be alert for signs of malnutrition.

Pain. Approximately 70 million Americans report persisting or intermittent pain, often underassessed. Adopt the comprehensive approach found on p. 59.

Health Promotion and Counseling: Evidence and Recommendations

Important Topics for Health Promotion and Counseling

- Optimal weight, nutrition, and diet
- Exercise

Optimal Weight, Nutrition, and Diet. Less than half of U.S. adults maintain a healthy weight (BMI ≥19 but <25). Obesity has increased in every segment of the population. More than 85% of people with type 2 diabetes and roughly 20% of those with hypertension or elevated cholesterol levels are overweight or obese. Increasing obesity in children contributes to rising rates of childhood diabetes. Diet recommendations hinge on assessment of the patient's motivation and readiness to lose weight and individual risk factors. Experts urge that everyone restrict salt intake to a half teaspoon a day. General national guidelines recommend:

- A 10% weight reduction over 6 months, or a decrease of 300 to 500 kcal/day, for people with BMIs between 27 and 35

- A weight loss goal of ½ to 1 pound per week because more rapid weight loss does not lead to better results at 1 year

Exercise. Thirty minutes of moderate activity (defined as walking 2 miles in 30 minutes, or its equivalent, on most days of the week) is recommended. Patients can increase exercise by such simple measures as parking further away from their place of work or using stairs instead of elevators.

Techniques of Examination

EXAMINATION TECHNIQUES	POSSIBLE FINDINGS
GENERAL SURVEY	
Apparent State of Health	Acutely or chronically ill, frail, robust, vigorous
Level of Consciousness. Is the patient awake, alert, and interactive?	If not, promptly assess level of consciousness (see p. 305)
Signs of Distress	
• Cardiac or respiratory distress	Clutching the chest, pallor, diaphoresis; labored breathing, wheezing, cough
• Pain	Wincing, sweating, protecting painful area
• Anxiety or depression	Anxious face, fidgety movements, cold and moist palms; inexpressive or flat affect, poor eye contact, psychomotor slowing
Skin Color and Obvious Lesions. See Chapter 6, The Skin, Hair, and Nails, for details.	Pallor, cyanosis, jaundice, rashes, bruises

EXAMINATION TECHNIQUES	POSSIBLE FINDINGS

Dress, Grooming, and Personal Hygiene

- Is the patient wearing any unusual jewelry? Where? Is there any body piercing or tattoo?

  Risk of hepatitis C

- Note patient's hair, fingernails, and use of cosmetics.

Facial Expression. Watch for eye contact. Is it natural? Sustained and unblinking? Averted quickly? Absent?

Stare of hyperthyroidism; flat or sad affect of depression. Decreased eye contact may be cultural or may suggest anxiety, fear, or sadness.

Odors of Body and Breath. Odors can be important diagnostic clues.

Breath odor of alcohol, acetone, uremia, or liver failure. Fruity odor of diabetes. (Never assume that alcohol on a patient's breath explains changes in mental status or neurologic findings.)

Posture, Gait, and Motor Activity

Preference to sit up in left-sided heart failure and to lean forward with arms braced in chronic obstructive pulmonary disease (COPD)

HEIGHT AND WEIGHT

Height. Measure the patient's height in stocking feet. Note the build—muscular or deconditioned, tall or short. Observe the body proportions.

Short stature in Turner's syndrome; elongated arms in Marfan's syndrome; loss of height in osteoporosis

Weight. Is the patient emaciated? Plump? If obese, is there central or dispersed distribution of fat? Weigh the patient with shoes off.

More than 50% of U.S. adults are overweight (BMI >25); nearly 25% are obese (BMI >30). These excesses are proven risk factors for diabetes, heart disease, stroke, hypertension, osteoarthritis, sleep apnea syndrome, and some forms of cancer.

Chapter 4 | Beginning the Physical Examination

EXAMINATION TECHNIQUES

POSSIBLE FINDINGS

Calculate the *body mass index* (BMI), which incorporates estimated but more accurate measurements of body fat than weight alone.

Methods to Calculate BMI

Unit of Measure	Method of Calculation
▸ *Weight in pounds,* height *in inches*	1. Body Mass Index Chart (see p. 54)
	2. $\dfrac{\left(\dfrac{\text{Weight (lbs)} \times 700^*}{\text{Height (inches)}}\right)}{\text{Height (inches)}}$
▸ *Weight in kilograms,* height *in meters squared*	3. $\dfrac{\text{Weight (kg)}}{\text{Height (m}^2\text{)}}$
▸ Either	4. BMI Calculator at Web site www.nhlbisupport.com/bmi

*Several organizations use 704.5, but the variation in BMI is negligible. Conversion formulas: 2.2 lb = 1 kg; 1.0 inch = 2.54 cm; 100 cm = 1 meter

Source: National Institutes of Health–National Heart, Lung and Blood Institute. Body Mass Index Calculator. Available at: www.nhlbisupport.com/bmi. Accessed June 25, 2011.

If the BMI is *above* 25, engage the patient in a 24-hour dietary recall and compare the intake of food groups and number of servings per day with current recommendations. Or, choose a screening tool and provide appropriate counseling or referral.

If the BMI falls *below* 17, be concerned about possible anorexia nervosa, bulimia, or other medical conditions (see Table 4-1, Eating Disorders and Excessively Low BMI, p. 61).

If the BMI is ≤35, measure the *waist circumference* just above the hip bones. The patient may have excess body fat if the waist measures ≥40 inches for men.

EXAMINATION TECHNIQUES

BMI Chart

	Normal						Overweight						Obese					
BMI	19	20	21	22	23	24	25	26	27	28	29	30	31	32	33	34	35
Height (inches)							Body Weight (pounds)											
58	91	96	100	105	110	115	119	124	129	134	138	143	148	153	158	162	167
59	94	99	104	109	114	119	124	128	133	138	143	148	153	158	163	168	173
60	97	102	107	112	118	123	128	133	138	143	148	153	158	163	168	174	179
61	100	105	111	116	122	127	132	137	143	148	153	158	164	169	174	180	185
62	104	109	115	120	126	131	136	142	147	153	158	164	169	175	180	185	191
63	107	113	118	124	130	135	141	145	152	158	163	169	174	180	185	191	197
64	110	116	122	128	134	140	145	151	157	163	169	174	180	185	192	197	204
65	114	120	126	132	138	144	150	156	162	168	174	180	186	192	198	204	210
66	118	124	130	136	142	148	155	161	167	173	179	186	192	198	204	210	216
67	121	127	134	140	146	153	159	166	172	178	185	191	198	204	211	217	223
68	125	131	138	144	151	158	164	171	177	184	190	197	203	210	216	223	230
69	128	135	142	149	155	162	169	176	182	189	196	203	209	216	223	230	236
70	132	139	146	153	160	167	174	181	188	189	196	203	209	216	223	230	236
71	136	143	150	157	165	172	179	186	193	200	208	215	222	229	236	243	250
72	140	147	154	162	169	177	184	191	199	206	213	221	228	235	242	250	258
73	144	151	159	166	174	182	189	197	204	212	219	227	235	242	250	257	265
74	148	155	163	171	179	186	194	202	210	218	225	233	241	249	256	264	272
75	152	160	168	176	184	192	200	208	216	224	232	240	248	256	264	272	279
76	156	164	172	180	189	197	205	213	221	230	238	246	254	263	271	279	287

Source: National Heart, Lung, and Blood Institute, National Institutes of Health. Body Mass Index Table. Available at: www.nhlbi.nih.gov/guidelines/obesity/bmi_tbl.pdf. Accessed June 25, 2011.

THE VITAL SIGNS: BLOOD PRESSURE, HEART RATE, RESPIRATORY RATE, AND TEMPERATURE

Blood Pressure. To measure blood pressure accurately, choose a cuff of appropriate size and ensure careful technique.

Selecting the Correct Blood Pressure Cuff

- Width of the inflatable bladder of the cuff should be about 40% of upper arm circumference (about 12–14 cm in the average adult).
- Length of inflatable bladder should be about 80% of upper arm circumference (almost long enough to encircle the arm)

Chapter 4 | Beginning the Physical Examination

EXAMINATION TECHNIQUES

Steps to Ensure Accurate Blood Pressure Recordings

- Ideally, ask the patient to avoid smoking or drinking caffeinated beverages for 30 minutes before the blood pressure is taken and to rest for at least 5 minutes.
- Make sure the examining room is quiet and comfortably warm.
- Make sure the arm selected is *free of clothing*. There should be no arteriovenous fistulas for dialysis, scarring from prior brachial artery cutdowns, or signs of lymphedema (seen after axillary node dissection or radiation therapy).
- Palpate the brachial artery to confirm that it has a viable pulse.
- Position the arm so that the brachial artery, at the antecubital crease, is *at heart level*—roughly level with the 4th interspace at its junction with the sternum.
- If the patient is seated, rest the arm on a table a little above the patient's waist; if standing, try to support the patient's arm at the midchest level.

Measuring Blood Pressure

- Center the inflatable bladder over the brachial artery. The lower border of the cuff should be about 2.5 cm above the antecubital crease. Secure the cuff snugly. Position the patient's arm so that it is slightly flexed at the elbow.
- To determine how high to raise the cuff pressure, first estimate the systolic pressure by palpation. As you feel the radial artery with the fingers of one hand, rapidly inflate the cuff until the radial pulse disappears. Read this pressure on the manometer and add 30 mm Hg to it. Use of this sum as the target for subsequent inflations prevents discomfort from unnecessarily high cuff pressures. It also avoids the occasional error caused by an auscultatory gap—a silent interval between the systolic and diastolic pressures.
- Deflate the cuff promptly.
- Now place the bell of a stethoscope lightly over the brachial artery, taking care to make an air seal with its full rim. Because the sounds to be heard *(Korotkoff sounds)* are relatively low in pitch, they are heard better with the *bell*.
- Inflate the cuff rapidly again to the level just determined, and then deflate it slowly, at a rate of about 2 to 3 mm Hg per second. Note the level at which you hear the sounds of at least two consecutive beats. This is the *systolic pressure*.
- Continue to lower the pressure slowly. The disappearance point, usually only a few mm Hg below the muffling point, is the best estimate of *diastolic pressure*.
- Read both the systolic and diastolic levels to the nearest 2 mm Hg. Wait 2 or more minutes and repeat. Average your readings. If the first two readings differ by more than 5 mm Hg, take additional readings.
- Take blood pressure in both arms at least once.
- In patients taking antihypertensive medications or with a history of fainting, postural dizziness, or possible depletion of blood volume, take the blood pressure in two positions—supine and standing (unless contraindicated). A fall in systolic pressure of 20 mm Hg or more, especially when accompanied by symptoms, indicates orthostatic (postural) hypotension.

EXAMINATION TECHNIQUES

In 2003, the Joint National Committee on Detection, Evaluation, and Treatment of High Blood Pressure (JNC) categorized four levels of systolic blood pressure (SBP) and diastolic blood pressure (DBP).

JNC VII Blood Pressure Classification for Adults

Category	Systolic (mm Hg)	Diastolic (mm Hg)
Normal	<120	<80
Prehypertension	120–139	80–89
Stage 1 Hypertension	140–159	90–99
Stage 2 Hypertension	≥160	≥100
If Diabetes or Renal Disease	<130	<80

When the systolic and diastolic levels fall in different categories, use the higher category. For example, 170/92 mm Hg is Stage 2 hypertension; 135/100 mm Hg is Stage 1 hypertension. In *isolated systolic hypertension,* systolic blood pressure is ≥140 mm Hg, and diastolic blood pressure is <90 mm Hg.

Heart Rate. The radial pulse is used commonly to assess heart rate. With the pads of your index and middle fingers, compress the radial artery until you detect a maximal pulsation. If the rhythm is regular, count the rate for 15 seconds and multiply by 4. If the rate is unusually fast or slow, count it for 60 seconds. When the rhythm is irregular, evaluate the rate by auscultation at the cardiac apex (the apical pulse).

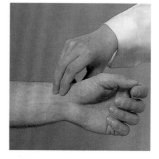

EXAMINATION TECHNIQUES

Rhythm.   Feel the radial pulse. Check the rhythm again by listening with your stethoscope at the cardiac apex. Is the rhythm regular or irregular? If irregular, try to identify a pattern: (1) Do early beats appear in a basically regular rhythm? (2) Does the irregularity vary consistently with respiration? (3) Is the rhythm totally irregular?

Respiratory Rate and Rhythm.   Observe the *rate, rhythm, depth,* and *effort of breathing.* Count the number of respirations in 1 minute either by visual inspection or by subtly listening over the patient's trachea with your stethoscope during examination of the head and neck or chest. Normally, adults take 14 to 20 breaths per minute in a quiet, regular pattern.

Temperature.   Average *oral temperature,* usually 37°C (98.6°F), fluctuates considerably from the early morning to the late afternoon or evening. *Rectal temperatures* are *higher* than oral temperatures by about 0.4 to 0.5°C (0.7 to 0.9°F) but also vary.

In contrast, *axillary temperatures* are *lower* than oral temperatures by approximately 1° but take 5 to 10 minutes to register and are considered less accurate than other measurements.

POSSIBLE FINDINGS

Palpation of an irregularly irregular rhythm reliably indicates *atrial fibrillation.* For all irregular patterns, an ECG is needed to identify the arrhythmia.

See Table 4-5, p. 65, Abnormalities in Rate and Rhythm of Breathing.

Fever or pyrexia refers to an elevated body temperature. *Hyperpyrexia* refers to extreme elevation in temperature, above 41.1°C (106°F), while *hypothermia* refers to an abnormally low temperature, below 35°C (95°F) rectally.

Causes of *fever* include infection, trauma (such as surgery or crush injuries), malignancy, blood disorders (such as acute hemolytic anemia), drug reactions, and immune disorders such as collagen vascular disease.

The chief cause of *hypothermia* is exposure to cold. Other predisposing causes include reduced movement as in paralysis, interference with vasoconstriction as from sepsis or excess alcohol, starvation, hypothyroidism, and hypoglycemia. Older adults are especially susceptible to hypothermia and also less likely to develop fever.

EXAMINATION TECHNIQUES	POSSIBLE FINDINGS

Oral temperatures: Choose either glass or electronic thermometer.

- *Glass thermometer:* Shake the thermometer down to 35°C (96°F) or below, insert it under the tongue, instruct the patient to close both lips, and wait 3 to 5 minutes. Then read the thermometer, reinsert for 1 minute, and read it again. Avoid breakage.

- *Electronic thermometer:* Carefully place the disposable cover over the probe and insert the thermometer under the tongue for about 10 seconds.

Tympanic membrane temperature: Make sure the external auditory canal is free of cerumen. Position the probe in the canal. Wait 2 to 3 seconds until the digital reading appears. This method measures core body temperature, which is higher than the normal oral temperature by approximately 0.8°C (11.4°F).

Rectal temperatures: Ask the patient to lie on one side with the hip flexed. Select a rectal thermometer with a stubby tip, lubricate it, and insert it about 3 cm to 4 cm (1½ inches) into the anal canal, in a direction pointing to the umbilicus. Remove it after 3 minutes, then read. Alternatively, use an electronic thermometer after lubricating the probe cover. Wait about 10 seconds for the digital temperature recording to appear.

Taking rectal temperatures is common practice in unresponsive patients at risk for biting down on the thermometer.

EXAMINATION TECHNIQUES

ACUTE AND CHRONIC PAIN

The experience of pain is complex and multifactorial. It involves sensory, emotional, and cognitive processing but may lack a specific physical etiology.

Chronic pain is defined in several ways: pain not associated with cancer or other medical conditions that persists for more than 3 to 6 months; pain lasting more than 1 month beyond the course of an acute illness or injury; or pain recurring at intervals of months or years. Chronic noncancer pain affects 5% to 33% of patients in primary care settings.

Adopt a comprehensive approach, carefully listening to the patient's description of the many features of pain and contributing factors. Accept the self-report, which experts state is the most reliable indicator of pain.

Location. Ask the patient to point to the pain. Lay terms may not be specific enough to localize the site of origin.

Severity. Use a consistent method to determine severity. Three scales are common: the Visual Analog Scale, and two scales using ratings from 1 to 10—the Numeric Rating Scale and the Faces Pain Scale.

Associated Features. Ask the patient to describe the pain and how it started. Pursue the seven features of pain, as you would with any symptom.

Attempted Treatments, Medications, Related Illnesses, and Impact on Daily Activities. Be sure to ask about any treatments that the patient has tried, including medications, physical therapy, and alternative medicines. A comprehensive medication history helps you to identify drugs that interact with analgesics and reduce their efficacy.

Identify any comorbid conditions such as arthritis, diabetes, HIV/AIDS, substance abuse, sickle cell disease, or psychiatric disorders. These can significantly affect the patient's experience of pain.

Health Disparities. Be aware of the well-documented health disparities in pain treatment and delivery of care, which range from lower use of analgesics in emergency rooms for African American and Hispanic patients to disparities in use of analgesics for cancer,

EXAMINATION TECHNIQUES

postoperative, and low back pain. Clinician stereotypes, language barriers, and unconscious clinician biases in decision making all contribute to these disparities. Critique your own communication style, seek information and best practice standards, and improve your techniques of patient education and empowerment.

Pain Management. Monitor the effectiveness of pain interventions, especially narcotics, by assessing the "four As": **A**nalgesia, **A**ctivities of daily living, **A**dverse effects, and **A**berrant drug-related behaviors. Risk of death from overdose of opioids rise four- to eight-fold for doses above 100 mg/day.

Recording Your Findings

Record the vital signs taken at the time of your examination. They are preferable to those taken earlier in the day by other providers. (Common abbreviations for blood pressure, heart rate, and respiratory rate are self-explanatory.)

Recording the Physical Examination—General Survey and Vital Signs

- "Mrs. Scott is a young, healthy-appearing woman, well-groomed, fit, and in good spirits. Height is 5'4", weight 135 lb, BP 120/80, HR 72 and regular, RR 16, temperature 37.5°C."

OR

- "Mr. Jones is an elderly man who looks pale and chronically ill. He is alert, with good eye contact, but cannot speak more than two or three words at a time because of shortness of breath. He has intercostal muscle retraction when breathing and sits upright in bed. He is thin, with diffuse muscle wasting. Height is 6'2", weight 175 lbs, BP 160/95, HR 108 and irregular, RR 32 and labored, temperature 101.2°F." (*Suggests COPD exacerbation.*)

Aids to Interpretation

Table 4-1   Eating Disorders and Excessively Low BMI

Anorexia Nervosa	Bulimia Nervosa
Refusal to maintain minimally normal body weight (or BMI above 17.5 kg/m^2)	Repeated binge eating followed by self-induced vomiting, misuse of laxatives, diuretics, or other medications; fasting; or excessive exercise
Fear of appearing fat	
Frequently starving but in denial; lacking insight	
Often brought in by family members	Often with normal weight
May present as failure to make expected weight gains in childhood or adolescence, amenorrhea in women, loss of libido or potency in men	Overeating at least twice a week during 3-month period; large amounts of food consumed in short period (~2 hrs)
Associated with depressive symptoms such as depressed mood, irritability, social withdrawal, insomnia, decreased libido	Preoccupation with eating; craving and compulsion to eat; lack of control over eating; alternating with periods of starvation
Additional features supporting diagnosis: self-induced vomiting or purging, excessive exercise, use of appetite suppressants and/or diuretics	Dread of fatness but may be obese
Biologic complications • *Neuroendocrine changes:* amenorrhea, hormonal alterations • *Cardiovascular disorders:* bradycardia, hypotension, dysrhythmias, cardiomyopathy • *Metabolic disorders:* hypokalemia, hypochloremic metabolic alkalosis, increased BUN, edema *Other:* dry skin, dental caries, delayed gastric emptying, constipation, anemia, osteoporosis	Subtypes of • *Purging:* bulimic episodes accompanied by self-induced vomiting or use of laxatives, diuretics, or enemas • *Nonpurging:* bulimic episodes accompanied by compensatory behavior such as fasting, exercise without purging Biologic complications; see changes listed for anorexia nervosa.

Sources: World Health Organization. The ICD-10 Classification of Mental and Behavioral Disorders: Diagnostic Criteria for Research. Geneva: World Health Organization, 1993; American Psychiatric Association. DSM-IV-TR: Diagnostic and Statistical Manual of Mental Disorders, 4th ed. Text Revision. Washington, DC: American Psychiatric Association, 2000. Halmi KA: Eating disorders: In: Kaplan HI, Sadock BJ, eds. Comprehensive Textbook of Psychiatry, 7th ed. Philadelphia: Lippincott Williams & Wilkins, 1663–1676, 2000. Mehler PS. Bulimia nervosa. N Engl J Med 2003;349(9):875–880.

Table 4-2 Nutrition Screening Checklist

Statement	Points
I have an illness or condition that made me change the kind and/or amount of food I eat.	Yes (2 pts) _____
I eat fewer than 2 meals per day.	Yes (3 pts) _____
I eat few fruits or vegetables, or milk products.	Yes (2 pts) _____
I have 3 or more drinks of beer, liquor, or wine almost every day.	Yes (2 pts) _____
I have tooth or mouth problems that make it hard for me to eat.	Yes (2 pts) _____
I don't always have enough money to buy the food I need.	Yes (4 pts) _____
I eat alone most of the time.	Yes (1 pt) _____
I take 3 or more different prescribed or over-the-counter drugs each day.	Yes (1 pt) _____
Without wanting to, I have lost or gained 10 pounds in the last 6 months.	Yes (2 pts) _____
I am not always physically able to shop, cook, and/or feed myself.	Yes (2 pts) _____
	TOTAL _____

Instructions: Check "yes" for each condition that applies, then total the nutritional score. For total scores between 3 and 5 points (moderate risk) or ≥6 points (high risk), further evaluation is needed (especially for the elderly).

Source: American Academy of Family Physicians. The Nutrition Screening Initiative. Available at: www.aafp.org/PreBuilt/NSI_DETERMINE.pdf. Accessed January 23, 2008.

Table 4-3 Nutrition Counseling: Sources of Nutrients

Nutrient	Food Source
Calcium	Dairy foods such as milk, natural cheeses, and yogurt Calcium-fortified cereals, fruit juice, soy milk, and tofu Dark green leafy vegetables like collard, turnip, and mustard greens; bok choy Sardines
Iron	Lean meat, dark turkey meat, liver Clams, mussels, oysters, sardines, anchovies Iron-fortified cereals Enriched and whole grain bread Spinach, peas, lentil, turnip greens, peas, and artichokes Dried prunes and raisins
Folate	Cooked dried beans and peas Oranges, orange juice Liver Black-eyed peas, lentils, okra, chick peas, peanuts Folate-fortified cereals
Vitamin D	Vitamin D–fortified milk Cod liver oil; salmon, mackerel, tuna Egg yolks, butter, margarine Vitamin D–fortified cereals

Source: Adapted from: Dietary Guidelines Committee, 2000 Report. Nutrition and Your Health: Dietary Guidelines for Americans. Washington, DC: Agricultural Research Service, U.S. Department of Agriculture, 2000; Choose MyPlate.gov. Available at http://www.choosemyplate.gov/index.html. Accessed June 24, 2011; Office of Dietary Supplements, National Institutes of Health. Dietary Supplement Fact Sheets: Calcium; Vitamin D. At http://ods.od.nih.gov/factsheets/list-all/. Accessed June 24, 2011.

Table 4-4. Patients With Hypertension: Recommended Changes in Diet

Dietary Change	Food Source
Increase foods high in potassium	Baked white or sweet potatoes
	White beans, beet greens, soybeans, spinach, lentils, kidney beans
	Bananas, plantains, many dried fruits, orange juice
	Tomato sauce, juice, and paste
Decrease foods high in sodium	Canned foods (soups, tuna fish) Pretzels, potato chips, pickles, olives
	Many processed foods (frozen dinners, ketchup, mustard)
	Batter-fried foods
	Table salt, including for cooking

Source: Adapted from Dietary Guidelines Committee. 2000 Report. Nutrition and Your Health: Dietary Guidelines for Americans. Washington, DC: Agricultural Research Service, U.S. Department of Agriculture, 2000. Choose MyPlate.gov. Available at http://www.choosemyplate.gov/index.html. Accessed June 24, 2011; Office of Dietary Supplements, National Institutes of Health. Dietary Supplement Fact Sheets: Calcium; Vitamin D. At http://ods.od.nih.gov/factsheets/list-all/. Accessed June 24, 2011.

	Abnormalities in Rate and Rhythm of Breathing
Inspiration Expiration / Time / Volume of air	**Normal.** In adults, 14–20 per min; in infants, up to 44 per min.
	Rapid Shallow Breathing (*Tachypnea*). Many causes, including restrictive lung disease, pleural chest pain, and an elevated diaphragm.
	Rapid Deep Breathing (*Hyperpnea, Hyperventilation*). Many causes, including exercise, anxiety, metabolic acidosis, brainstem injury. *Kussmaul breathing,* due to metabolic acidosis, is deep, but rate may be fast, slow, or normal.
	Slow Breathing (*Bradypnea*). May be secondary to diabetic coma, drug-induced respiratory depression, increased intracranial pressure.
Hyperpnea Apnea	**Cheyne-Stokes Breathing.** Rhythmically alternating periods of hyperpnea and apnea. In infants and the aged, may be normal during sleep; also accompanies brain damage, heart failure, uremia, drug-induced respiratory depression.
	Ataxic (*Biot's*) Breathing. Unpredictable irregularity of depth and rate. Causes include brain damage and respiratory depression.
Sighs	**Sighing Breathing.** Breathing punctuated by frequent sighs. When associated with other symptoms, it suggests the hyperventilation syndrome. Occasional sighs are normal.

CHAPTER 5

Behavior and Mental Status

Empathic listening, careful observation, and skilled history taking help patients to reveal their deepest concerns and experiences. Clinicians often miss clues to trauma, mental illness, and harmful dysfunctional behaviors. The prevalence of mental health disorders in the U.S. population is 30%, yet only approximately 20% of affected patients receive treatment. Even for patients who obtain care, evidence suggests that adherence to treatment guidelines in primary care offices is <50%.

Often, patients have health symptoms that mirror medical illnesses. Thirty percent of symptoms last more than 6 weeks and are "medically unexplained," masking anxiety, depression, or even somatoform disorders. See Table 5-1, Somatoform Disorders: Types and Approach, pp. 76–78. Depression and anxiety are highly correlated with substance abuse, for example, and clinicians are advised to look for overlap in these conditions. "Difficult patients" are frequently those with multiple unexplained symptoms and underlying psychiatric conditions that are amenable to therapy. Without better "dual diagnosis," patient health, function, and quality of life are at risk.

Mental Health Disorders and Unexplained Symptoms in Primary Care Settings

Mental Health Disorders in Primary Care

- Approximately 20% of primary care outpatients have mental disorders, but up to 50% to 75% of these disorders are undetected and untreated.
- Prevalence of mental disorders in primary care settings is roughly:
  - Anxiety—20%
  - Mood disorders including dysthymia, depressive, and bipolar disorders—25%
  - Depression—10%
  - Somatoform disorder—10% to 15%
  - Alcohol and substance abuse—15% to 20%

(continued)

Mental Health Disorders and Unexplained Symptoms in Primary Care Settings (continued)

Explained and Unexplained Symptoms

- Physical symptoms account for approximately 50% of office visits.
- Roughly one-third of physical symptoms are unexplained; in 20% to 25% of patients, physical symptoms become chronic or recurring.
- In patients with *unexplained symptoms,* the prevalence of depression and anxiety exceeds 50% and increases with the total number of reported physical symptoms, making detection and "dual diagnosis" important clinical goals.

Common Functional Syndromes

- Co-occurrence rates for *common functional syndromes* such as irritable bowel syndrome, fibromyalgia, chronic fatigue, temporomandibular joint disorder, and multiple chemical sensitivity reach 30% to 90%, depending on the disorders compared.
- The prevalence of *symptom overlap* is high in the common functional syndromes: namely, complaints of fatigue, sleep disturbance, musculoskeletal pain, headache, and gastrointestinal problems.
- The common functional syndromes also overlap in rates of functional impairment, psychiatric comorbidity, and response to cognitive and antidepressant therapy.

For unexplained conditions lasting beyond 6 weeks, experts recommend brief screening questions with high sensitivity and specificity, followed by more detailed investigation when indicated due to high rates of coexisting depression and anxiety.

Patient Identifiers for Mental Health Screening

- Medically unexplained physical symptoms—more than half have a depressive or anxiety disorder
- Multiple physical or somatic symptoms or "high symptom count"
- High severity of the presenting somatic symptom
- Chronic pain
- Symptoms for more than 6 weeks
- Physician rating as a "difficult encounter"
- Recent stress
- Low self-rating of overall health
- High use of health care services
- Substance abuse

The Health History

Common or Concerning Symptoms

- Changes in attention, mood, or speech
- Changes in insight, orientation, or memory
- Anxiety, panic, ritualistic behavior, and phobias
- Delirium or dementia

Your assessment of mental status begins with the patient's first words. As you gather the health history, you will quickly observe the patient's level of *alertness* and *orientation, mood, attention,* and *memory*. You will learn about the patient's *insight* and *judgment,* as well as any *recurring or unusual thoughts or perceptions*. For some, you will need to conduct a more formal evaluation of mental status.

Many of the terms used to describe the mental status examination are familiar to you from social conversation. Take the time to learn their precise meanings in the context of the formal evaluation of mental status (see below).

Terminology: The Mental Status Examination

Level of Consciousness	Alertness or State of Awareness of the Environment
Attention	The ability to focus or concentrate over time on one task or activity
Memory	The process of registering or recording information. *Recent or short-term memory* covers minutes, hours, or days; *remote or long-term memory* refers to intervals of years.
Orientation	Awareness of personal identity, place, and time; requires both memory and attention
Perceptions	Sensory awareness of objects in the environment and their interrelationships; also refers to internal stimuli (e.g., dreams)
Thought processes	The logic, coherence, and relevance of the patient's thoughts, or *how* people think
Thought content	*What* the patient thinks about, including level of insight and judgment
Insight	Awareness that symptoms or disturbed behaviors are normal or abnormal
Judgment	Process of comparing and evaluating alternatives; reflects values that may or may not be based on reality and social conventions or norms

(continued)

Terminology: The Mental Status Examination (continued)

Level of Consciousness	Alertness or State of Awareness of the Environment
Affect	An observable, usually episodic, feeling tone expressed through voice, facial expression, and demeanor
Mood	A more sustained emotion that may color a person's view of the world (affect is to mood as weather is to climate)
Language	A complex symbolic system for expressing, receiving, and comprehending words; essential for assessing other mental functions
Higher cognitive functions	Assessed by vocabulary, fund of information, abstract thinking, calculations, construction of objects with two or three dimensions

Assess level of consciousness, general appearance and mood, and ability to pay attention, remember, understand, and speak.

See Table 5-2, Disorders of Mood, pp. 78–79.

Assess the patient's responses to illness and life circumstances, which often tell you about his or her insight and judgment. Test orientation and memory.

Explore any unusual thoughts, preoccupations, beliefs, or perceptions as they arise during the interview.

See Table 5-3, Anxiety Disorders, pp. 80–81, and Table 5-4, Selected Psychotic Disorders, p. 82.

All patients with documented or suspected brain lesions, psychiatric symptoms, or reports from family members of vague or changed behavioral symptoms need further systematic assessment.

See Table 20-2, Delirium and Dementia, pp. 391–392.

Health Promotion and Counseling: Evidence and Recommendations

Important Topics for Health Promotion and Counseling

- Screening for depression and suicidality
- Screening for alcohol, prescription drug, and substance abuse

Mood Disorders and Depression. Lifetime prevalence of *major depression* meeting formal diagnostic criteria in the United States is approximately 7%. Primary care providers fail to diagnose major depression in up to 50% of affected patients, often missing early clues such as *low self-esteem*, *anhedonia* (lack of pleasure in daily activities), *sleep disorders*, and *difficulty concentrating* or *making decisions*. Failure to diagnose depression can have fatal consequences—suicide rates in patients with major depression are eight times higher than in the general population. Ask, "Over the past 2 weeks, have you felt down, depressed, or hopeless?" and "Over the past 2 weeks, have you felt little interest or pleasure in doing things?"

Suicide. Suicide rates are highest among men 75 years and older and are increasing among teenagers and young adults. More than half of patients committing suicide have visited their physicians in the prior month. More than 90% of suicide deaths occur in patients with depression or other mental health disorders or substance abuse. Risk factors include suicidal or homicidal ideation, intent, or plan; access to the means for suicide; current symptoms of psychosis or severe anxiety; any history of psychiatric illness (especially linked to a hospital admission); substance abuse; personality disorder; and prior history or family history of suicide. Patients with these risk factors should be immediately referred for psychiatric care and possibly hospitalization.

Alcohol, Prescription Drug, and Substance Abuse. The comorbidity of alcohol and substance abuse with mental health disorders and suicide are extensive. Alcohol, tobacco, and illicit drugs account for more illness, deaths, and disabilities than any other preventable condition. Lifetime prevalence of alcohol and illicit drug use in the United States is 13% and 3%. In recent U.S. surveys, 8% of those 12 years or older, or 19 million people, reported use of illicit drugs in the prior 30 days. An estimated 3% are dependent on or abuse illicit drugs; of these, 60% use marijuana. Prescription drug abuse now kills more people than illicit substances. Because screening for alcohol and drug use is part of *every* patient history, review the screening questions recommended in Chapter 3, Interviewing and the Health History.

Techniques of Examination

The Mental Status Examination

- Appearance and behavior
- Speech and language
- Mood
- Thoughts and perceptions
- Cognition, including memory, attention, information and vocabulary, calculations, abstract thinking, and constructional ability

| EXAMINATION TECHNIQUES | POSSIBLE FINDINGS |

Observe patient's mental status throughout your interaction. Test specific functions if indicated during the interview or physical examination.

APPEARANCE AND BEHAVIOR

Assess *the following:*

- *Level of Consciousness.* Observe alertness and response to verbal and tactile stimuli.

  Normal consciousness, lethargy, obtundation, stupor, coma (see p. 304–305)

- *Posture and Motor Behavior.* Observe pace, range, character, and appropriateness of movements.

  Restlessness, agitation, bizarre postures, immobility, involuntary movements

- *Dress, Grooming, and Personal Hygiene*

  Fastidiousness, neglect

- *Facial Expressions.* Assess during rest and interaction.

  Anxiety, depression, elation, anger, responses to imaginary people or objects, withdrawal

- *Manner, Affect, and Relation to People and Things*

SPEECH AND LANGUAGE

Note quantity, rate, loudness, clarity, and fluency of speech. If indicated, test for aphasia.

Aphasia, dysphonia, dysarthria, changes with mood disorders

Testing for Aphasia

Word Comprehension	Ask patient to follow a one-stage command, such as "Point to your nose." Try a two-stage command: "Point to your mouth, then your knee."
Repetition	Ask patient to repeat a phrase of one-syllable words (the most difficult repetition task): "No ifs, ands, or buts."
Naming	Ask patient to name the parts of a watch.
Reading Comprehension	Ask patient to read a paragraph aloud.
Writing	Ask patient to write a sentence.

Chapter 5 | Behavior and Mental Status

| EXAMINATION TECHNIQUES | POSSIBLE FINDINGS |

MOOD

Ask about the patient's spirits. Note nature, intensity, duration, and stability of any abnormal mood. If indicated, assess risk of suicide.

Happiness, elation, depression, anxiety, anger, indifference

THOUGHT AND PERCEPTIONS

Thought Processes. Assess logic, relevance, organization, and coherence.

Derailments, flight of ideas, incoherence, confabulation, blocking

Thought Content. Ask about and explore any unusual or unpleasant thoughts.

Obsessions, compulsions, delusions, feelings of unreality

Perceptions. Ask about any unusual perceptions (e.g., seeing or hearing things).

Illusions, hallucinations

Insight and Judgment. Assess patient's insight into the illness and level of judgment used in making decisions or plans.

Recognition or denial of mental cause of symptoms; bizarre, impulsive, or unrealistic judgment

COGNITIVE FUNCTIONS

If indicated, assess:

Orientation to time, place, and person

Disorientation

Attention

- *Digit span*—ability to repeat a series of numbers forward and then backward
- *Serial 7s*—ability to subtract 7 repeatedly, starting with 100
- *Spelling backward* of a five-letter word, such as W-O-R-L-D

Poor performance of digit span, serial 7s, and spelling backward are common in dementia and delirium but have other causes, too.

Remote Memory (e.g., birthdays, anniversaries, social security number, schools, jobs, wars)

Impaired in late stages of dementia

EXAMINATION TECHNIQUES	POSSIBLE FINDINGS

Recent Memory (e.g., events of the day)

New Learning Ability—ability to repeat three or four words after a few minutes of unrelated activity

Recent memory and new learning ability impaired in dementia, delirium, and amnestic disorders

HIGHER COGNITIVE FUNCTIONS

If indicated, assess:

Information and Vocabulary. Note range and depth of patient's information, complexity of ideas expressed, and vocabulary used. For the fund of information, ask names of presidents, other political figures, or large cities.

These attributes reflect intelligence, education, and cultural background. They are limited by mental retardation but are fairly well preserved in early dementia.

Calculating Abilities, such as addition, subtraction, and multiplication

Poor calculation in mental retardation and dementia

Abstract Thinking—ability to respond abstractly to questions about
- The meaning of *proverbs*, such as "A stitch in time saves nine"
- The *similarities* of beings or things, such as a cat and a mouse or a piano and a violin

Concrete responses (observable details rather than concepts) are common in mental retardation, dementia, and delirium. Responses are sometimes bizarre in schizophrenia.

Constructional Ability. Ask patient:

Impaired ability common in dementia and with parietal lobe damage

- To copy figures such as circle, cross, diamond, and box, and two intersecting pentagons, or
- To draw a clock face with numbers and hands

SPECIAL TECHNIQUE

Mini-Mental State Examination (MMSE). This brief test is useful in screening for cognitive dysfunction and dementia and following their course over time. For more detailed information regarding the MMSE, contact the Publisher, Psychological Assessment Resources, Inc., 16204 North Florida Avenue, Lutz, Florida 33549. Some sample questions are given on the next page.

EXAMINATION TECHNIQUES

MMSE Sample Items

Orientation to Time
"What is the date?"

Registration
"Listen carefully; I am going to say three words. You say them back after I stop. Ready? Here they are . . .
HOUSE (pause), CAR (pause), LAKE (pause). Now repeat those words back o me." [Repeat up to five times, but score only the first trial.]

Naming
"What is this?" [Point to a pencil or pen.]

Reading
"Please read this and do what it says." [Show examinee the words on the stimulus form.]
CLOSE YOUR EYES

Reproduced by special permission of the Publisher, Psychological Assessment Resources, Inc., 16204 North Florida Avenue, Lutz, FL 33549, from the Mini Mental State Examination, by Marshal Folstein and Susan Folstein, Copyright 1975, 1998, 2001 by Mini Mental LLC, Inc. Published 2001 by Psychological Assessment Resources, Inc. Further reproduction is prohibited without permission of PAR, Inc. The MMSE can be purchased from PAR, Inc.

Recording Your Findings

Recording Behavior and Mental Status

"Mental Status: The patient is alert, well-groomed, and cheerful. Speech is fluent and words are clear. Thought processes are coherent, insight is good. The patient is oriented to person, place, and time. Serial 7s accurate; recent and remote memory intact. Calculations intact."
OR
"Mental Status: The patient appears sad and fatigued; clothes are wrinkled. Speech is slow and words are mumbled. Thought processes are coherent, but insight into current life reverses is limited. The patient is oriented to person, place, and time. Digit span, serial 7s, and calculations accurate, but responses delayed. Clock drawing is good." (Suggests depression)

Aids to Interpretation

Table 5-1 Somatoform Disorders: Types and Approach to Symptoms

Types of Somatoform Disorders

Somatoform Disorders*

Disorder	Features
Somatization disorder	Chronic multisystem disorder characterized by complaints of pain, gastrointestinal and sexual dysfunction, and pseudoneurologic symptoms. Onset is usually early in life, and psychosocial and vocational achievements are limited.
Conversion disorder	Syndrome of symptoms of deficits mimicking neurologic or medical illness in which psychological factors are judged to be of etiologic importance
Pain disorder	Clinical syndrome characterized predominantly by pain in which psychological factors are judged to be of etiologic importance
Hypochondriasis	Chronic preoccupation with the idea of having a serious disease. The preoccupation is usually poorly amenable to reassurance
Body dysmorphic disorder	Preoccupation with an imagined or exaggerated defect in physical appearance

Other Somatoform-like Disorders

Factitious disorder	Intentional production or feigning of physical or psychological signs when external reinforcers (e.g., avoidance of responsibility, financial gain) are not clearly present
Malingering	Intentional production or feigning of physical or psychological signs when external reinforcers (e.g., avoidance of responsibility, financial gain) are present
Dissociative disorders	Disruptions of consciousness, memory, identity, or perception judged to be due to psychological factors

Approach to Somatic and Unexplained Symptoms

Stepped Care Approach to Somatic Symptoms in Primary Care†

Is the somatic symptom likely to be…	Clinician action might be…
Acutely serious? (<5% of cases)	Expedited diagnostic workup
Minor/self-limited? (70%–75% of cases)	Address patient expectations Symptom-specific therapy Follow-up in 2–6 weeks

Table 5-1: Somatoform Disorders: Types and Approach to Symptoms *(continued)*

Is the somatic symptom likely to be …	Clinician action might be …
Chronic or recurrent? (20%–25% of cases)	Screen for depression and anxiety
Caused or aggravated by a depressive or anxiety disorder?	Antidepressant therapy and/or cognitive–behavioral therapy (CBT)
Due to a functional somatic syndrome?	Syndrome-specific therapy Antidepressant therapy and/or CBT
Persistent and medically unexplained?	Regular, time-limited clinic visits Consider mental health referral Symptom management strategies, if evidence-based (e.g., behavioral treatments, pain self-management programs, pain or other specialty clinics, complementary and alternative medicine) Rehabilitative rather than disability approach

Management Guidelines for Patients With Medically Unexplained Symptoms‡

General Aspects	Show empathy and understanding for the complaints and frustrating experiences the patient has had so far (e.g., explain that medically unexplained symptoms are common). Develop a good patient–physician relationship; try to be the "coordinator" of diagnostic procedures and care.
Diagnosis	Explore not only the history of complaints and former treatments, but any impairment, anxiety, and psychosocial issues. Use screeners and self-report questionnaires to enhance detection; use symptom diaries to assess course and factors influencing symptoms. When the patient presents with a new symptom, examine the relevant organ system. Provide the results of investigations to give clear reassurance that there is no serious physical disease. Avoid unnecessary diagnostic tests or surgical procedures.
Treatment	Provide regularly scheduled visits (e.g., every 4–6 weeks), especially in the case of a history of very frequent healthcare utilization. Explain that treatment is coping, not curing (when pathology cannot be found or does not explain degree of complaints).

(continued)

Table 5-1 Somatoform Disorders: Types and Approach to Symptoms (continued)

Is the somatic symptom likely to be…	Clinician action might be…
Referral	Suggest coping strategies like regular physical activity, relaxation, distraction. If referral is necessary to start psychotherapy or psychopharmacotherapy, prepare the patient for the treatment and provide reassurance that you will continue to be the patient's doctor.

Sources: *Schiffer RB. Psychiatric disorders in medical practice. In: Goldman L, Ausiello D, eds. Cecil Textbook of Medicine. 22nd ed. Philadelphia: Saunders 2004, pp. 2628–2639; †Kroenke K. Patients presenting with somatic complaints: epidemiology, psychiatric comorbidity, and management. Int J Methods Psychiatr Res 2003;12(1):34–43. ‡Reif W, Martin A, Rauh E, et al. Evaluation of general practitioners' training: how to manage patients with unexplained physical symptoms. Psychosomatics 2006;47(4):304–311.

Table 5-2 Disorders of Mood

Major Depressive Episode	Manic Episode
At least five of the symptoms listed below (including one of the first two) must be present during the same 2-week period; they must represent a change from the person's previous state.	A distinct period of abnormally and persistently elevated, expansive, or irritable mood must be present for at least a week (any duration if hospitalization is necessary). During this time, at least three of the symptoms listed below have been persistent and significant. (Four symptoms are required if the mood is only irritable.)
• Depressed mood (may be an irritable mood in children and adolescents) most of the day, nearly every day	
• Markedly diminished interest or pleasure in almost all activities most of the day, nearly every day	• Inflated self-esteem or grandiosity • Decreased need for sleep (feels rested after sleeping 3 hours)
• Significant weight gain or loss (not dieting) or increased or decreased appetite nearly every day	• More talkative than usual or pressure to keep talking

Table 5-2 Disorders of Mood (continued)

Major Depressive Episode	Manic Episode
• Insomnia or hypersomnia nearly every day • Psychomotor agitation or retardation nearly every day • Fatigue or loss of energy nearly every day • Feelings of worthlessness or inappropriate guilt nearly every day • Inability to think or concentrate or indecisiveness nearly every day • Recurrent thoughts of death or suicide, or a specific plan for or attempt at suicide The symptoms cause significant distress or impair social, occupational, or other important functions. In severe cases, hallucinations and delusions may occur.	• Flight of ideas or racing thoughts • Distractibility • Increased goal-directed activity (either socially at work or school, or sexually) or psychomotor agitation • Excessive involvement in pleasurable high-risk activities (buying sprees, foolish business ventures, sexual indiscretions) The disturbance is severe enough to impair social or occupational functions or relationships. It may necessitate hospitalization for the protection of self or others. In severe cases, hallucinations and delusions may occur.
Mixed Episode	**Hypomanic Episode**
A mixed episode, which must last at least 1 week, meets the criteria for both major and manic depressive episodes.	The mood and symptoms resemble those in a manic episode but are less impairing, do not require hospitalization, do not include hallucinations or delusions, and have a shorter minimum duration—4 days.
Dysthymic Disorder	**Cyclothymic Episode**
A depressed mood and symptoms for most of the day, for more days than not, over at least 2 years (1 year in children and adolescents). Freedom from symptoms lasts no more than 2 months at a time.	Numerous periods of hypomanic and depressive symptoms that last for at least 2 years (1 year in children and adolescents). Freedom from symptoms lasts no more than 2 months at a time.

Tables 5-2 to 5-4 are based, with permission, on the Diagnostic and Statistical Manual of Mental Disorders, 4th ed., Text Revision [DSM IV-TR]. Washington, DC: American Psychiatric Association, 2000. For further details and criteria, the reader should consult this manual, its successor, or comprehensive textbooks of psychiatry.

Table 5-3 Anxiety Disorders

Panic Disorder. Recurrent, unexpected panic attacks, at least one of which has been followed by a month or more of persistent concern about further attacks, worry over their implications or consequences, or a significant change in behavior in relation to the attacks.

A *panic attack* is a discrete period of intense fear or discomfort that develops abruptly and peaks within 10 minutes. It involves at least four of the following symptoms: (1) palpitations, pounding heart, or accelerated heart rate; (2) sweating; (3) trembling or shaking; (4) shortness of breath or a sense of smothering; (5) a feeling of choking; (6) chest pain or discomfort; (7) nausea or abdominal distress; (8) feeling dizzy, unsteady, lightheaded, or faint; (9) feelings of unreality or depersonalization; (10) fear of losing control or going crazy; (11) fear of dying; (12) paresthesias (numbness or tingling); and (13) chills or hot flushes.

Agoraphobia. Anxiety about being in places or situations where escape may be difficult or embarrassing or help for sudden symptoms unavailable. Such situations are avoided, require a companion, or cause marked anxiety.

Specific Phobia. A marked, persistent, and excessive or unreasonable fear that is cued by the presence or anticipation of a specific object or situation, such as dogs, injections, or flying. The person recognizes the fear as excessive or unreasonable, but exposure to the cue provokes immediate anxiety. Avoidance or fear impairs the person's normal routine, occupational or academic functioning, or social activities or relationships.

Social Phobia. A marked, persistent fear of one or more social or performance situations that involve exposure to unfamiliar people or to scrutiny by others. Those afflicted fear that they will act in embarrassing or humiliating ways, as by showing their anxiety. Exposure creates anxiety and possibly a panic attack, and the person avoids precipitating situations. He or she recognizes the fear as excessive or unreasonable. Normal functioning, social activities, or relationships are impaired.

Table 5-3 Anxiety Disorders *(continued)*

Obsessive–Compulsive Disorder. Obsessions or compulsions that cause marked anxiety or distress. Although recognized as excessive or unreasonable, they are time-consuming and interfere with the person's normal routine and relationships.

Acute Stress Disorder. Exposure to a traumatic event that involved actual or threatened death or serious injury to self or others, leading to intense fear, helplessness, or horror. During or immediately after this event, the person has at least three dissociative symptoms: (1) a subjective sense of numbing, detachment, or absence of emotional responsiveness; (2) a reduced awareness of surroundings, as in a daze; (3) feelings of unreality; (4) feelings of depersonalization; and (5) amnesia for an important part of the event. The event is persistently reexperienced, as in thoughts, images, dreams, illusions, and flashbacks. The person is anxious, shows increased arousal, and avoids stimuli that evoke memories of the event. Causes marked distress or impairs social, occupational, or other important functions. Symptoms occur within 4 weeks of the event and last from 2 days to 4 weeks.

Posttraumatic Stress Disorder. The event, fearful response, and persistent reexperiencing of the traumatic event resemble acute stress disorder. Hallucinations may occur. The person has increased arousal, tries to avoid stimuli related to the trauma, and has numbing of general responsiveness. Causes marked distress and impaired social or occupational function, and lasts for more than a month.

Generalized Anxiety Disorder. Lacks a specific traumatic event or focus for concern. Excessive anxiety and worry are hard to control and generalize to a number of events or activities. At least three of the following symptoms are associated: (1) feeling restless, keyed up, or on edge; (2) being easily fatigued; (3) difficulty in concentrating or mind going blank; (4) irritability; (5) muscle tension; and (6) difficulty in falling or staying asleep, or restless, unsatisfying sleep. Causes significant distress or impairs daily function.

Table 5-4 Selected Psychotic Disorders

Schizophrenia. Impairs major functioning at work or school, in interpersonal relations, or in self-care. Performance of one or more of these functions must decrease for a significant time to a level markedly below prior achievement. Person displays at least two of the following for a significant part of 1 month: (1) delusions; (2) hallucinations; (3) disorganized speech; (4) grossly disorganized or catatonic behavior; and (5) negative symptoms such as a flat affect, alogia (lack of content in speech), or avolition (lack of interest, drive, and ability to set and pursue goals). Continuous signs of the disturbance must persist for at least 6 months.

Subtypes of this disorder include paranoid, disorganized, and catatonic schizophrenia.

Schizophreniform Disorder. Symptoms are similar to those of schizophrenia but last <6 months. Functional impairment need not be present.

Schizoaffective Disorder. Features both a major mood disturbance and schizophrenia. Mood disturbance (depressive, manic, or mixed) present during most of the illness and must, for a time, be concurrent with symptoms of schizophrenia and demonstrate delusions or hallucinations for at least 2 weeks without prominent mood symptoms.

Delusional Disorder. Nonbizarre delusions involve situations in real life, such as having a disease, and persists for at least a month. Functioning is not markedly impaired and behavior is not obviously odd or bizarre. Symptoms of schizophrenia, except for tactile and olfactory hallucinations, are not present.

Brief Psychotic Disorder. At least one of the following psychotic symptoms must be present: delusions, hallucinations, disordered speech such as frequent derailment or incoherence, or grossly disorganized or catatonic behavior. Disturbance lasts ≥1 day but <1 month, and person returns to prior functional level.

CHAPTER

6

The Skin, Hair, and Nails

The Health History

Common or Concerning Symptoms

- Hair loss
- Rash
- Growths

Health Promotion and Counseling: Evidence and Recommendations

Important Topics for Health Promotion and Counseling

- Skin cancers: types and risk factors
- Avoidance of excessive sun exposure

Counsel patients to avoid unnecessary sun exposure, tanning beds, and sunlamps and to use sunscreen with at least SPF-15. It is helpful to show patients pictures of *basal cell carcinomas, squamous cell carcinomas* and *melanomas* (pp. 94–95).

Teach the ABCDE screen for dysplastic nevi/melanomas: **A**symmetry, irregular **B**orders, variation in **C**olor, **D**iameter ≥6 mm, and **E**volution or change in size, symptoms, or morphology. Survey skin at 3-year intervals for patients 20 to 40 years of age and annually for patients older than 40 years. For those older than age 50 or with dysplastic nevi or history of melanoma, encourage monthly self-examination and do regular clinical screening.

Techniques of Examination

| EXAMINATION TECHNIQUES | POSSIBLE FINDINGS |

SKIN

Examine the entire skin surface under good lighting.

Inspect and palpate any growths.

Note:

- Color — Cyanosis, jaundice, carotenemia, changes in melanin

- Moisture — Dry, oily

- Temperature — Cool, warm

- Texture — Smooth, rough

- Mobility—ease with which a fold of skin can be moved — Decreased if edema

- Turgor—speed with which the fold returns into place — Decreased if dehydration

Note any lesions and their:

- Anatomical location and distribution — Generalized, localized

- Patterns and shapes — Linear, clustered, dermatomal

- Type — Macule, papule, pustule, bulla, tumor

- Color — Red, white, brown, heliotrope

Chapter 6 | The Skin, Hair, and Nails

EXAMINATION TECHNIQUES	POSSIBLE FINDINGS

HAIR

Inspect and palpate the hair.

Note:
- Quantity — Thin, thick
- Distribution — Patchy or total alopecia
- Texture — Fine, coarse

NAILS

Inspect and palpate the fingernails and toenails.

Note:
- Color — Cyanosis, pallor
- Shape — Clubbing
- Any lesions — Paronychia, onycholysis

Recording Your Findings

Recording the Physical Examination—The Skin

> "Color pink. Skin warm and moist. Nails without clubbing or cyanosis. No suspicious nevi, rash, petechiae, or ecchymoses."

Aids to Interpretation

Table 6-1 Color Changes in the Skin

Color/Mechanism	Selected Causes
Brown: Increased melanin (greater than a person's genetic norm)	Sun exposure Pregnancy (melasma) Addison's disease
Blue (cyanosis): Increased deoxyhemoglobin from hypoxia:	
• Peripheral	Anxiety or cold environment
• Central (arterial)	Heart or lung disease
Abnormal hemoglobin	Methemoglobinemia, sulfhemoglobinemia
Red: Increased visibility of oxyhemoglobin from:	
• Dilated superficial blood vessels or increased blood flow in skin	Fever, blushing, alcohol intake, local inflammation
• Decreased use of oxygen in skin	Cold exposure (e.g., cold ears)
Yellow:	
Increased bilirubin of jaundice (sclera looks yellow)	Liver disease, hemolysis of red blood cells
Carotenemia (sclera does not look yellow)	Increased carotene intake from yellow fruits and vegetables
Pale:	
Decreased melanin	Albinism, vitiligo, tinea versicolor
Decreased visibility of oxyhemoglobin from:	
• Decreased blood flow to skin	Syncope or shock
• Decreased amount of oxyhemoglobin	Anemia
Edema (may mask skin pigments)	Nephrotic syndrome

Chapter 6 | The Skin, Hair, and Nails

Table 6-2 Primary Skin Lesions

Flat, Nonpalpable Lesions With Changes in Skin Color

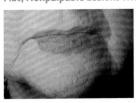

Macule—Small flat spot, up to 1.0 cm
Examples:
- Hemangioma
- Vitiligo

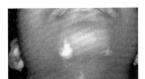

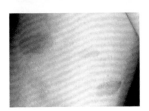

Patch—Flat spot, 1.0 cm or larger
Example: Café-au-lait spot

Palpable Elevations: Solid Bumps

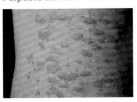

Papule—Up to 1.0 cm
Example: An elevated nevus

(continued)

Table 6-2 Primary Skin Lesions (continued)

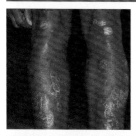

Plaque—Elevated superficial lesion 1.0 cm or larger, often formed by coalescence of papules
Example: Psoriasis

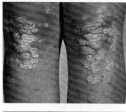

Nodule—Knot-like lesion larger than 0.5 cm, deeper and more firm than a papule
Example: Dermatofibroma

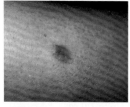

Cyst—Nodule filled with expressible material, either liquid or semisolid
Example: Epidermal inclusion cyst

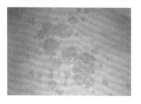

Wheal—A somewhat irregular, relatively transient, superficial area of localized skin edema
Examples: Mosquito bite, hives (urticaria)

Table 6-2 Primary Skin Lesions *(continued)*

Palpable Elevations With Fluid-Filled Cavities

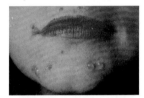

Vesicle—Up to 1.0 cm; filled with serous fluid
Example: Herpes simplex

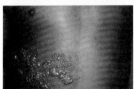

Example: Herpes zoster

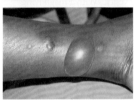

Bulla—1.0 cm or larger; filled with serous fluid
Example: Insect bite

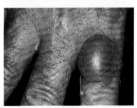

Example: Insect bite

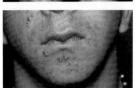

Pustule—Filled with pus (yellow proteinaceous fluid filled with neutrophils)
Example: Acne

(continued)

Table 6-2 Primary Skin Lesions (continued)

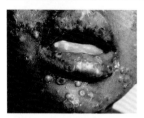

Example: Small pox

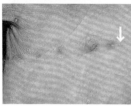

Burrow—A minute, slightly raised tunnel in the epidermis, commonly found on the finger webs and on the sides of the fingers. It looks like a short (5–15 mm), linear or curved gray line and may end in a tiny vesicle. With a magnifying lens, look for the *burrow* of the mite that causes scabies.
Example: Scabies

Table 6-3 Secondary Skin Lesions

May arise from primary lesions, overtreatment, excess scratching

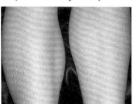

Scale—A thin flake of dead, exfoliated epidermis
Example: Ichthyosis vulgaris

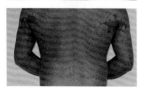

Example: Dry skin

Table 6-3 Secondary Skin Lesions (continued)

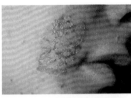

Crust—The dried residue of skin exudates such as serum, pus, or blood
Example: Impetigo

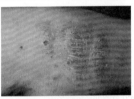

Lichenification—Visible and palpable thickening of the epidermis and roughening of the skin with increased visibility of the normal skin furrows (often from chronic rubbing)
Example: Neurodermatitis

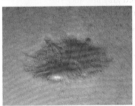

Scars—Increased connective tissue that arises from injury or disease
Example: Hypertrophic scar from steroid injections

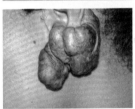

Keloids—Hypertrophic scarring that extends beyond the borders of the initiating injury
Example: Keloid—ear lobe

Sources of photos: *Hemangioma, Café-au-Lait Spot, Elevated Nevus, Psoriasis [bottom], Dermatofibroma, Herpes Simplex, Insect Bite [bottom], Impetigo, Lichenification*—Hall JC. Sauer's Manual of Skin Diseases, 9th ed. Philadelphia: Lippincott Williams & Wilkins, 2006; *Vitiligo, Psoriasis [top], Epidermal Inclusion Cyst, Urticaria, Insect Bite [top], Acne, Ichthyosis, Psoriasis, Acne Scar, Keloids*—Goodheart HP. Goodheart's Photoguide of Common Skin Disorders: Diagnosis and Management, 2nd ed. Philadelphia: Lippincott Williams & Wilkins, 2003; *Small Pox*—Ostler HB, Mailbach HI, Hoke AW, Schwab IR. Diseases of the Eye and Skin: A Color Atlas. Philadelphia: Lippincott Williams & Wilkins, 2004.

Table 6-4　Secondary Skin Lesions—Depressed

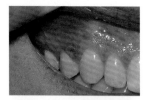

Erosion—Nonscarring loss of the superficial epidermis; surface is moist but does not bleed
Example: Aphthous stomatitis, moist area after the rupture of a vesicle, as in chickenpox

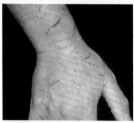

Excoriation—Linear or punctate erosions caused by scratching
Example: Cat scratches

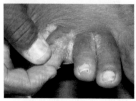

Fissure—A linear crack in the skin, often resulting from excessive dryness
Example: Athlete's foot

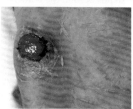

Ulcer—A deeper loss of epidermis and dermis; may bleed and scar
Examples: Stasis ulcer of venous insufficiency, syphilitic chancre

---

Sources of photos: *Erosion, Excoriation, Fissure*—Goodheart HP. Goodheart's Photoguide of Common Skin Disorders: Diagnosis and Management, 2nd ed. Philadelphia: Lippincott Williams & Wilkins, 2003; *Ulcer*—Hall JC. Sauer's Manual of Skin Diseases, 9th ed. Philadelphia: Lippincott Williams & Wilkins, 2006.

Table 6-5 Vascular and Purpuric Lesions of the Skin

Lesion	Features: Appearance; Distribution; Significance
Cherry Angioma 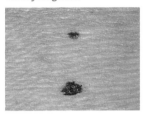	• Bright or ruby red, may become purplish with age; 1–3 mm; round, flat, sometimes raised; may be surrounded by a pale halo • Found on trunk or extremities • Not significant; increase in size and number with aging
Spider Angioma 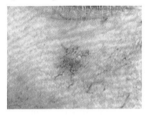	• Fiery red; very small to 2 cm; central body, sometimes raised, radiating with erythema • Face, neck, arms, and upper trunk, but almost never below the waist • Seen in liver disease, pregnancy, vitamin B deficiency; normal in some people
Spider Vein 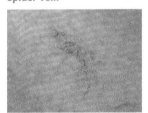	• Bluish; varies from very small to several inches; may resemble a spider or be linear, irregular, or cascading • Most often on the legs, near veins; also on anterior chest • Often accompanies increased pressure in the superficial veins, as in varicose veins
Petechia/Purpura 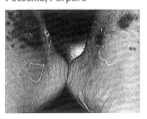	• Deep red or reddish purple; fades over time; 1–3 mm or larger; rounded, sometimes irregular, flat • Varied distribution • Seen if blood outside the vessels; may suggest a bleeding disorder or, if petechiae, emboli to skin

(continued)

| Table 6-5 | **Vascular and Purpuric Lesions of the Skin** *(continued)* |

Lesion	Features: Appearance; Distribution; Significance
Ecchymosis 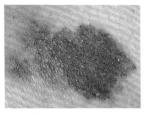	• Purple or purplish blue, fading to green, yellow, and brown over time; larger than petechiae; rounded, oval, or irregular • Varied distribution • Seen if blood outside the vessels; often secondary to bruising or trauma; also seen in bleeding disorders

Table 6-6 Skin Tumors

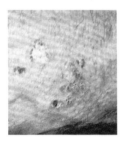

Actinic Keratoses Superficial, flattened papules covered by a dry scale. Often multiple; may be round or irregular; pink, tan, or grayish. Appear on sun-exposed skin of older, fair-skinned persons. Considered dysplastic or precancerous: 1 out of 1,000 per year develop into *squamous cell carcinoma* (look for continued growth, induration, redness at the base, and ulceration). Typically on face and hands.

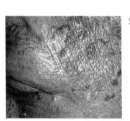

Seborrheic Keratoses Common, benign, whitish-yellowish to brown, raised papules or plaques that feel slightly greasy, velvety or warty; have a "stuck-on" appearance. Typically multiple and symmetrical, distributed on the trunk of older people, also on the face and elsewhere. In blacks, may appear as small, deeply pigmented papules on cheeks and temples (dermatosis papulosa nigra).

Table 6-6 Skin Tumors (continued)

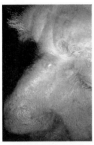

Basal Cell Carcinoma Though malignant, grows slowly and almost never metastasizes. Most common in fair-skinned adults 40 years or older; usually on the face. Initial translucent red macule or papule may develop a depressed center and firm elevated border. Telangiectatic vessels often visible.

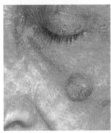

Squamous Cell Carcinoma Usually on sun-exposed skin of fair-skinned adults 60 years or older. May develop in an actinic keratosis. Usually grows more quickly than a basal cell carcinoma, is firmer, and looks redder. The face and the dorsum of the hand are often affected.

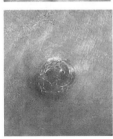

Kaposi's Sarcoma in AIDS May appear in many forms: macules, papules, plaques, or nodules almost anywhere on the body. Lesions are often multiple and may involve internal structures.

Sources of photos: *Basal Cell Carcinoma:* Rapini R. *Squamous Cell Carcinoma, Actinic Keratosis, and Seborrheic Keratosis*—Hall JC. Sauer's Manual of Skin Diseases, 9th ed. Philadelphia: Lippincott Williams & Wilkins, 2006; *Kaposi's Sarcoma in AIDS*— DeVita VT Jr, Hellman S, Rosenberg SA [eds]. AIDS: Etiology, Diagnosis, Treatment, and Prevention. Philadelphia: JB Lippincott, 1985.

Table 6-7 Benign and Malignant Nevi

Benign

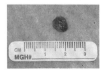

Diameter <6 mm
Symmetric; regular borders; even in color

Malignant Melanoma: "ABCDE"

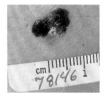

Asymmetric

Borders irregular

Color varied
Diameter >6 mm
Evolution or change in size, symptoms or morphology

Courtesy of American Cancer Society; American Academy of Dermatology.

Table 6-8 — Hair Loss

Alopecia Areata Clearly demarcated round or oval patches of hair loss, usually affecting young adults and children. There is no visible scaling or inflammation.

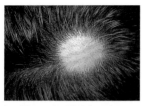
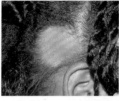

Trichotillomania Hair loss from pulling, plucking, or twisting hair. Hair shafts are broken and of varying lengths. More common in children, often in settings of family or psychosocial stress.

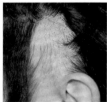
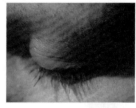

Tinea Capitis ("Ringworm") Round scaling patches of alopecia. Hairs are broken off close to the surface of the scalp. Usually caused by fungal infection from *Trichophyton tonsurans* from humans, *microsporum canis* from dogs or cats. Mimics seborrheic dermatitis.

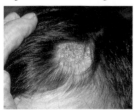
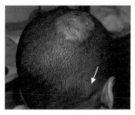

Sources of photos: *Alopecia Areata [top], Trichotillomania [top]*—Hall JC. Sauer's Manual of Skin Diseases, 9th ed. Philadelphia: Lippincott Williams & Wilkins, 2006; *Alopecia Areata [bottom], Tinea Capitis*—Goodheart HP. Goodheart's Photoguide of Common Skin Disorders: Diagnosis and Management, 2nd ed. Philadelphia: Lippincott Williams & Wilkins, 2003; *Trichotillomania [bottom]*—Ostler HB, Mailbach HI, Hoke AW, Schwab IR. Diseases of the Eye and Skin: A Color Atlas. Philadelphia: Lippincott Williams & Wilkins, 2004.

Table 6-9 Findings in or Near the Nails

Clubbing

Dorsal phalanx rounded and bulbous; convexity of nail plate increased. Angle between plate and proximal nail fold increased to 180° or more. Proximal nail folds feel spongy. Many causes, including chronic hypoxia and lung cancer.

Paronychia

Inflammation of proximal and lateral nail folds, acute or chronic. Folds red, swollen, may be tender.

Onycholysis

Painless separation of nail plate from nail bed, starting distally. Many causes.

Terry's Nails

Whitish with a distal band of reddish brown. Seen in aging and some chronic diseases.

Leukonychia

White spots caused by trauma. They grow out with nail(s).

Transverse White Lines

Curved white lines similar to curve of lunula. They follow an illness and grow out with nails.

CHAPTER 7

The Head and Neck

The Health History

Common or Concerning Symptoms

- Headache
- Change in vision
- Double vision, or diplopia
- Hearing loss, earache, tinnitus
- Vertigo
- Nosebleed, or epistaxis
- Sore throat, hoarseness
- Swollen glands
- Goiter

THE HEAD

Headache is a common symptom that always requires careful evaluation because a small fraction of headaches arise from life-threatening conditions. Elicit a full description of the headache and all seven attributes of the patient's pain (see p. 3).

See Table 7-1, Primary Headaches, p. 111, and Table 7-2, Secondary Headaches, pp. 112–114. *Tension* and *migraine headaches* are the most common recurring headaches.

Is the headache one-sided or bilateral? Steady or throbbing? Continuous or comes and goes? Ask the patient to *point to the area of pain or discomfort*. Assess *chronologic pattern* and *severity*.

Tension headaches often arise in the temporal areas; cluster headaches may be retro-orbital.

Changing or progressively severe headaches increase the likelihood of *tumor, abscess,* or other *mass lesion*. Extremely severe headaches suggest *subarachnoid hemorrhage* or *meningitis*.

Headache Warning Signs

- Progressively frequent or severe over a 3-month period
- Sudden onset like a "thunderclap" or "the worst headache of my life"
- New onset after age 50 years
- Aggravated or relieved by change in position
- Precipitated by Valsalva maneuver
- Associated symptoms of fever, night sweats, or weight loss
- Presence of cancer, HIV infection, or pregnancy
- Recent head trauma
- Associated papilledema, neck stiffness, or focal neurologic deficits

---

- Ask about associated symptoms, such as nausea and vomiting, and neurologic symptoms such as change in vision or motor-sensory deficits.

    Visual aura or scintillating scotomas may accompany *migraine*. Nausea and vomiting are common with migraine but also occur with *brain tumor* and *subarachnoid hemorrhage*.

- Ask if coughing, sneezing, or changing the position of the head affects (better, worse, or none) the headache.

    Such maneuvers may increase pain from brain tumor and acute sinusitis.

- Ask about family history.

    Family history is often positive in patients with migraine.

THE EYES

Ask "How is your vision?" If the patient reports a change in vision, pursue the related details:

Gradual blurring, often from refractive errors; also in hyperglycemia.

- Is the onset sudden or gradual?

    Sudden visual loss suggests *retinal detachment, vitreous hemorrhage,* or *occlusion of the central retinal artery*.

- Is the problem worse during close work or at distances?

    Difficulty with close work suggests *hyperopia* (farsightedness) or *presbyopia* (aging vision); difficulty with distances suggests *myopia* (nearsightedness).

- Is there blurring of the entire field of vision or only parts? Is blurring central, peripheral, or only on one side?

    Slow central loss occurs in *nuclear cataract* and *macular degeneration;* peripheral loss in advanced *open-angle glaucoma;* one-sided loss in *hemianopsia* and quadrantic defects (p. 115).

- Has the patient seen lights flashing across the field of vision? Vitreous floaters?

These symptoms suggest detachment of vitreous from retina. Prompt eye consultation is indicated.

Ask about *pain* in or around the eyes, *redness*, and *excessive tearing* or *watering*.

Eye pain in *acute glaucoma* and *optic neuritis*.

Check for *diplopia*, or double vision.

Diplopia in brainstem or cerebellum lesions, also from weakness or paralysis of one or more extraocular muscles.

THE EARS

Ask "How is your hearing?"

See Table 7-8, Patterns of Hearing Loss, p. 121.

Does the patient have special difficulty understanding people as they talk? Does a noisy environment make a difference?

Sensorineural loss leads to difficulty understanding speech, often complaining that others mumble; noisy environments worsen hearing. In *conductive loss*, noisy environments may help.

For complaints of *earache*, or *pain in the ear*, ask about associated fever, sore throat, cough, and concurrent upper respiratory infection.

Consider *otitis externa* if pain in the ear canal; *otitis media* if pain associated with respiratory infection.

Tinnitus is an internal musical ringing or rushing or roaring noise, often unexplained.

When associated with hearing loss and vertigo, tinnitus suggests *Ménière's disease*.

Ask about *vertigo*, the perception that the patient or the environment is rotating or spinning.

Vertigo in labrynthitis (inner ear), CN VII lesions, brainstem lesions

THE NOSE AND SINUSES

Rhinorrhea, or drainage from the nose, frequently accompanies *nasal congestion*. Ask further about *sneezing*, watery eyes, throat discomfort, and *itching* in the eyes, nose, and throat.

Causes include viral infections, *allergic rhinitis* ("hay fever"), and *vasomotor rhinitis*. Itching favors an allergic cause.

For *epistaxis,* or bleeding from the nose, identify the source carefully—is bleeding from the nose or has the patient coughed up or vomited blood? Assess the site of bleeding, its severity, and associated symptoms.

Local causes of epistaxis include trauma (especially nose-picking), inflammation, drying and crusting of the nasal mucosa, tumors, and foreign bodies. Anticoagulants, NSAIDs, and coagulopathies may contribute.

THE MOUTH, THROAT, AND NECK

Sore throat or *pharyngitis* is a frequent complaint. Ask about fever, swollen glands, and any associated cough.

Fever, pharyngeal exudates, and anterior cervical lymphadenopathy, especially without cough, suggest *streptococcal pharyngitis,* or "strep throat" (p. 125).

Hoarseness may arise from overuse of the voice, allergies, smoking, or inhaled irritants.

Also present in *viral laryngitis,* hypothyroidism, laryngeal disease, or when extrapharyngeal lesions press on the laryngeal nerves

Assess thyroid function. Ask about *goiter, temperature intolerance,* and *sweating.*

With goiter, thyroid function may be increased, decreased, or normal. Cold intolerance in *hypothyroidism*; heat intolerance, palpitations, and involuntary weight loss in *hyperthyroidism*

Health Promotion and Counseling: Evidence and Recommendations

Important Topics for Health Promotion and Counseling

- Loss of vision: cataracts, macular degeneration, glaucoma
- Hearing loss
- Oral health

Disorders of vision shift with age. Healthy young adults generally have refractive errors. Up to 25% of adults older than 65 years have refractive errors; *cataracts, macular degeneration,* and *glaucoma* also become more prevalent. Glaucoma is the leading cause of blindness in African Americans and the second leading cause of blindness overall. Glaucoma causes gradual vision loss, with damage to the optic nerve, loss of visual fields, beginning usually at the periphery, and pallor and increasing size of the optic cup (enlarging to more than half the diameter of the optic disc).

More than a third of adults older than 65 years have *detectable hearing deficits.* Questionnaires and handheld audioscopes work well for periodic screening.

Be sure to promote *oral health:* Up to half of all children 5 to 17 years of age have one to eight cavities, and the average U.S. adult has 10 to 17 decayed, missing, or filled teeth. More than half of all adults older than 65 years have no teeth! Inspect the oral cavity for decayed or loose teeth, inflammation of the gingiva, and signs of periodontal disease (bleeding, pus, receding gums, and bad breath). Counsel patients to use fluoride-containing toothpastes, brush, floss, and seek dental care at least annually.

Techniques of Examination

EXAMINATION TECHNIQUES	POSSIBLE FINDINGS

THE HEAD

Examine the:

- Hair, including quantity, distribution, and texture

  Coarse and sparse in *hypothyroidsm,* fine in *hyperthyroidism*

- Scalp, including lumps or lesions

  Pilar cysts, psoriasis, pigmented nevi

- Skull, including size and contour

  Hydrocephalus, skull depression from trauma

- Face, including symmetry and facial expression

  Facial paralysis; flat affect of depression, moods such as anger, sadness

- Skin, including color, texture, hair distribution, and lesions

  Pale, fine, hirsute, acne, skin cancer

THE EYES

Test visual acuity in each eye.

Diminished acuity

Assess visual fields, if indicated.

Hemianopsia, quadrantic defects in cerebrovascular accidents (CVAs). See Table 7-3, Visual Field Defects, p. 115.

EXAMINATION TECHNIQUES	POSSIBLE FINDINGS
Inspect the:	See Table 7-4, Physical Findings In and Around the Eye, pp. 116–117.
• Position and alignment of eyes	Exophthalmos, strabismus
• Eyebrows	Seborrheic dermatitis
• Eyelids	Sty, chalazion, ectropion, ptosis, xanthelasma
• Lacrimal apparatus	Swollen lacrimal sac
• Conjunctiva and sclera	Red eye, conjunctivitis, jaundice, episcleritis
• Cornea, iris, and lens	Corneal opacity, cataract
Examine pupils for:	
• Size, shape, and symmetry	Miosis, mydriasis, anisocoria
• Reactions to light, direct and consensual	Absent in paralysis of CN III
• The near reaction: pupillary constriction with gaze shift to near objection; with convergence and accommodation (lens becomes more convex)	Useful in tonic (Adie's) versus Argyll Robertson pupils: constriction slows in tonic pupil; absent in Argyll Robertson pupils of syphilis; poor convergence in hyperthyroidism

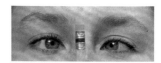

THE NEAR REACTION

Assess the extraocular muscles by observing:

• The corneal reflections from a midline light	Asymmetric reflection if deviation in ocular alignment
• The six cardinal directions of gaze	Cranial nerve palsy, strabismus, nystagmus, lid lag of hyperthyroidism

Chapter 7 | The Head and Neck

| EXAMINATION TECHNIQUES | POSSIBLE FINDINGS |

Superior rectus (III) — Inferior oblique (III) — Superior rectus (III)
Lateral rectus (VI) — Medial rectus (III) — Lateral rectus (VI)
Inferior rectus (III) — Superior oblique (IV) — Inferior rectus (III)

Inspect the fundi with an ophthalmoscope.

Tips for Using the Ophthalmoscope

- Darken the room. Turn the lens disc to the large round beam of white light. *Lower the brightness of the light beam* to make the examination more comfortable for the patient.
- Turn the lens disc to the 0 diopter (a diopter measures the power of a lens to converge or diverge light).
- Hold the ophthalmoscope *in your right hand and use your right eye* to examine *the patient's right eye*; hold it *in your left hand and use your left eye* to examine *the patient's left eye* to avoid bumping the patient's nose.
- Brace the ophthalmoscope firmly against the medial aspect of your bony orbit, with the handle tilted laterally at about a 20-degree slant from the vertical. Instruct the patient to look slightly up and over your shoulder at a point directly ahead on the wall.
- Place yourself about 15 inches away from the patient and *at an angle 15 degrees lateral to the patient's line of vision*. Look for the orange glow in the pupil—the *red reflex*. Note any opacities interrupting the red reflex. No red reflex suggests an opacity of the lens (cataract) or possibly the vitreous.
- Place the thumb of your other hand across the patient's eyebrow. Keeping the light beam focused on the red reflex, move in at a 15-degree angle toward the pupil until you almost touch the patient's eyelashes. Adjust the position of your ophthalmoscope and angle of vision *as a unit* until you see the fundus.

Inspect the fundi for the following:

- Red reflex

    Cataracts, artificial eye

- Optic disc

    Papilledema, glaucomatous cupping, optic atrophy. See Table 7-5, Abnormalities of the Optic Disc, p. 118, and Table 7-6, Ocular Fundi: Diabetic Retinopathy, p. 119.

EXAMINATION TECHNIQUES	POSSIBLE FINDINGS

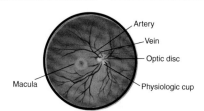

- Arteries, veins, and AV crossings

  AV nicking, copper wiring in hypertensive changes

- Adjacent retina (note any lesions)

  Hemorrhages, exudates, cotton-wool patches, microaneurysms, pigmentation

- Macular area

  Macular degeneration

- Anterior structures

  Vitreous floaters, cataracts

Tips for Examining the Optic Disc and Retina

- *Locate the optic disc.* Look for the round yellowish-orange structure.
- Now, *bring the optic disc into sharp focus* by adjusting the lens of your ophthalmoscope.
- *Inspect the optic disc.* Note the following features:
  - *The sharpness or clarity of the disc outline*
  - *The color of the disc*
  - *The size of the central physiologic cup* (an enlarged cup suggests chronic open-angle glaucoma)
  - *Venous pulsations* in the retinal veins as they emerge from the central portion of the disc (loss of venous pulsations from elevated intracranial pressure may occur in head trauma, meningitis)
- *Inspect the retina.* Distinguish arteries from veins based on the features listed below.

	Arteries	**Veins**
Color	Light red	Dark red
Size	Smaller (⅔ to ¾ the diameter of veins)	Larger
Light Reflex (*reflection*)	Bright	Inconspicuous or absent

(continued)

Chapter 7 | The Head and Neck

| EXAMINATION TECHNIQUES | POSSIBLE FINDINGS |

Tips for Examining the Optic Disc and Retina (continued)

- Follow the vessels peripherally in each of four directions.
- Inspect the *fovea* and surrounding *macula*. Macular degeneration types include *dry atrophic* (more common but less severe) and *wet exudative* (neovascular). Undigested cellular debris, called *drusen*, may be hard or soft.
- Assess for any *papilledema* from increased intracranial pressure leading to swelling of the optic nerve head.

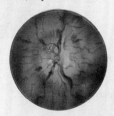

PAPILLEDEMA

THE EARS

Examine on each side:

The Auricle

Inspect the auricle.   Keloid, epidermoid cyst

If you suspect otitis:

- Move the auricle up and down, and press on the tragus.   Pain in otitis externa ("the tug test")

- Press firmly behind the ear.   Possible tenderness in otitis media and mastoiditis

Ear Canal and Drum

Pull the auricle up, back, and slightly out. Inspect, through an otoscope speculum:

- The canal   Cerumen; swelling and erythema in otitis externa

- The eardrum   Red bulging drum in acute otitis media; serous otitis media, tympanosclerosis, perforations. See Table 7-7, Abnormalities of the Eardrum, p. 120.

| EXAMINATION TECHNIQUES | POSSIBLE FINDINGS |

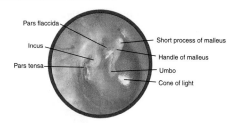

Hearing

Assess auditory acuity to whispered or spoken voice.

If hearing is diminished, use a 512-Hz tuning fork to:

- Test *lateralization* (Weber test). Place vibrating and tuning fork on vertex of skull and check hearing.

  These tests help distinguish between sensorineural and conduction hearing loss.

  See Table 7-8, Patterns of Hearing Loss, p. 121.

- Compare *air and bone conduction* (*Rinne test*). Place vibrating and tuning fork on mastoid bone, then remove and check hearing.

THE NOSE AND SINUSES

Inspect the external nose.

Inspect, through a speculum, the:

- Nasal mucosa that covers the septum and turbinates, noting its color and any swelling

  Swollen and red in viral rhinitis, swollen and pale in allergic rhinitis; polyps; ulcer from cocaine use

- Nasal septum for position and integrity

  Deviation, perforation

Palpate the frontal and maxillary sinuses.

Tender in acute sinusitis

| EXAMINATION TECHNIQUES | POSSIBLE FINDINGS |

THE MOUTH AND PHARYNX

Inspect the:

- Lips — Cyanosis, pallor, cheilosis. See also Table 7-9, Abnormalities of the Lips, p. 122.

- Oral mucosa — Aphthous ulcers (canker sores)

- Gums — Gingivitis, periodontal disease

- Teeth — Dental caries, tooth loss

- Roof of the mouth — Torus palatinus

- Tongue, including: — See Table 7-10, Abnormalities of the Tongue, pp. 123–124.

  - Papillae — Glossitis

  - Symmetry — Deviation to one side from paralysis of CN XII from CVA

  - Any lesions — Cancer

- Floor of the mouth — Cancer

- Pharynx, including: — See Table 7-11, Abnormalities of the Pharynx, p. 125.

  - Color or any exudate — Pharyngitis

  - Presence and size of tonsils — Exudates, tonsillitis, peritonsillar abscess

  - Symmetry of the soft palate as patient says "ah" — Soft palate fails to rise in paralysis of CN X from CVA

THE NECK

Inspect the neck. — Scars, masses, torticollis

Palpate the lymph nodes. — Cervical lymphadenopathy from inflammation, malignancy, HIV

EXAMINATION TECHNIQUES	POSSIBLE FINDINGS
Inspect and palpate the position of the trachea.	Deviated trachea from neck mass or pneumothorax

Inspect the thyroid gland:

- At rest

  Goiter, nodules. See Table 7-12, Abnormalities of the Thyroid Gland, p. 126.

- As patient swallows water

From behind patient, palpate the thyroid gland, including the isthmus and the lateral lobes:

Goiter, nodules, tenderness of thyroiditis

- At rest

- As patient swallows water

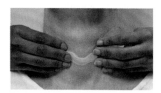

Alternate Sequence. After examining the thyroid gland from behind the patient, you may proceed to musculoskeletal examination of the neck and upper back and check for costovertebral angle tenderness.

Recording Your Findings

Recording the Physical Examination—The Head, Eyes, Ears, Nose, and Throat (HEENT)

HEENT: Head—The skull is normocephalic/atraumatic (NC/AT). Hair with average texture. *Eyes*—Visual acuity 20/20 bilaterally. Sclera white; conjunctiva pink. Pupils constrict 4 mm to 2 mm, equally round and reactive to light and accommodations. Disc margins sharp; no hemorrhages or exudates; no arteriolar narrowing. *Ears*—Acuity good to whispered voice. Tympanic membranes (TMs) with good cone of light. Weber midline. AC > BC. *Nose*—Nasal mucosa pink, septum midline; no sinus tenderness. *Throat (or Mouth)*—Oral mucosa pink; dentition good; pharynx without exudates. *Neck*—Trachea midline. Neck supple; thyroid isthmus palpable, lobes not felt. *Lymph Nodes*—No cervical, axillary, epitrochlear, inguinal adenopathy.

Aids to Interpretation

Table 7-1 Primary Headaches

Problem	Common Characteristics	Associated Symptoms, With Provoking and Relieving Factors
Tension	**Location:** Variable **Quality:** Pressing or tightening pain; mild to moderate intensity **Onset:** Gradual **Duration:** Minutes to days	Sometimes photophobia, phonophobia; nausea absent ↑ by sustained muscle tension, as in driving or typing ↓ possibly by massage, relaxation
Migraine • *With aura* • *Without aura* • *Variants*	**Location:** Unilateral in ~70%; bifrontal or global in ~30% **Quality:** Throbbing or aching, variable in severity **Onset:** Fairly rapid, peaks in 1–2 hr **Duration:** 4–72 hr	Nausea, vomiting, photophobia, phonophobia, visual auras (flickering zig-zagging lines), motor auras affecting hand or arm, sensory auras (numbness, tingling usually precede headache) ↑ by alcohol, certain foods, tension, noise, bright light. More common premenstrually. ↓ by quiet dark room, sleep
Cluster	**Location:** Unilateral, usually behind or around the eye **Quality:** Deep, continuous, severe **Onset:** Abrupt, peaks within minutes **Duration:** Up to 3 hr	Lacrimation, rhinorrhea, miosis, ptosis, eyelid edema, conjunctival infection ↑ sensitivity to alcohol during some episodes

Table 7-2 Secondary Headaches

Problem	Common Characteristics	Associated Symptoms, With Provoking and Relieving Factors
Analgesic Rebound	**Location:** Previous headache pattern **Quality:** Variable **Onset:** Variable **Duration:** Depends on prior headache pattern	Depends on prior headache pattern ↑ by fever, carbon monoxide, hypoxia, withdrawal of caffeine, other headache triggers ↓ —depends on cause
Headaches From Eye Disorders *Errors of Refraction (farsightedness and astigmatism, but not nearsightedness)*	**Location:** Around and over the eyes; may radiate to the occipital area **Quality:** Steady, aching, dull **Onset:** Gradual **Duration:** Variable	Eye fatigue, "sandy" sensation in eyes, redness of the conjunctiva ↑ by prolonged use of the eyes, particularly for close work ↓ by rest of the eyes
Acute Glaucoma	**Location:** In and around one eye **Quality:** Steady, aching, often severe **Onset:** Often rapid **Duration:** Variable, may depend on treatment	Diminished vision, sometimes nausea and vomiting ↑ —sometimes by drops that dilate the pupils
Headache From Sinusitis	**Location:** Usually above eye (frontal sinus) or over maxillary sinus **Quality:** Aching or throbbing, variable in severity; consider possible migraine **Onset:** Variable **Duration:** Often several hours at a time, recurring over days or longer	Local tenderness, nasal congestion, tooth pain, discharge, and fever ↑ by coughing, sneezing, or jarring the head ↓ by nasal decongestants, antibiotics

Table 7-2 Secondary Headaches (continued)

Problem	Common Characteristics	Associated Symptoms, With Provoking and Relieving Factors
Meningitis	**Location:** Generalized **Quality:** Steady or throbbing, very severe **Onset:** Fairly rapid **Duration:** Variable, usually days	Fever, stiff neck
Subarachnoid Hemorrhage	**Location:** Generalized **Quality:** Severe, "the worst of my life" **Onset:** Usually abrupt; prodromal symptoms may occur **Duration:** Variable, usually days	Nausea, vomiting, possibly loss of consciousness, neck pain
Brain Tumor	**Location:** Varies with the location of the tumor **Quality:** Aching, steady, variable in intensity **Onset:** Variable **Duration:** Often brief	↑ by coughing, sneezing, or sudden movements of the head
Cranial Neuralgias: Trigeminal Neuralgia (CN V)	**Location:** Cheek, jaws, lips, or gums; trigeminal nerve divisions 2 and 3 > 1 **Quality:** Shocklike, stabbing, burning, severe **Onset:** Abrupt, paroxysmal **Duration:** Each jab lasts seconds but recurs at intervals of seconds or minutes	Exhaustion from recurrent pain ↑ by touching certain areas of the lower face or mouth; chewing, talking, brushing teeth

(continued)

Table 7-2 Secondary Headaches *(continued)*

Problem	Common Characteristics	Associated Symptoms, With Provoking and Relieving Factors
Giant Cell (Temporal) Arteritis	**Location:** Near the involved artery, often the temporal, also the occipital; age-related **Quality:** Throbbing, generalized, persistent, often severe **Onset:** Gradual or rapid **Duration:** Variable	Tenderness of the adjacent scalp; fever (in ~50%), fatigue, weight loss; new headache (~60%), jaw claudication (~50%), visual loss or blindness (~15%–20%), polymyalgia rheumatica (~50%) ↑ by movement of neck and shoulders
Postconcussion Headache	**Location:** Injured area, but not necessarily **Quality:** Generalized, dull, aching, constant **Onset:** Within hours to 1–2 days of the injury **Duration:** Weeks, months, or even years	Poor concentration, problems with memory, vertigo, irritability, restlessness, fatigue ↑ by mental and physical exertion, straining, stooping, emotional excitement, alcohol ↓ by rest

Table 7-3   Visual Field Defects

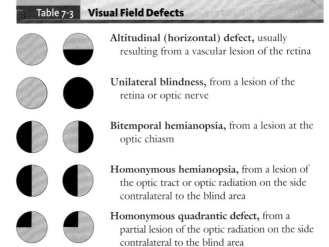

Altitudinal (horizontal) defect, usually resulting from a vascular lesion of the retina

Unilateral blindness, from a lesion of the retina or optic nerve

Bitemporal hemianopsia, from a lesion at the optic chiasm

Homonymous hemianopsia, from a lesion of the optic tract or optic radiation on the side contralateral to the blind area

Homonymous quadrantic defect, from a partial lesion of the optic radiation on the side contralateral to the blind area

LEFT   RIGHT

(from patient's viewpoint)

Table 7-4	Physical Findings in and Around the Eye

Eyelids

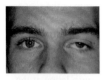

Ptosis. A drooping upper eyelid that narrows the palpebral fissure from a muscle or nerve disorder

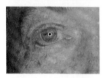

Ectropion. Outward turning of the margin of the lower lid, exposing the palpebral conjunctiva

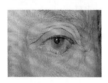

Entropion. Inward turning of the lid margin, causing irritation of the cornea or conjunctiva

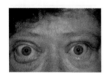

Lid Retraction and Exophthalmos. A wide-eyed stare suggests hyperthyroidism. Note the rim of sclera between the upper lid and the iris. *Retracted* lids and "*lid lag*" when eyes move from up to down markedly increase the likelihood of hyperthyroidism, especially when accompanied by fine tremor, moist skin, and heart rate >90 beats per minute. *Exophthalmos* describes protrusion of the eyeball, a common feature of Graves' ophthalmopathy, triggered by autoreactive T lymphocytes.

Chapter 7 | The Head and Neck

| Table 7-4 | **Physical Findings in and Around the Eye** *(continued)* |

In and Around the Eye

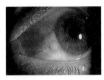
Pinguecula. Harmless yellowish nodule in the bulbar conjunctiva on either side of the iris; associated with aging

Episcleritis. A localized ocular redness from inflammation of the episcleral vessels

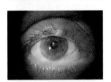
Sty. A pimplelike infection around a hair follicle near the lid margin

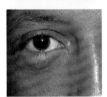
Chalazion. A beady nodule in either eyelid caused by a chronically inflamed meibomian gland

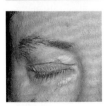
Xanthelasma. Yellowish plaque seen in lipid disorders

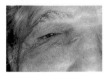
Inflammation of the Lacrimal Sac (Dacryocystitis). From inflammation or obstruction of the lacrimal duct

Table 7-5   Abnormalities of the Optic Disc

	Process	Appearance
Normal	Tiny disc vessels give normal color to the disc.	Disc is yellowish orange to creamy pink. Disc vessels are tiny. Disc margins are sharp (except perhaps nasally).
Papilledema	Venous stasis leads to engorgement and swelling.	Disc is pink, hyperemic. Disc vessels are more visible, more numerous, and curve over the borders of the disc. Disc is swollen, with margins blurred.
Glaucomatous Cupping	Increased pressure within the eye leads to increased cupping (backward depression of the disc) and atrophy.	The base of the enlarged cup is pale.
Optic Atrophy	Death of optic nerve fibers leads to loss of the tiny disc vessels.	Disc is white. Disc vessels are absent.

Table 7-6 Ocular Fundi: Diabetic Retinopathy

Nonproliferative Retinopathy, Moderately Severe

Note tiny red dots or microaneurysms, also the ring of hard exudates (white spots) located superotemporally. Retinal thickening or edema in the area of hard exudates can impair visual acuity if it extends to center of macula. Detection requires specialized stereoscopic examination.

Nonproliferative Retinopathy, Severe

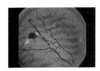

In superior temporal quadrant, note large retinal hemorrhage between two cotton-wool patches, beading of the retinal vein just above, and tiny tortuous retinal vessels above the superior temporal artery, termed *intraretinal microvascular abnormalities*.

Proliferative Retinopathy, With Neovascularization

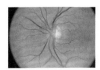

Note new preretinal vessels arising on disc and extending across disc margins. Visual acuity is still normal, but the risk of severe visual loss is high. Photocoagulation can reduce this risk by >50%.

Proliferative Retinopathy, Advanced

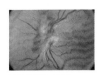

Same eye as above, but 2 years later and without treatment. Neovascularization has increased, now with fibrous proliferations, distortion of the macula, and reduced visual acuity.

Source of photos: Nonproliferative Retinopathy, Moderately Severe; Proliferative Retinopathy, With Neovascularization; Nonproliferative Retinopathy, Severe; Proliferative Retinopathy, Advanced—Early Treatment Diabetic Retinopathy Study Research Group. Courtesy of MF Davis, MD, University of Wisconsin, Madison. Source: Frank RB. Diabetic retinopathy. N Engl J Med 2004;350:48–58.

Table 7-7 Abnormalities of the Eardrum

Perforation

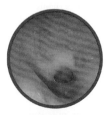

Hole in the eardrum that may be central or marginal
Usually from *otitis media* or trauma

Tympanosclerosis

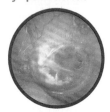

A chalky white patch
Scar of an old otitis media; of little or no clinical consequence

Serous Effusion

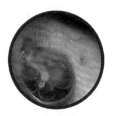

Amber fluid behind the eardrum, with or without air bubbles
Associated with viral upper respiratory infections or sudden changes in atmospheric pressure (diving, flying)

Acute Otitis Media With Purulent Effusion

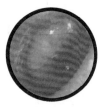

Red, bulging drum, loss of landmarks
Associated with bacterial infection

Table 7-8	**Patterns of Hearing Loss**	
	Conductive Loss	**Sensorineural Loss**
Impaired Understanding of Words	Minor	Often troublesome
Effect of Noisy Environment	May help	Increases the hearing difficulty
Usual Age of Onset	Childhood, young adulthood	Middle and later years
Ear Canal and Drum	Often a visible abnormality	Problem not visible
Weber Test (in Unilateral Hearing Loss)	Lateralizes to the impaired ear	Lateralizes to the good ear
Rinne Test	$BC \geq AC$	$AC > BC$
Causes Include	Plugged ear canal, *otitis media*, immobile or perforated drum, otosclerosis, foreign body	Sustained loud noise, drugs, inner ear infections, trauma, hereditary disorder, aging, acoustic neuroma

Table 7-9 Abnormalities of the Lips

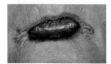
Angular cheilitis. Softening and cracking of the angles of the mouth

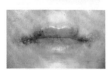
Herpes simplex. Painful vesicles, followed by crusting; also called **cold sore** or **fever blister**

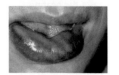
Angioedema. Diffuse, tense, subcutaneous swelling, usually allergic in cause

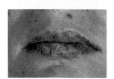
Hereditary hemorrhagic telangiectasia. Red spots, significant because of associated bleeding from nose and GI tract

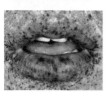
Peutz-Jeghers syndrome. Brown spots of the lips and buccal mucosa, significant because of their association with intestinal polyposis

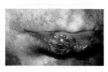
Syphilitic chancre. A firm lesion that ulcerates and may crust

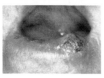
Carcinoma of the lip. A thickened plaque or irregular nodule that may ulcerate or crust; malignant

Table 7-10 Abnormalities of the Tongue

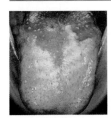
Geographic tongue. Scattered areas in which the papillae are lost, giving a maplike appearance; harmless

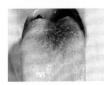
Hairy tongue. Results from elongated papillae that may look yellowish, brown, or black; harmless

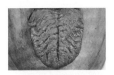
Fissured tongue. May appear with aging; harmless

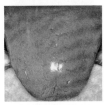
Smooth tongue. Results from loss of papillae, caused by vitamin B or iron deficiency or possibly chemotherapy

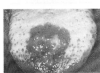
Candidiasis. May show a thick, white coat, which, when scraped off, leaves a raw red surface; tongue may also be red; antibiotics, corticosteroids, AIDS may predispose

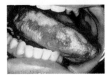
Hairy leukoplakia. White raised, feathery areas, usually on sides of tongue. Seen in HIV/AIDS

(continued)

Table 7-10 Abnormalities of the Tongue (continued)

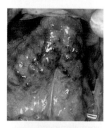

Varicose veins. Dark round spots in the undersurface of the tongue, associated with aging; also called **caviar lesions**

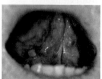

Aphthous ulcer (canker sore). Painful, small, whitish ulcer with a red halo; heals in 7–10 days

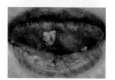

Mucous patch of syphilis. Slightly raised, oval lesion, covered by a grayish membrane

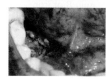

Carcinoma of the tongue or floor of the mouth. A malignancy that should be considered in any nodule or nonhealing ulcer at the base or edges of the mouth

Table 7-11 Abnormalities of the Pharynx

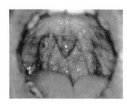

Pharyngitis, mild to moderate. Note redness and vascularity of the pillars and uvula.

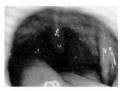

Pharyngitis, diffuse. Note redness is diffuse and intense. Cause may be viral or, if patient has fever, bacterial. If patient has no fever, exudate, or cervical lymphadenopathy, viral infection is more likely.

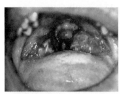

Exudative pharyngitis. A sore red throat with patches of white exudate on the tonsils is associated with streptococcal pharyngitis and some viral illnesses.

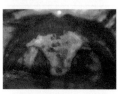

Diphtheria. An acute infection caused by *Corynebacterium diphtheriae*. The throat is dull red, and a gray exudate appears on the uvula, pharynx, and tongue.

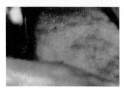

Koplik's spots. These small white specks that resemble grains of salt on a red background are an early sign of measles.

Table 7-12 Abnormalities of the Thyroid Gland

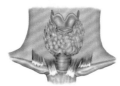

Diffuse enlargement. May result from Graves' disease, Hashimoto's thyroiditis, endemic goiter (iodine deficiency), or sporadic goiter

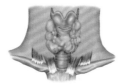

Multinodular goiter. An enlargement with two or more identifiable nodules, usually metabolic in cause

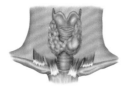

Single nodule. May result from a cyst, a benign tumor, or cancer of the thyroid, or may be one palpable nodule in a clinically unrecognized multinodular goiter

CHAPTER 8

The Thorax and Lungs

The Health History

Common or Concerning Symptoms

- Chest pain
- Shortness of breath (dyspnea)
- Wheezing
- Cough
- Blood-streaked sputum (hemoptysis)

Complaints of *chest pain* or *chest discomfort* raise the specter of heart disease but often arise from conditions in the thorax and lungs. For this important symptom, keep the possible causes below in mind. Also see Table 8-1, Chest Pain, pp. 137–138.

- The myocardium — Angina pectoris, myocardial infarction
- The pericardium — Pericarditis
- The aorta — Dissecting aortic aneurysm
- The trachea and large bronchi — Bronchitis
- The parietal pleura — Pericarditis, pneumonia
- The chest wall, including the musculoskeletal system and skin — Costochondritis, herpes zoster
- The esophagus — Reflux esophagitis, esophageal spasm
- Extrathoracic structures such as the neck, gallbladder, stomach — Cervical arthritis, biliary colic, gastritis

For patients who are *short of breath*, focus on such *pulmonary complaints* as:

- dyspnea and wheezing   See Table 8-2, Dyspnea, pp. 139–140.

- cough and hemoptysis   See Table 8-3, Cough and Hemoptysis, pp. 141–143.

Health Promotion and Counseling: Evidence and Recommendations

Despite declines in smoking over the past several decades, 21% of Americans still smoke. Regularly counsel all adults, pregnant women, parents, and adolescents who smoke to stop. Include "the five **A**s" and assess readiness to quit, using the Stages of Change Model.

Assessing Readiness to Quit Smoking: Brief Interventions Models

5 As Model	Stages of Change Model
Ask about tobacco use	**Precontemplation**—"I don't want to quit."
Advise to quit	**Contemplation**—"I am concerned but not ready to quit now."
Assess willingness to make a quit attempt	**Preparation**—"I am ready to quit."
Assist in quit attempt	**Action**—"I just quit."
Arrange follow-up	**Maintenance**—"I quit 6 months ago."

Provide *flu shots* to everyone age 6 months or older and especially to those with chronic pulmonary conditions, nursing home residents, household contacts, and health care personnel.

Recommend *pneumococcal vaccine* to adults 65 years and older, smokers between the ages of 16 and 64 years, and those with increased risk of pneumococcal infection.

Chapter 8 | The Thorax and Lungs

Techniques of Examination

EXAMINATION TECHNIQUES	POSSIBLE FINDINGS

SURVEY OF THORAX

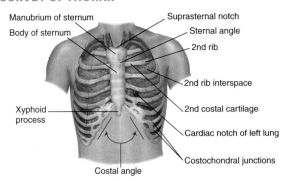

Inspect the thorax and its respiratory movements.

Note:

• Rate, rhythm, depth, and effort of breathing	Tachypnea, hyperpnea, Cheyne–Stokes breathing
• Inspiratory retraction of the supraclavicular areas	Occurs in chronic obstructive pulmonary disease (COPD), asthma, upper airway obstruction
• Inspiratory contraction of the sternomastoids	Indicates severe breathing difficulty
Observe shape of patient's chest.	Normal or barrel chest (see Table 8-4, Deformities of the Thorax, pp. 144–145)

Listen to patient's breathing for:

• Rate and rhythm of breathing	14–16 breaths/minute in adults (see Chapter 4, pp. 57, 65)
• Stridor	Stridor in upper airway obstruction from foreign body or epiglottitis
• Wheezes	Expiratory wheezing in asthma and COPD

| EXAMINATION TECHNIQUES | POSSIBLE FINDINGS |

THE POSTERIOR CHEST

Inspect the chest for:

- Deformities or asymmetry — Kyphoscoliosis

- Abnormal inspiratory retraction of the interspaces — Retraction in airway obstruction

- Impairment or unilateral lag in respiratory movement — Disease of the underlying lung or pleura, phrenic nerve palsy

Palpate the chest for:

- Tender areas — Fractured ribs

- Assessment of visible abnormalities — Masses, sinus tracts

- Chest expansion — Impairment, both sides in COPD and restrictive lung disease

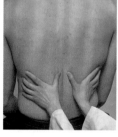

- Tactile fremitus as the patient says "aa" or "blue moon" — Local or generalized decrease or increase

Chapter 8 | The Thorax and Lungs

EXAMINATION TECHNIQUES

Percuss the chest in the areas illustrated, comparing one side with the other at each level, using the side-to-side "ladder pattern."

POSSIBLE FINDINGS

Dullness when fluid or solid tissue replaces normally air-filled lung; *hyperresonance* in emphysema or pneumothorax

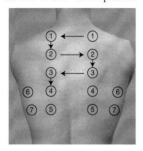
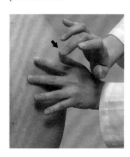

Percussion Notes and Their Characteristics

	Relative Intensity, Pitch, and Duration	Examples
Flat	Soft/high/short	Large pleural effusion
Dull	Medium/medium/medium	Lobar pneumonia
Resonant	Loud/low/long	Normal lung, simple chronic bronchitis
Hyperresonant	Louder/lower/longer	Emphysema, pneumothorax
Tympanitic	Loud/high (timbre is musical)	Large pneumothorax

Percuss level of diaphragmatic dullness on each side and **estimate** diaphragmatic descent after patient takes full inspiration.

Pleural effusion or a *paralyzed diaphragm* raises level of dullness.

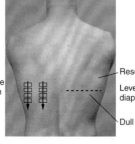

EXAMINATION TECHNIQUES	POSSIBLE FINDINGS
Listen to chest with stethoscope in the "ladder" pattern, again comparing sides.	See Table 8-5, Physical Findings in Selected Chest Disorders, p. 146.
• Evaluate the breath sounds.	Vesicular, bronchovesicular, or bronchial breath sounds; decreased breath sounds from decreased airflow
• Note any adventitious (added) sounds.	Crackles (fine and coarse) and continuous sounds (wheezes and rhonchi)
Observe qualities of breath sound, timing in the respiratory cycle, and location on the chest wall. Do they clear with deep breathing or coughing?	Clearing after cough suggests atelectasis

Characteristics of Breath Sounds

	Duration	Intensity and Pitch of Expiratory Sound	Example Locations
Vesicular	Insp > Exp	Soft/low	Most of the lungs
Bronchovesicular	Insp = Exp	Medium/medium	1st and 2nd interspaces, interscapular area
Bronchial	Exp > Insp	Loud/high	Over the manubrium
Tracheal	Insp = Exp	Very loud/high	Over the trachea

Duration is indicated by the length of the line, intensity by the width of the line, and pitch by the slope of the line.

Chapter 8 | The Thorax and Lungs

EXAMINATION TECHNIQUES | **POSSIBLE FINDINGS**

Adventitious or Added Breath Sounds

Crackles (or Rales)	Wheezes and Rhonchi
▶ **Discontinuous**	▶ **Continuous**
▶ Intermittent, nonmusical, and brief	▶ ≥250 msec, musical, prolonged (but not necessarily persisting throughout the respiratory cycle)
▶ Like dots in time	▶ Like dashes in time
▶ *Fine crackles:* Soft, high-pitched, very brief (5–10 msec)	▶ *Wheezes:* Relatively high-pitched (≥400 Hz) with hissing or shrill quality
▶ *Coarse crackles:* Somewhat louder, lower in pitch, brief (20–30 msec)	▶ *Rhonchi:* Relatively low-pitched (≤200 Hz) with snoring quality

Assess transmitted voice sounds, bronchial breath sounds heard in abnormal places. Ask patient to:

- Say "ninety-nine" and "ee."

  Bronchophony if sounds become louder; egophony if "ee" to "A" change to lobar consolidation

- Whisper "ninety-nine" or "one-two-three."

  Whispered pectoriloquy

Transmitted Voice Sounds

Through Normally Air-Filled Lung	Through Airless Lung*
Usually accompanied by vesicular breath sounds and normal tactile fremitus	Usually accompanied by bronchial or bronchovesicular breath sounds and increased tactile fremitus
Spoken words muffled and indistinct	Spoken words louder, clearer (*bronchophony*)
Spoken "ee" heard as "ee"	Spoken "ee" heard as "ay" (*egophony*)
Whispered words faint and indistinct, if heard at all	Whispered words louder, clearer (*whispered pectoriloquy*)

*As in lobar pneumonia and toward the top of a large pleural effusion

| EXAMINATION TECHNIQUES | POSSIBLE FINDINGS |

Alternate Sequence. While the patient is still sitting, you may inspect the breasts and examine the axillary and epitrochlear lymph nodes, and examine the temporomandibular joint and the musculoskeletal system of the upper extremities.

THE ANTERIOR CHEST

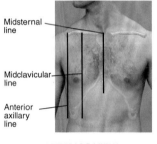

ANTERIOR VIEW

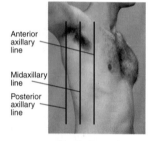

RIGHT ANTERIOR OBLIQUE VIEW

Inspect the chest for:

- Deformities or asymmetry

  Pectus excavatum

- Intercostal retraction

  From obstructed airways

- Impaired or lagging respiratory movement

  Disease of the underlying lung or pleura, phrenic nerve palsy

Palpate the chest for:

- Tender areas

  Tender pectoral muscles, costochondritis

- Assessment of visible abnormalities

  Flail chest

- Respiratory expansion

- Tactile fremitus

EXAMINATION TECHNIQUES

Percuss the chest in the areas illustrated.

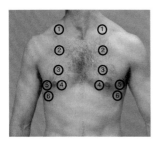

Listen to the chest with stethoscope. Note:

- Breath sounds

- Adventitious sounds

- If indicated, transmitted voice sounds

SPECIAL TECHNIQUES

CLINICAL ASSESSMENT OF PULMONARY FUNCTION

Walk with patient down the hall or up a flight of stairs. Observe the rate, effort, and sound of breathing, and inquire about symptoms. Or do a "6-minute walk test."

FORCED EXPIRATORY TIME

Ask the patient to take a deep breath in and then breathe out as quickly and completely as possible, with mouth open. Listen over trachea with diaphragm of stethoscope, and time audible expiration. Try to get three consistent readings, allowing rests as needed.

POSSIBLE FINDINGS

Normal cardiac dullness may disappear in emphysema.

Older adults walking 8 feet in <3 seconds are less likely to be disabled than those taking >5 to 6 seconds.

If the patient understands and cooperates well, a forced expiratory time of 6 to 8 seconds strongly suggests COPD

Recording Your Findings

Recording the Physical Examination—The Thorax and Lungs

"Thorax is symmetric with good expansion. Lungs resonant. Breath sounds vesicular; no rales, wheezes, or rhonchi. Diaphragms descend 4 cm bilaterally."
OR
"Thorax symmetric with moderate kyphosis and increased anteroposterior (AP) diameter, decreased expansion. Lungs are hyperresonant. Breath sounds distant with delayed expiratory phase and scattered expiratory wheezes. Fremitus decreased; no bronchophony, egophony, or whispered pectoriloquy. Diaphragms descend 2 cm bilaterally." *(Suggests COPD)*

Chapter 8 | The Thorax and Lungs

Aids to Interpretation

Table 8-1 Chest Pain

Problem and Location	Quality, Severity, Timing, and Associated Symptoms
Cardiovascular	
Angina Pectoris Retrosternal or across the anterior chest, sometimes radiating to the shoulders, arms, neck, lower jaw, or upper abdomen	• Pressing, squeezing, tight, heavy, occasionally burning • Mild to moderate severity, sometimes perceived as discomfort rather than pain • Usually 1–3 min but up to 10 min; prolonged episodes up to 20 min • Sometimes with dyspnea, nausea, swelling
Myocardial Infarction Same as in angina	• Same as in angina • Often but not always a severe pain • 20 min to several hours • Associated with nausea, vomiting, sweating, weakness
Pericarditis *Precordial:* May radiate to the tip of the shoulder and to the neck	• Sharp, knifelike quality • Often severe • Persistent timing • Symptoms of the underlying illness; relieved by leaning forward
Retrosternal	• Crushing quality • Severe • Persistent timing • Symptoms of the underlying illness
Dissecting Aortic Aneurysm Anterior chest, radiating to the neck, back, or abdomen	• Ripping, tearing quality • Very severe • Abrupt onset, early peak, persistent for hours or more • Associated syncope, hemiplegia, paraplegia

(continued)

Table 8-1	Chest Pain (continued)
Problem and Location	**Quality, Severity, Timing, and Associated Symptoms**
Pulmonary	
Tracheobronchitis Upper sternal or on either side of the sternum	• Burning qualtiy • Mild to moderate severity • Variable timing • Associated cough
Pleural Pain Chest wall overlying the process	• Sharp, knifelike quality • Often severe • Persistent timing • Associated symptoms of the underlying illness
Gastrointestinal and Other	
Reflex Esophagitis Retrosternal, may radiate to the back	• Burning quality, may be squeezing • Mild to severe • Variable timing • Associated with regurgitation, dysphagia
Diffuse Esophageal Spasm Retrosternal, may radiate to the back, arms, and jaw	• Usually squeezing quality • Mild to severe • Variable timing • Associated dysphagia
Chest Wall Pain Often below the left breast or along the costal cartilages; also elsewhere	• Stabbing, sticking, or dull aching quality • Variable severity • Fleeting timing, hours or days • Often with local tenderness
Anxiety	• Pain may be sharp, intense, or severe • Can mimic angina • Associated with stress of anxiety

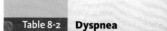

Table 8-2   Dyspnea

Problem	Timing	Provoking and Relieving Factors
Left-Sided Heart Failure *(left ventricular failure or mitral stenosis)*	Dyspnea may progress slowly or suddenly, as in acute pulmonary edema	↑ by exertion, lying down ↓ by rest, sitting up, though dyspnea may become persistent *Associated Symptoms:* Often cough, orthopnea, paroxysmal nocturnal dyspnea; sometimes wheezing
Chronic Bronchitis *(may be seen with COPD)*	Chronic productive cough followed by slowly progressive dyspnea	↑ by exertion, inhaled irritants, respiratory infections ↓ by expectoration, rest though dyspnea may become persistent *Associated Symptoms:* Chronic productive cough, recurrent respiratory infections; wheezing possible
Chronic Obstructive Pulmonary Disease (COPD)	Slowly progressive; relatively mild cough later	↑ by exertion ↓ by rest, though dyspnea may become persistent *Associated Symptoms:* Cough with scant mucoid sputum
Asthma	Acute episodes, then symptom-free periods; nocturnal episodes common	↑ by allergens, irritants, respiratory infections, exercise, emotion ↓ by separation from aggravating factors *Associated Symptoms:* Wheezing, cough, tightness in chest

(continued)

Table 8-2 Dyspnea (continued)

Problem	Timing	Provoking and Relieving Factors
Acute Pulmonary Embolism	Sudden onset of dyspnea	*Associated Symptoms:* Often none; retrosternal oppressive pain if occlusion is massive; pleuritic pain, cough, and hemoptysis may follow an embolism if pulmonary infarction ensues; symptoms of anxiety
Pneumonia	Acute illness; timing varies with causative agent	*Associated Symptoms:* Pleuritic pain, cough, sputum, fever, though not necessarily present
Diffuse Interstitial Lung Diseases *(sarcoidosis, neoplasms, asbestosis, idiopathic pulmonary fibrosis)*	Progressive; varies in rate of development depending on cause	↑ by exertion ↓ by rest, though dyspnea may become persistent *Associated Symptoms:* Often weakness, fatigue; cough less common than in other lung diseases
Spontaneous Pneumothorax	Sudden onset of dyspnea	*Associated Symptoms:* Pleuritic pain, cough

Table 8-3 Cough and Hemoptysis

Problem	Cough, Sputum, Associated Symptoms, and Setting
Acute Inflammation	
Laryngitis	*Cough and Sputum:* Dry, or with variable amounts of sputum *Associated Symptoms and Setting:* Acute, fairly minor illness with hoarseness. May be associated with viral nasopharyngitis
Tracheobronchitis	*Cough and Sputum:* Dry or productive of sputum *Associated Symptoms and Setting:* An acute, often viral illness, with burning retrosternal discomfort
Mycoplasma and Viral Pneumonias	*Cough:* Dry and hacking *Sputum:* Often mucoid *Associated Symptoms and Setting:* An acute febrile illness, often with malaise, headache, and possibly dyspnea
Bacterial Pneumonias	*Cough and Sputum:* With pneumococcal infection, mucoid or purulent; may be blood streaked, diffusely pinkish, or rusty. With *Klebsiella,* similar to pneumococcal, or sticky red and jellylike. *Associated Symptoms and Setting:* An acute illness with chills, high fever, dyspnea, and chest pain; often preceded by acute upper respiratory infection. *Klebsiella* often in older alcoholic men.
Chronic Inflammation	
Postnasal Drip	*Cough:* Chronic *Sputum:* Mucoid or mucopurulent *Associated Symptoms and Setting:* Repeated attempts to clear the throat. Postnasal drip, discharge in posterior pharynx. Associated with chronic rhinitis, with or without sinusitis

(continued)

Table 8-3	**Cough and Hemoptysis** (continued)
Problem	**Cough, Sputum, Associated Symptoms, and Setting**
Chronic Bronchitis	*Cough:* Chronic *Sputum:* Mucoid to purulent; may be blood-streaked or even bloody *Associated Symptoms and Setting:* Often long history of cigarette smoking. Recurrent superimposed infections; often wheezing and dyspnea.
Bronchiectasis	*Cough:* Chronic *Sputum:* Purulent, often copious and foul smelling; may be blood-streaked or bloody *Associated Symptoms and Setting:* Recurrent bronchopulmonary infections common; sinusitis may coexist
Pulmonary Tuberculosis	*Cough and Sputum:* Dry, mucoid or purulent; may be blood-streaked or bloody *Associated Symptoms and Setting:* Early, no symptoms. Later, anorexia, weight loss, fatigue, fever, and night sweats.
Lung Abscess	*Cough and Sputum:* Purulent and foul smelling; may be bloody *Associated Symptoms and Setting:* A febrile illness. Often poor dental hygiene and a prior episode of impaired consciousness
Asthma	*Cough and Sputum:* Thick and mucoid, especially near end of an attack *Associated Symptoms and Setting:* Episodic wheezing and dyspnea, but cough may occur alone. Often a history of allergy

Table 8-3 Cough and Hemoptysis (continued)

Problem	Cough, Sputum, Associated Symptoms, and Setting
Gastroesophageal Reflux	*Cough and Sputum:* Chronic, especially at night or early morning *Associated Symptoms and Setting:* Wheezing, especially at night (often mistaken for asthma), early morning hoarseness, repeated attempts to clear throat. Often with history of heartburn and regurgitation
Neoplasm	*Cough:* Dry to productive
Cancer of the Lung	*Sputum:* May be blood-streaked or bloody *Associated Symptoms and Setting:* Usually a long history of cigarette smoking
Cardiovascular Disorders	
Left Ventricular Failure or Mitral Stenosis	*Cough:* Often dry, especially on exertion or at night *Sputum:* May progress to pink and frothy, as in pulmonary edema, or to frank hemoptysis *Associated Symptoms and Setting:* Dyspnea, orthopnea, paroxysmal nocturnal dyspnea
Pulmonary Emboli	*Cough:* Dry to productive *Sputum:* May be dark, bright red, or mixed with blood *Associated Symptoms and Setting:* Dyspnea, anxiety, chest pain, fever; factors that predispose to deep venous thrombosis
Irritating Particles, Chemicals, or Gases	*Cough and Sputum:* Variable. There may be a latent period between exposure and symptoms. *Associated Symptoms and Setting:* Exposure to irritants; eye, nose, and throat symptoms

Table 8-4 Deformities of the Thorax

Cross-Section of Thorax

Normal Adult

The thorax is wider than it is deep; lateral diameter is greater than anteroposterior (AP) diameter.

Barrel Chest

Has increased AP diameter, seen in normal infants and normal aging; also in COPD.

 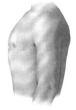

Traumatic Flail Chest

If multiple ribs are fractured, can see paradoxical movements of the thorax. Descent of the diaphragm decreases intrathoracic pressure on inspiration. The injured area may cave inward; on expiration, it moves outward.

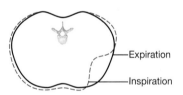

Funnel Chest
(Pectus Excavatum)

Depression in the lower portion of the sternum. Related compression of the heart and great vessels may cause murmurs.

 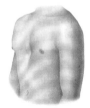

Table 8-4 Deformities of the Thorax (continued)

Cross-Section of Thorax
Pigeon Chest
(Pectus Carinatum)

Sternum is displaced anteriorly, increasing the AP diameter; costal cartilages adjacent to the protruding sternum are depressed.

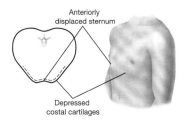

Thoracic Kyphoscoliosis

Abnormal spinal curvatures and vertebral rotation deform the chest, making interpretation of lung findings difficult.

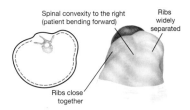

Table 8-5 Physical Findings in Selected Chest Disorders

	Trachea	Percussion Note	Breath Sounds	Transmitted Voice Sounds	Adventitious Sounds
Chronic Bronchitis	Midline	Resonant	Normal	Normal	None, or wheezes, rhonchi, crackles
Left Heart Failure (Early)	Midline	Resonant	Normal	Normal	Late inspiratory crackles in lower lungs; possible wheezes
Consolidation*	Midline	Dull	Bronchial	Increased[†]	Late inspiratory crackles
Atelectasis (Lobar Obstruction)	May be shifted *toward* involved side	Dull	Usually absent	Usually absent	None
Pleural Effusion	May be shifted *away*	Dull	Decreased to absent	Decreased to absent	Usually none, possible pleural rub
Pneumothorax	May be shifted *away*	Hyperresonant or tympanitic	Decreased to absent	Decreased to absent	Possible pleural rub
COPD	Midline	Hyperresonant	Decreased to absent	Decreased	None or the wheezes and rhonchi of chronic bronchitis
Asthma	Midline	Resonant to hyperresonant	May be obscured by wheezes	Decreased	Wheezes, perhaps crackles

*As in lobar pneumonia, pulmonary edema, or pulmonary hemorrhage
[†]With increased tactile fremitus, bronchophony, egophony, whispered pectoriloquy

CHAPTER 9

The Cardiovascular System

The Health History

Common or Concerning Symptoms

- Chest pain
- Palpitations
- Shortness of breath: dyspnea, orthopnea, or paroxysmal nocturnal dyspnea
- Swelling or edema

As you assess reports of *chest pain or discomfort*, keep serious adverse events in mind, such as *angina pectoris, myocardial infarction,* or even a *dissecting aortic aneurysm*. Ask also about any associated palpitations, orthopnea, paroxysmal nocturnal dyspnea (PND), and edema.

- *Palpitations* are an unpleasant awareness of the heartbeat.

- *Shortness of breath* may represent dyspnea, orthopnea, or PND.

  - *Dyspnea* is an uncomfortable awareness of breathing that is inappropriate for a given level of exertion.

  - *Orthopnea* is dyspnea that occurs when the patient is lying down and improves when the patient sits up. It suggests *left ventricular heart failure* or *mitral stenosis;* it also may accompany *obstructive pulmonary disease*.

  - *PND* describes episodes of sudden dyspnea and orthopnea that awaken the patient from sleep, usually 1 to 2 hours after going to bed, prompting the patient to sit up, stand up, or go to a window for air.

- *Edema* refers to the accumulation of excessive fluid in the interstitial tissue spaces; it appears as swelling. *Dependent edema* appears in the feet and lower legs when sitting or in the sacrum when bedridden.

Health Promotion and Counseling: Evidence and Recommendations

Important Topics for Health Promotion and Counseling

- Screening for cardiovascular risk factors
  - *Step 1:* Screen for global risk factors
  - *Step 2:* Calculate 10-year and long-term CVD risk using online calculators
  - *Step 3:* Track individual risk factors—hypertension, diabetes, dyslipidemias, metabolic syndrome, smoking, family history and obesity
- Promoting lifestyle modification and risk factor reduction

Cardiovascular disease is the leading cause of death for both men and women in the United States. *Primary prevention,* in those without evidence of cardiovascular disease, and *secondary prevention,* in those with known cardiovascular events (e.g., myocardial infarction, heart failure), remain important clinical priorities. Use education and counseling to help your patients maintain optimal levels of blood pressure, cholesterol, weight, and exercise and to reduce risk factors for cardiovascular disease and stroke.

The American Heart Association recommends a new goal for 2020, "ideal cardiovascular health," namely:

- Total cholesterol <200 mg/dL (untreated)
- Lean body mass
- BP <120/<80 (untreated)
- Fasting glucose <100 mg/dL (untreated)
- Abstinence from smoking
- Physical activity goal: ≥150 min/wk moderate intensity, ≥75 min/wk vigorous intensity, or combination
- Healthy diet

Only 3% of U.S. adults have optimal health behaviors for all 7 goals. Women and African Americans have emerged as groups at especially high risk.

CVD Screening Steps

Step 1: Screen for Global Risk Factors. Begin routine screening at age 20 for combined individual risk factors or "global" risk of CVD and any family history or premature heart disease. See the recommended screening intervals listed below.

Major Cardiovascular Risk Factors and Screening Frequency

Risk Factor	Screening Frequency	Goal
Family history of premature CVD (at age <55 years in first-degree male relatives and <65 years in first-degree female relatives)	Update regularly	
Cigarette smoking	At each visit	Cessation
Poor diet	At each visit	Improved overall eating pattern
Physical inactivity	At each visit	30 min moderate intensity daily
Obesity, especially central adiposity	At each visit	BMI 20–25 kg/m^2; waist circumference 40 inches in men, ≤35 inches in women
Hypertension	At each visit	<140/90 <135/85 if African American with HTN and without end-organ or CVD <130/80 if diabetes or African American with HTN and end-organ or CVD <125/75 if renal disease
Dyslipidemias	Every 5 years if low risk Every 2 years if risk factors	See ATP III guidelines
Diabetes	Every 3 years beginning at age 45 More frequently at any age if risk factors	HgA1C ≥6.5%, at risk if 5.7%–6.4%
Pulse	At each visit	Identify and treat atrial fibrillation

Source: Adapted from: Pearson TA, Blair SN, Daniels SR et al. AHA Guidelines for Primary Prevention of Cardiovascular Disease and Stroke: 2002Update. Consensus Panel Guide to Com prehensive Risk Reduction for Adult Patients without Coronary or Other Atherosclerotic Vascular Diseases. Circulation 2002;106:388–391; Flack JM, Sica DA, Bakris G et al. Management of high blood pressure in blacks. An update of the International Society on Hypertension in Blacks Consensus Statement. Hypertension 2010;56:780–800; American Diabetes Association. Standards of medical care in diabetes–2011. Diabetes Care 2001;34:S1–S61.

Step 2: Calculate 10-year and Long-Term CVD Risk Using Online Calculators. For Step 2, assemble risk factor data and calculate multivariable global risk assessment. This is easily accomplished by accessing well-validated online calculators that provide 10-year CVD risk assessments that can also be used to guide treatment of dyslipidemias.

- Framingham 10-year and 30-year risk calculator: http://www.framinghamheartstudy.org/risk/gencardio.html

- Stroke risk calculator (Cleveland Clinic): http://my.clevelandclinic.org/p2/stroke-risk-calculator.aspx

Step 3: Track Individual Risk Factors–Hypertension, Diabetes, Dyslipidemias, Metabolic Syndrome, Obesity, Smoking, and Family History.

Hypertension. The U.S. Preventive Services Task Force recommends *screening all people 18 years or older for high blood pressure*. Use the blood pressure classification of the Seventh Report of the Joint National Committee on Prevention, Detection, Evaluation, and Treatment of High Blood Pressure (JNC 7).

JNC 7: Classification and Management of Blood Pressure for Adults

Normal	<120/80 mm Hg
Prehypertension	120–139/80–89 mm Hg
Stage 1 Hypertension	140–159/90–99 mm Hg
Stage 2 Hypertension	>160/>100 mm Hg
If diabetes or kidney disease	<130/80 mm Hg

Diabetes. Use the screening and diagnostic criteria below.

American Diabetes Association 2011: Criteria for Diabetes Screening and Diagnosis

Screening Criteria

Healthy adults with no risk factors: Begin at age 45 years, repeat at 3 year intervals

Adults with BMI ≥25 kg/m^2 and additional risk factors:
- Physical inactivity
- First-degree relative with diabetes

(continued)

American Diabetes Association 2011: Criteria for Diabetes Screening and Diagnosis (continued)

- Members of a high-risk ethnic population–African American, Latino American, Asian American, Pacific Islander
- Mothers of infants ≥9 lb or diagnosed with GDM
- Hypertension ≥140/90 mm Hg or on therapy for hypertension
- HDL cholesterol <35 mg/dL and/or triglycerides >250 mg/dL
- Women with polycystic ovary syndrome
- A1C ≥5.7%, impaired glucose tolerance, or impaired fasting glucose on previous testing
- Other conditions associated with insulin resistance such as severe obesity, acanthosis nigricans
- History of cardiovascular disease

Diagnostic Criteria	Diabetes	Prediabetes
A1C	≤6.5%	5.7%–6.4%
Fasting plasma glucose (on at least 2 occasions)	≥126 mg/dL	100–125 mg/dL
2-hour plasma glucose (oral tolerance test)	≥200 mg/dL	140–199 mg/dL
Random glucose if classic symptoms	≥200 mg/dL	

Dyslipidemias. LDL is the primary target of cholesterol-lowering therapy. Ten-year risk categories are as follows:

- *High risk* (10-year CVD risk >20%): established CVD and CHD risk equivalents

- *Moderately high risk* (10-year CVD risk 10% to 20%): multiple or ≥2 risk factors

- *Low risk* (10-year CVD risk <10%): 0 to 1 risk factor

For high-risk people, the recommended LDL goal is <70 mg/dL and intensive lipid therapy is a *therapeutic option*.

ATP III Guidelines: 10-Year Risk and LDL Goals

10-Year Risk Category	LDL Goal (mg/dL)	Consider Drug Therapy if LDL (mg/dL)
High risk (>20%)	<100 Optional goal: <70	>100 (<100: consider drug options, including further 30%–40% reduction in LDL)
Moderately high risk (10%–20%)	<130 Optional goal: <100	≥130 100–129: consider drug options to achieve goal of <100
Moderate risk (<10%)	<130	≥160
Lower risk (0–1 risk factor)	<160	>190 (160–189: drug therapy *optional*)

Source: Adapted from National Cholesterol Education Panel Report. Implications of recent clinical trials for the National Cholesterol Education Program Adult Treatment Panel III Guidelines. Grundy SM, Cleeman JI, Merz NB, et al., for the Coordinating Committee of the National Cholesterol Education Program. Circulation 2004;119:227–239.

The Metabolic Syndrome. The *metabolic syndrome* consists of a cluster of risk factors which confer and increased risk of both CVD and diabetes. In 2009, the International Diabetes Association and other societies harmonized diagnostic criteria as the presence of three or more of the five risk factors listed below.

Metabolic Syndrome: 2009 Diagnostic Criteria

Waist circumference	Men ≥102 cm, women ≥88 cm
Fasting plasma glucose	≥100 mg/dL or being treated for elevated glucose
HDL cholesterol	Men <40 mg/dL, women <50 mg/dL, or being treated
Triglycerides	≥150 mg/dL, or being treated
Blood pressure	≥130/≥85, or being treated

Source: Alberti K, Eckel RH, Grundy SM et al. Harmonizing the metabolic syndrome: a joint interim statement of the Internal Diabetes Federation Task Force on Epidemiology and Prevention; National Heart, Lung and Blood Institute; American Heart Association; World Heart Federation; Internal Atherosclerosis Society; and Internal Association for the Study of Obesity. Circulation 2009;120:1620–1645.

Other Risk Factors: Smoking, Family History, and Obesity.

In adult smokers, 33% of deaths are related to CVD. *Smoking* increases the risk of coronary heart disease by two- to fourfold. Among adults, 13% report a *family history* of heart attack before age 50, which roughly doubles the risk the risk of heart attack. *Obesity,* or BMI more than 30, contributed to 112,000 excess adult deaths compared to normal weight in recent data and was associated with 13% of CVD deaths in 2004.

Promoting Lifestyle Modification and Risk Factor Reduction.

The JNC 7 and AHA encourage well-studied effective lifestyle modification and risk interventions to prevent hypertension, CHD, and stroke.

Lifestyle Modifications for Cardiovascular Health

- Optimal weight (BMI of 18.5–24.9 kg/m^2)
- Salt intake <½ teaspoon or 1500 mg/day of sodium
- Regular aerobic exercise (e.g., brisk walking) for at least 30 min/day, most days of the week
- Moderate alcohol consumption of 2 or fewer drinks per day for men and 1 drink or fewer per day for women
- Diet rich in fruits, vegetables, and low-fat dairy products with reduced saturated and total fat
- Dietary intake of >3,500 mg of potassium
- Optimal blood pressure control (see p. 150)
- Lipid management
- Diabetes management so that fasting glucose level is <100 mg/dL and HgA1C is <7%
- Complete smoking cessation
- Conversion of atrial fibrillation to normal sinus rhythm or, if chronic, anticoagulation

---

Techniques of Examination

EXAMINATION TECHNIQUES	POSSIBLE FINDINGS

HEART RATE AND BLOOD PRESSURE

If not already done, measure the radial or apical pulse.

Estimate systolic blood pressure by palpation and **add** 30 mm Hg. Use this sum as the target for further cuff inflations.	This step helps you to detect an auscultatory gap and avoid recording an inappropriately low systolic blood pressure.

| EXAMINATION TECHNIQUES | POSSIBLE FINDINGS |

Measure *blood pressure* with a sphygmomanometer. If indicated, recheck it.

Orthostatic (postural) hypotension with position change from supine to standing, SBP↓ ≥20 mm Hg; HR↑ ≥20 beats/min

JUGULAR VEINS

Identify *jugular venous pulsations* and their highest point in the neck. Start with head of the bed at 30 degrees; adjust angle of the bed as necessary.

Study the waves of venous pulsation. Note the *a* wave of atrial contraction and the *v* wave of venous filling.

Absent *a* waves in *atrial fibrillation*; prominent *v* waves in *tricuspid regurgitation*

Measure *jugular venous pressure* (JVP)—the vertical distance between this highest point and the sternal angle, normally <3 to 4 cm.

Elevated JVP in right-sided heart failure; decreased JVP in hypovolemia from dehydration or gastrointestinal bleeding

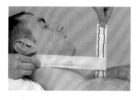

CAROTID PULSE

Assess the amplitude and contour of the carotid upstroke.

A *delayed* upstroke in *aortic stenosis*; a *bounding* upstroke in *aortic insufficiency*

Check for variations in pulse amplitude.

See pulsus alternans and paradoxical pulse, p. 159

Listen for bruits.

Carotid bruits suggest atherosclerotic narrowing and increase stroke risk.

Chapter 9 | The Cardiovascular System

EXAMINATION TECHNIQUES | POSSIBLE FINDINGS

THE HEART

Sequence of the Cardiac Examination

Patient Position	Examination
Supine, with the head elevated 30 degrees	Inspect and palpate the precordium: the 2nd interspaces; the right ventricle; and the left ventricle, including the apical impulse (diameter, location, amplitude, duration).
Left lateral decubitus	Palpate the apical impulse if not previously detected. Listen at the apex with the *bell of the stethoscope for low-pitched extra sounds* (S_3, opening snap, diastolic rumble of mitral stenosis).
Supine, with the head elevated 30 degrees	Listen at the 2nd right and left interspaces, along the left sternal border, and across to the apex with the *diaphragm*.
	Listen with the bell at the right sternal border for tricuspid murmurs and sounds.
Sitting, leaning forward, after full exhalation	Listen along the left sternal border and at the apex for the soft decrescendo diastolic murmur of *aortic insufficiency*.

INSPECTION AND PALPATION

Inspect and palpate the anterior chest for heaves, lifts, or thrills.

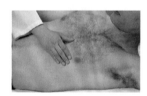

Identify the *apical impulse*. Turn patient to left as necessary. Note:

- Location of impulse

  Displaced to left in pregnancy

- Diameter

  Increased diameter, amplitude, and duration in left ventricular dilatation from *congestive heart failure* (CHF) or *ischemic cardiomyopathy*

- Amplitude—usually *tapping*

  Sustained in left ventricular hypertrophy; diffuse in CHF

- Duration

EXAMINATION TECHNIQUES	POSSIBLE FINDINGS

Feel for a right ventricular impulse in left parasternal and epigastric areas.

Prominent impulses suggest right ventricular enlargement.

Palpate left and right second interspaces close to sternum. Note any thrills in these areas.

Pulsations of great vessels; accentuated S_2; thrills of *aortic* or *pulmonic stenosis*

AUSCULTATION

Listen to heart by "inching" your stethoscope from the base to the apex (or apex to base) in the areas illustrated.

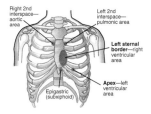

Use the *diaphragm* in the areas illustrated above for relatively *high-pitched sounds* like S_1, S_2.

Also murmurs of *aortic and mitral regurgitation*; *pericardial friction rubs*

Use the *bell* for *low-pitched sounds* at the lower left sternal border and apex.

S_3, S_4, murmur of *mitral stenosis*

Listen at each area for:

See Table 9-1, Heart Sounds, p. 161; Table 9-2, Variations in the First Heart Sound—S_1, p. 162; Table 9-3, Variations in the Second Heart Sound—S_2, pp. 163–164.

- S_1

- S_2. Is splitting normal in left 2nd and 3rd interspaces?

Physiologic (inspiratory) or pathologic (expiratory) splitting

- Extra sounds in systole

Systolic clicks

- Extra sounds in diastole

S_3, S_4

- Systolic murmurs

Midsystolic, pansystolic, late systolic murmurs

- Diastolic murmurs

Early, mid-, or late diastolic murmurs

Chapter 9 | The Cardiovascular System

EXAMINATION TECHNIQUES | POSSIBLE FINDINGS

ASSESSING AND DESCRIBING MURMURS

Identify, if murmurs are present, their:

- Timing in the cardiac cycle (systole, diastole). It is helpful to palpate the carotid upstroke while listening to any murmur—murmurs occurring simultaneously with the upstroke are systolic.

    See Table 9-4, Heart Murmurs, p. 165.

- Shape

    Plateau, crescendo, decrescendo

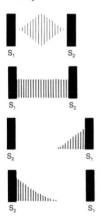

A *crescendo–decrescendo murmur* first rises in intensity, then falls (e.g., aortic stenosis).

A *plateau murmur* has the same intensity throughout (e.g., mitral regurgitation).

A *crescendo murmur* grows louder (e.g., mitral stenosis).

A *decrescendo murmur* grows softer (e.g., aortic regurgitation).

- Location of maximal intensity

    Murmurs loudest at the *base* are often aortic; at the *apex*, they are often mitral.

- Radiation

- Pitch

    High, medium, low

- Quality

    Blowing, harsh, musical, rumbling

- Intensity on a 6-point scale

    See "Gradations of Murmurs" on next page.

Listen at the apex with patient turned toward left side for low-pitched sounds.

Left-sided S_3, and diastolic murmur of *mitral stenosis*

| EXAMINATION TECHNIQUES | POSSIBLE FINDINGS |

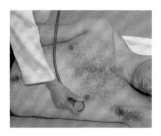

Listen down left sternal border to the apex as patient sits, leaning forward, with breath held after exhalation.

Diastolic decrescendo murmur of *aortic regurgitation*

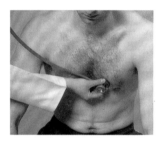

Gradations of Murmurs

Grade	Description
Grade 1	Very faint, heard only after listener has "tuned in"; may not be heard in all positions
Grade 2	Quiet, but heard immediately after placing the stethoscope on the chest
Grade 3	Moderately loud
Grade 4	Loud, *with palpable thrill*
Grade 5	Very loud, *with thrill*. May be heard when the stethoscope is partly off the chest
Grade 6	Very loud, *with thrill*. May be heard with stethoscope entirely off the chest

SPECIAL TECHNIQUES

| EXAMINATION TECHNIQUES | POSSIBLE FINDINGS |

PULSUS ALTERNANS

Feel pulse for alternation in amplitude. Lower pressure of blood pressure cuff slowly to systolic level while you listen with stethoscope over brachial artery.

Alternating amplitude of pulse or sudden doubling of Korotkoff sounds indicates *pulsus alternans*—a sign of left ventricular heart failure.

PARADOXICAL PULSE

Lower pressure of blood pressure cuff slowly and note two pressure levels: (1) where Korotkoff sounds are first heard and (2) where they first persist through the respiratory cycle. These levels are normally not more than 3 to 4 mm Hg apart.

A drop of >10 mm Hg during inspiration signifies a paradoxical pulse. Consider obstructive pulmonary disease, pericardial tamponade, or constrictive pericarditis.

AIDS TO IDENTIFY SYSTOLIC MURMURS

Valsalva Maneuver
Ask patient to strain down.

In suspected *mitral valve prolapse (MVP)*, listen to the timing of click and murmur.

Ventricular filling decreases, the systolic click of MVP is earlier, and the murmur lengthens.

To distinguish *aortic stenosis (AS)* from *hypertrophic cardiomyopathy (HC)*, listen to the intensity of the murmur.

In AS, the murmur decreases; in HC, it often increases.

Squatting and Standing
In suspected *MVP*, listen for the click and murmur in both positions.

Squatting increases ventricular filling and delays the click and murmur. Standing reverses the changes.

Try to distinguish *AS* from *HC* by listening to the murmur in both positions.

Squatting increases murmur of AS and decreases murmur of HC. Standing reverses the changes.

Recording Your Findings

Recording the Physical Examination—The Cardiovascular Examination

"The jugular venous pulse (JVP) is 3 cm above the sternal angle with the head of the bed elevated to 30 degrees. Carotid upstrokes are brisk, without bruits. The point of maximal impulse (PMI) is tapping, 7 cm lateral to the midsternal line in the 5th intercostal space. Crisp S_1 and S_2. At the base, S_2 is greater than S_1 and physiologically split, with $A_2 > P_2$. At the apex, S_1 is greater than S_2 and constant. No murmurs or extra sounds."

OR

"The JVP is 5 cm above the sternal angle with the head of the bed elevated to 50 degrees. Carotid upstrokes are brisk; a bruit is heard over the left carotid artery. The PMI is diffuse, 3 cm in diameter, palpated at the anterior axillary line in the 5th and 6th intercostal spaces. S_1 and S_2 are soft. S_3 present at the apex. High-pitched, harsh 2/6 holosystolic murmur best heard at the apex, radiating to the axilla. No S_4 or diastolic murmurs." *(Suggests CHF with possible left carotid stenosis and mitral regurgitation.)*

Aids to Interpretation

Table 9-1 Heart Sounds

Finding	Possible Causes
S_1 accentuated	Tachycardia, states of high cardiac output; mitral stenosis
S_1 diminished	First-degree heart block; reduced left ventricular contractility; immobile mitral valve, as in mitral regurgitation
Systolic clicks(s)	Mitral valve prolapse (as in E_1 above)
S_2 accentuated in right 2nd interspace	Systemic hypertension, dilated aortic root
S_2 diminished or absent in right 2nd interspace	Immobile aortic valve, as in calcific aortic stenosis
P_2 accentuated	Pulmonary hypertension, dilated pulmonary artery, atrial septal defect
P_2 diminished or absent	Aging, pulmonic stenosis
Opening snap	Mitral stenosis
S_3	Physiologic (usually in children and young adults); volume overload of ventricle, as in mitral regurgitation or heart failure
S_4	Excellent physical conditioning (trained athletes); resistance to ventricular filling because of decreased compliance, left ventricular hypertrophy from pressure overload, as in hypertensive heart disease or aortic stenosis

Table 9-2	Variations in the First Heart Sound—S_1
Normal Variations	S_1 is softer than S_2 at the *base* (right and left 2nd interspaces).
	S_1 is often but not always louder than S_2 at the *apex*.
Accentuated S_1	Occurs in (1) tachycardia, rhythms with a short PR interval, and high cardiac output states (e.g., exercise, anemia, hyperthyroidism), and (2) mitral stenosis.
Diminished S_1	Occurs in first-degree heart block, calcified mitral valve of mitral regurgitation, and ↓ left ventricular contractility in heart failure or coronary heart disease.
Varying S_1	S_1 varies in complete heart block and any totally irregular rhythm (e.g., atrial fibrillation).
Split S_1	Normally heard along the *lower left sternal border* if audible tricuspid component. If S_1 sounds split at apex, consider an S_4, an aortic ejection sound, an early systolic click, right bundle branch block, and premature ventricular contractions.

| Table 9-3 | **Variations in the Second Heart Sound—S_2 During Inspiration and Expiration** |

Physiologic Splitting

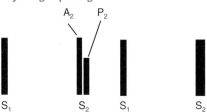

Heard in the 2nd or 3rd left interspace: the pulmonic component of S_2 is usually too faint to be heard at the apex or aortic area, where S_2 is single and derived from aortic valve closure alone. Accentuated by inspiration; usually disappears on exertion.

Pathologic Splitting

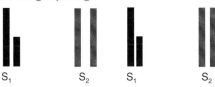

Wide splitting of S_2 persists throughout respiration; arises from delayed closure of the pulmonic valve (e.g., by pulmonic stenosis or right bundle branch block); also from early closure of the aortic valve, as in mitral regurgitation.

Fixed Splitting

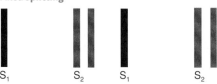

Does not vary with respiration, as in atrial septal defect, right ventricular failure.

(continued)

Table 9-3	**Variations in the Second Heart Sound—S_2 During Inspiration and Expiration** *(continued)*

Paradoxical or Reversed Splitting

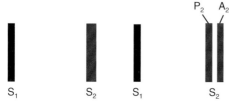

Appears on expiration and disappears on inspiration. Closure of the aortic valve is abnormally delayed, so A_2 follows P_2 on expiration, as in left bundle branch block.

More on A_2 and P_2

Increased Intensity of A_2, 2nd Right Interspace (where only A_2 can usually be heard) occurs in systemic hypertension because of the increased ejection pressure. It also occurs when the aortic root is dilated, probably because the aortic valve is then closer to the chest wall.

Decreased or Absent A_2, 2nd Right Interspace is noted in calcific aortic stenosis because of immobility of the valve. If A_2 is inaudible, no splitting is heard.

Increased Intensity of P_2. When P_2 is equal to or louder than A_2, pulmonary hypertension may be suspected. Other causes include a dilated pulmonary artery and an atrial septal defect. When a split S_2 is heard widely, even at the apex and the right base, P_2 is accentuated.

Decreased or Absent P_2 is most commonly due to the increased anteroposterior diameter of the chest associated with aging. It can also result from pulmonic stenosis. If P_2 is inaudible, no splitting is heard.

Table 9-4 Heart Murmurs

	Likely Causes
Midsystolic	Innocent murmurs (no valve abnormality)
	Physiologic murmurs (from ↑ flow across a semilunar valve, as in pregnancy, fever, anemia)
	Aortic stenosis
	Murmurs that mimic aortic stenosis—aortic sclerosis, bicuspid aortic valve, dilated aorta, and pathologically ↑ systolic flow across aortic valve
	Hypertrophic cardiomyopathy
	Pulmonic stenosis
Pansystolic	Mitral regurgitation
	Tricuspid regurgitation
	Ventricular septal defect
Late Systolic	Mitral valve prolapse, often with click (C)
Early Diastolic	Aortic regurgitation
Middiastolic and Presystolic	Mitral stenosis—note opening snap (OS)
Continuous Murmurs and Sounds	Patent ductus arteriosus—harsh, machinery-like
	Pericardial friction rub—a scratchy sound with 1–3 components
	Venous hum—continuous, above midclavicles, loudest in diastole

CHAPTER 10

The Breasts and Axillae

The Health History

Common or Concerning Symptoms

- Breast lump or mass
- Breast pain or discomfort
- Nipple discharge

Ask, "Do you examine your breasts?" . . . "How often?" Ask about any discomfort, pain, or lumps in the breasts. Also ask about any discharge from the nipples, change in breast contour, dimpling, swelling, or puckering of the skin over the breasts.

Health Promotion and Counseling: Evidence and Recommendations

Important Topics for Health Promotion and Counseling

- Palpable masses of the breast
- Assessing risk of breast cancer
- Breast cancer screening
- Breast self-examination (BSE)

Palpable Masses of the Breast. Breast masses show marked variation in etiology, from fibroadenomas and cysts seen in younger women, to abscess or mastitis, to primary breast cancer. All breast masses warrant careful evaluation, and definitive diagnostic measures should be pursued.

Palpable Masses of the Breast

Age	Common Lesion	Characteristics
15–25	Fibroadenoma	Usually smooth, rubbery, round, mobile, nontender
25–50	Cysts	Usually soft to firm, round, mobile; often tender
	Fibrocystic changes	Nodular, ropelike
	Cancer	Irregular, firm, may be mobile or fixed to surrounding tissue
Over 50	Cancer until proven otherwise	As above
Pregnancy/ lactation	Lactating adenomas, cysts, mastitis, and cancer	As above

Adapted from Schultz MZ, Ward BA, Reiss M. Breast diseases. In: Noble J, Greene HL, Levinson W, et al., eds: Primary Care Medicine, 2nd ed. St. Louis: Mosby, 1996. See also Venet L, Strax P, Venet W, et al. Adequacies and inadequacies of breast examinations by physicians in mass screenings. Cancer 1971;28(6):1546–1551.

Assessing Risk of Breast Cancer. Although 70% of affected women have no known predisposing factors, selected risk factors are well established. Use the Breast Cancer Risk Assessment Tool of the National Cancer Institute (http://www.cancer.gov/bcrisktool) or other available clinical models, such as the Gail model, to individualize risk factor assessment for your patients. Ask women beginning in their 20s about any family history of breast or ovarian cancer, or both, on the maternal or paternal side, to help assess risk of BRCA1 or BRCA2 gene mutation. (See http: astor.som.jhmi.edu/Bayesmendel/brcapro.html). See also Table 10-1, Breast Cancer in Women: Factors That Increase Relative Risk, p. 175.

Breast Cancer Screening. The American Cancer Society recommendations, listed below, vary slightly from those of the U.S. Preventive Services Task Force.

- Yearly *mammography* for women 40 years of age and older. For women at increased risk, many clinicians advise initiating screening mammography between ages 30 and 40, then every 2 to 3 years until 50 years of age.

Chapter 10 | The Breasts and Axillae

- *Clinical breast examination* (CBE) by a health care professional every 3 years for women between 20 and 39 years of age, and annually after 40 years of age

- Regular *breast self-examination* (BSE), in conjunction with mammography and CBE, to help promote health awareness

Techniques of Examination

| EXAMINATION TECHNIQUES | POSSIBLE FINDINGS |

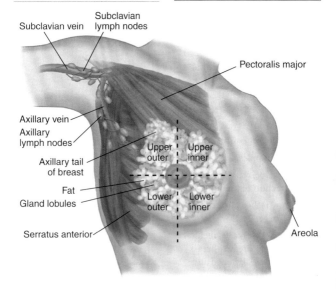

THE FEMALE BREAST

Inspect the breasts in four positions.

Note:

- Size and symmetry

    See Table 10-2, Visible Signs of Breast Cancer, pp. 176–177, development, asymmetry.

- Contour

    Flattening, dimpling

EXAMINATION TECHNIQUES	POSSIBLE FINDINGS

- Appearance of the skin

Edema (peau d'orange) in breast cancer

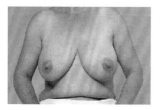

ARMS AT SIDES

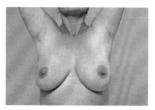

ARMS OVER HEAD

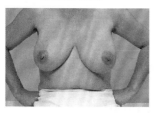

HANDS PRESSED AGAINST HIPS

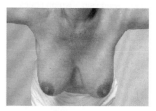

LEANING FORWARD

Inspect the nipples.

- Compare their size, shape, and direction of pointing.

Inversion, retraction, deviation

- Note any rashes, ulcerations, or discharge.

Paget's disease of the nipple, galactorrhea

⌐ Palpate the breasts, including augmented breasts. Breast tissue should be flattened and the patient supine. Palpate a rectangular area extending from the clavicle to the inframammary fold, and from the midsternal line to the posterior axillary line and well into the axilla for the tail of Spence.

| EXAMINATION TECHNIQUES | POSSIBLE FINDINGS |

Note:

- Consistency

  Physiologic nodularity

- Tenderness

  Infection, premenstrual tenderness

- Nodules. If present, note *location, size, shape, consistency, delimitation, tenderness,* and *mobility*.

  Cyst, fibroadenoma, cancer

Use *vertical strip pattern* (currently the best validated technique) or a circular or wedge pattern. Palpate in *small, concentric circles*.

- For *the lateral portion of the breast,* ask the patient to roll onto the opposite hip, place her hand on her forehead, but keep shoulders pressed against the bed or examining table.

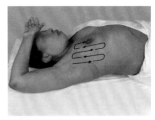

- For *the medial portion of the breast,* ask the patient to lie with her shoulders flat against the bed or examining table, place her hand at her neck, and lift up her elbow until it is even with her shoulder.

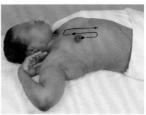

Palpate each nipple

Thickening in cancer

Palpate and inspect along the incision lines of mastectomy.

Local recurrences of breast cancer

| EXAMINATION TECHNIQUES | POSSIBLE FINDINGS |

THE MALE BREAST

♀/♂ Inspect and palpate the nipple and areola.

Gynecomastia, mass suspicious for cancer, fat

AXILLAE

Inspect for rashes, infection, and pigmentation.

Hidradenitis suppurativa, acanthosis nigricans

Palpate the axillary nodes, including the central, pectoral, lateral, and subscapular groups.

Lymphadenopathy

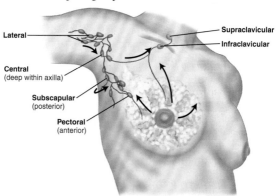

ARROWS INDICATE DIRECTION OF LYMPH FLOW

SPECIAL TECHNIQUE

BREAST DISCHARGE

Compress the areola in a spokelike pattern around the nipple. Watch for discharge.

Type and source of discharge may be identified.

♀/♂ BREAST SELF-EXAMINATION

Patient Instructions for the Breast Self-Examination (BSE)

Supine

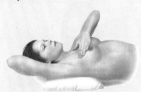

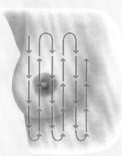

1. Lie down with a pillow under your right shoulder. Place your right arm behind your head.
2. Use the finger pads of the three middle fingers on your left hand to feel for lumps in the right breast. The finger pads are the top third of each finger.
3. Press firmly enough to know how your breast feels. A firm ridge in the lower curve of each breast is normal. If you're not sure how hard to press, talk with your health care provider, or try to copy the way the doctor or nurse does it.
4. Press firmly on the breast in an up-and-down or "strip" pattern.

You can also use a circular or wedge pattern, but be sure to use the same pattern every time. Check the entire breast area, and remember how your breast feels from month to month.

5. Repeat the examination on your left breast, using the finger pads of the right hand.
6. If you find any changes, see your doctor right away.

(continued)

Patient Instructions for the Breast Self-Examination (BSE) *(continued)*

Standing

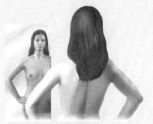
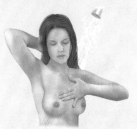

1. While standing in front of a mirror with your hands pressing firmly down on your hips, look at your breasts for any changes of size, shape, contour, or dimpling, or redness or scaliness of the nipple or breast skin. (The pressing down on the hips position contracts the chest wall muscles and enhances any breast changes.)

2. Examine each underarm while sitting up or standing and with your arm only slightly raised so you can easily feel in this area. Raising your arm straight up tightens the tissue in this area and makes it harder to examine.

Adapted from the American Cancer Society, updated September 2010. Available at http://www.cancer.org/Cancer/BreastCancer/MoreInformation/BreastCancerEarlyDetection/breast-cancer-early-detection-a-c-s-recs-b-s-e. Accessed December 3, 2010.

Recording Your Findings

Recording the Physical Examination—Breasts and Axillae

"Breasts symmetric and smooth, without masses. Nipples without discharge." (Axillary adenopathy usually included after Neck in section on Lymph Nodes; see p. 123.)
OR
"Breasts pendulous with diffuse fibrocystic changes. Single firm 1 × 1 cm mass, mobile and nontender, with overlying peau d'orange appearance in right breast, upper outer quadrant at 11 o'clock, 2 cm from the nipple." *(Suggests possible breast cancer.)*

Aids to Interpretation

Table 10-1	Breast Cancer in Women: Factors That Increase Relative Risk
Relative Risk	**Factor**
>4.0	• Female • Age (65+ versus <65 years, although risk increases across all ages until age 80) • Certain inherited genetic mutations for breast cancer (BRCA1 and/or BRCA2) • Two or more first-degree relatives with breast cancer diagnosed at an early age • Personal history of breast cancer • High breast tissue density • Biopsy-confirmed atypical hyperplasia
2.1–4.0	• One first-degree relative with breast cancer • High-dose radiation to chest • High bone density (postmenopausal)
1.1–2.0	
Factors that affect circulating hormones	• Late age at first full-term pregnancy (>30 years) • Early menarche (<12 years) • Late menopause (>55 years) • No full-term pregnancies • Never breast-fed a child • Recent oral contraceptive use • Recent and long-term use of hormone replacement therapy • Obesity (postmenopausal)
Other factors	• Personal history of endometrium, ovary, or colon cancer • Alcohol consumption • Height (tall) • High socioeconomic status • Jewish heritage

Source: American Cancer Society. Breast Cancer Facts and Figures 2009–2010, p. 11. Available at: www.cancer.org/acs/groups/content/cnho/documents/document/f861009final90809pdf.pdf. Accessed July 31, 2012.

Table 10-2 Visible Signs of Breast Cancer

Retraction Signs

Fibrosis from breast cancer produces retraction signs: dimpling, changes in contour, and retraction or deviation of the nipple. Other causes of retraction include fat necrosis and mammary duct ectasia.

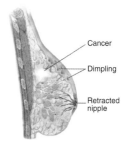

Skin Dimpling

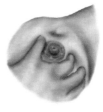

Abnormal Contours

Look for any variation in the normal convexity of each breast, and compare one side with the other.

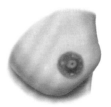

Nipple Retraction and Deviation

A retracted nipple is flattened or pulled inward. It may also be broadened and feel thickened. The nipple may deviate, or point in a different direction, typically toward the underlying cancer.

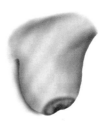

| Table 10-2 | **Visible Signs of Breast Cancer** *(continued)* |

Edema of the Skin

From lymphatic blockade, appearing as thickened skin with enlarged pores—the so-called *peau d'orange* (orange peel) *sign*.

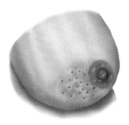

Paget's Disease of the Nipple

An uncommon form of breast cancer that usually starts as a scaly, eczemalike lesion. The skin may also weep, crust, or erode. A breast mass may be present. Suspect Paget's disease in any persisting dermatitis of the nipple and areola.

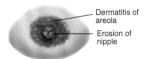

- Dermatitis of areola
- Erosion of nipple

CHAPTER 11

The Abdomen

The Health History

Common or Concerning Symptoms

Gastrointestinal Disorders	Urinary and Renal Disorders
• Abdominal pain, acute and chronic • Indigestion, nausea, vomiting including blood, loss of appetite, early satiety • Dysphagia and/or odynophagia • Change in bowel function • Diarrhea, constipation • Jaundice	• Suprapubic pain • Dysuria, urgency, or frequency • Hesitancy, decreased stream in males • Polyuria or nocturia • Urinary incontinence • Hematuria • Kidney or flank pain • Ureteral colic

PATTERNS AND MECHANISMS OF ABDOMINAL PAIN

Be familiar with three broad categories:

Visceral pain—occurs when hollow abdominal organs such as the intestine or biliary tree contract unusually forcefully or are distended or stretched.

Visceral pain in the right upper quadrant (RUQ) from liver distention against its capsule in *alcoholic hepatitis*

- May be difficult to localize

- Varies in quality; may be gnawing, burning, cramping, or aching

- When severe, may be associated with sweating, pallor, nausea, vomiting, restlessness.

Parietal pain—from inflammation of the parietal peritoneum.

- Steady, aching

- Usually more severe

- Usually more precisely localized over the involved structure than visceral pain

Visceral periumbilical pain in *early acute appendicitis* from distention of inflamed appendix gradually changes to parietal pain in the right lower quadrant (RLQ) from inflammation of the adjacent parietal peritoneum.

Referred pain—occurs in more distant sites innervated at approximately the same spinal levels as the disordered structure.

Pain of duodenal or pancreatic origin may be referred to the back; pain from the biliary tree—to the right shoulder or right posterior chest.

Pain from the chest, spine, or pelvis may be referred to the abdomen.

Pain from *pleurisy* or *acute myocardial infarction* may be referred to the upper abdomen.

THE GASTROINTESTINAL TRACT

Ask patients to *describe the abdominal pain in their own words*, especially timing of the pain (acute or chronic); then ask them to *point to the pain*.

Pursue important details:

"Where does the pain start?"
"Does it radiate or travel?"
"What is the pain like?"
"How severe is it?"
"How about on a scale of 1 to 10?"
"What makes it better or worse?"

Elicit any *symptoms associated with the pain*, such as fever or chills; ask their sequence.

Upper Abdominal Pain, Discomfort, or Heartburn. Ask about chronic or recurrent upper abdominal discomfort, or *dyspepsia*. Related symptoms include bloating, nausea, upper abdominal fullness, and heartburn.

Find out just what your patient means. Possibilities include:

- Bloating from excessive gas, especially with frequent belching, abdominal distention, or flatus, the passage of gas by rectum

- *Nausea and vomiting*

- Unpleasant *abdominal fullness* after normal meals or *early satiety*, the inability to eat a full meal

- *Heartburn*

Consider diabetic gastroparesis, anticholinergic drugs, gastric outlet obstruction, gastric cancer. Early satiety may signify *hepatitis*.

Suggests *gastroesophageal reflux disease (GERD)*

Lower Abdominal Pain or Discomfort—Acute and Chronic. If acute, is the pain sharp and continuous or intermittent and cramping?

Right lower quadrant (RLQ) pain, or pain migrating from periumbilical region in *appendicitis*; in women with RLQ pain, possible *pelvic inflammatory disease, ectopic pregnancy*

Left lower quadrant (LLQ) pain in *diverticulitis*

If chronic, is there a change in bowel habits? Alternating diarrhea and constipation?

Colon cancer; irritable bowel syndrome

Other GI Symptoms

- Anorexia

    Liver disease, pregnancy, diabetic ketoacidosis, adrenal insufficiency, uremia, anorexia nervosa

- Dysphagia or difficulty swallowing

    If solids and liquids, neuromuscular disorders affecting motility. If only solids, consider structural conditions like Zenker's diverticulum, Schatzki's ring, stricture, neoplasm

- Odynophagia, or painful swallowing

    Radiation; caustic ingestion, infection from *cytomegalovirus*, herpes simplex, HIV

- Diarrhea, acute (<2 weeks) and chronic

    Acute infection (viral, salmonella, shigella, etc.); chronic in *Crohn's disease*, ulcerative colitis; oily diarrhea *(steatorrhea)*—in pancreatic insufficiency. See Table 11-1, Diarrhea, pp. 194–195.

- Constipation

    Medications, especially anticholinergic agents and opioids; *colon cancer*

- Melena, or black tarry stools

    GI bleed

- Jaundice from increased levels of bilirubin: Intrahepatic jaundice can be *hepatocellular,* from damage to the hepatocytes, or *cholestatic,* from impaired excretion caused by damaged hepatocytes or intrahepatic bile ducts

    Impaired excretion of conjugated bilirubin in *viral hepatitis, cirrhosis, primary biliary cirrhosis,* drug-induced cholestasis

Extrahepatic jaundice arises from obstructed extrahepatic bile ducts, commonly the cystic and common bile ducts

| Ask about the color of *the urine and stool*. | Dark urine from increased conjugated bilirubin excreted in urine; acholic clay-colored stool when excretion of bilirubin into intestine is obstructed |

Risk Factors for Liver Disease

- *Hepatitis A:* Travel or meals in areas with poor sanitation, ingestion of contaminated water or foodstuffs
- *Hepatitis B:* Parenteral or mucous membrane exposure to infectious body fluids such as blood, serum, semen, and saliva, especially through sexual contact with an infected partner or use of shared needles for injection drug use
- *Hepatitis C:* Illicit intravenous drug use or blood transfusion
- *Alcoholic hepatitis* or *alcoholic cirrhosis:* Interview the patient carefully about alcohol use
- *Toxic liver damage* from medications, industrial solvents, environmental toxins or some anesthetic agents
- *Extrahepatic biliary obstruction* that may result from gallbladder disease or surgery
- *Hereditary disorders* reported in the Family History

THE URINARY TRACT

| Ask about *pain on urination*, usually a burning sensation, sometimes termed *dysuria* (also refers to difficulty voiding). | Bladder infection

Also, consider bladder stones, foreign bodies, tumors, and *acute prostatitis.* In women, internal burning in *urethritis,* external burning in *vulvovaginitis* |

Other associated symptoms include:

| • *Urgency,* an unusually intense and immediate desire to void | May lead to urge incontinence |

- *Urinary frequency,* or abnormally frequent voiding

- Fever or chills; blood in the urine

| • Any pain in the abdomen, flank, or back | Dull, steady pain in *pyelonephritis;* severe colicky pain in ureteral obstruction from renal stone |

In men, *hesitancy* in starting the urine stream, *straining to void, reduced caliber and force of the urine stream,* or *dribbling* as they complete voiding.

Prostatitis, urethritis

Assess any:

- *Polyuria,* a significant increase in 24-hour urine volume

  Diabetes mellitus, diabetes insipidus

- *Nocturia,* urinary frequency at night

  Bladder obstruction

- *Urinary incontinence,* involuntary loss of urine:

  See Table 11-2, Urinary Incontinence, pp. 196–197.

  - From coughing, sneezing, lifting

    Stress incontinence (poor urethral sphincter tone)

  - From urge to void

    Urge incontinence (detrusor overactivity)

  - From bladder fullness with leaking but incomplete emptying

    Overflow incontinence (anatomic obstruction, impaired neural innervation to bladder)

Health Promotion and Counseling: Evidence and Recommendations

Important Topics for Health Promotion and Counseling

- Screening for alcohol abuse
- Risk factors for hepatitis A, B, and C
- Screening for colon cancer

Alcohol Abuse. Assessing *use of alcohol* is an important clinician responsibility. Focus on detection, counseling, and, for significant impairment, specific treatment recommendations. Use the four CAGE questions to screen for alcohol dependence or abuse in all adolescents and adults, including pregnant women (see Chapter 3, p. 46). Brief counseling interventions have been shown to reduce alcohol consumption by 13% to 34% over 6 to 12 months.

Hepatitis. Protective measures against *infectious hepatitis* include counseling about transmission:

- *Hepatitis A:* Transmission is fecal–oral. Illness occurs approximately 30 days after exposure. Hepatitis A vaccine is recommended for children after age 1 and groups at risk: travelers to endemic areas; food handlers; military personnel; caretakers of children; Native Americans and Alaska Natives; selected health care, sanitation, and laboratory workers; homosexual men; and injection drug users.

- *Hepatitis B:* Transmission occurs during contact with infected body fluids, such as blood, semen, saliva, and vaginal secretions. Infection increases risk of fulminant hepatitis, chronic infection, and subsequent cirrhosis and hepatocellular carcinoma. Provide counseling and serologic screening for patients at risk. Hepatitis B vaccine is recommended for infants at birth and groups at risk: all young adults not previously immunized, injection drug users and their sexual partners, people at risk for sexually transmitted infections, travelers to endemic areas, recipients of blood products as in hemodialysis, and health care workers with frequent exposure to blood products. Many of these groups also should be screened for HIV infection, especially pregnant women at their first prenatal visit.

- *Hepatitis C:* Hepatitis C, now the most common form, is spread by blood exposure and is associated with injection drug use. No vaccine is available.

Colorectal Cancer. The U.S. Preventive Services Task Force made the recommendations below in 2008.

Screening for Colorectal Cancer

Assess Risk: Begin screening at age 20 years. If high risk, refer for more complex management. If average risk at age 50 (high-risk conditions absent), offer the screening options listed.

- **Common high-risk conditions** (25% of colorectal cancers)
  - Personal history of colorectal cancer or adenoma
  - First-degree relative with colorectal cancer or adenomatous polyps
  - Personal history of breast, ovarian, or endometrial cancer
  - Personal history of ulcerative or Crohn's colitis

(continued)

> **Screening for Colorectal Cancer** (continued)
>
> - **Hereditary high-risk conditions** (6% of colorectal cancers)
>   - Familial adenomatous polyposis
>   - Hereditary nonpolyposis colorectal cancer
> - **Screening recommendations—U.S. Preventive Services Task Force 2008**
> - **Adults age 50 to 75 years**—options
>   - High-sensitivity fecal occult blood testing (FOBT) annually
>   - Sigmoidoscopy every 5 years with FOBT every 3 years
>   - Screening colonoscopy every 10 years
> - **Adults age 76 to 85 years**—do not screen routinely, as gain in life-years is small compared to colonoscopy risks, and screening benefits not seen for 7 years; use individual decision making if screening for the first time
> - **Adults older than age 85**—do not screen, as "competing causes of mortality preclude a mortality benefit that outweighs harms"

Detection rates for colorectal cancer and insertion depths of colonoscopy are roughly as follows: 25% to 30% at 20 cm; 50% to 55% at 35 cm; 40% to 65% at 40 cm to 50 cm. Full colonoscopy or air contrast barium enema detects 80% to 95% of colorectal cancers.

Techniques of Examination

EXAMINATION TECHNIQUES	POSSIBLE FINDINGS

THE ABDOMEN

○—— Inspect the abdomen, including:

- Skin

  Scars, striae, veins, ecchymoses (in intra- or retroperitoneal hemorrhages)

- Umbilicus

  Hernia, inflammation

- Contours for shape, symmetry, enlarged organs or masses

  Bulging flanks of ascites, suprapubic bulge, large liver or spleen, tumors

- Any peristaltic waves

  Increase in GI obstruction

- Any pulsations

  Increased in aortic aneurysm

Chapter 11 | The Abdomen

EXAMINATION TECHNIQUES	POSSIBLE FINDINGS
Auscultate the abdomen for:	
• Bowel sounds	Increased or decreased motility
• Bruits	Bruit of renal artery stenosis
• Friction rubs	Liver tumor, splenic infarct

Bowel Sounds and Bruits

Change	Seen With
Increased bowel sounds	Diarrhea
	Early intestinal obstruction
Decreased, then absent bowel sounds	Adynamic ileus
	Peritonitis
High-pitched tinkling bowel sounds	Intestinal fluid
	Air under tension in a dilated bowel
High-pitched rushing bowel sounds with cramping	Intestinal obstruction
Hepatic bruit	Carcinoma of the liver
	Alcoholic hepatitis
Arterial bruits	Partial obstruction of the aorta or renal, iliac or femoral arteries

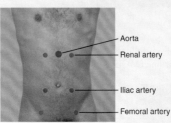

Percuss the abdomen for patterns of tympany and dullness.	Ascites, GI obstruction, pregnant uterus, ovarian tumor
Palpate all quadrants of the abdomen:	See Table 11-3, Abdominal Tenderness, p. 197.

| EXAMINATION TECHNIQUES | POSSIBLE FINDINGS |

- Lightly for guarding, rebound, and tenderness

"Acute abdomen" or peritonitis if:

- *Firm, boardlike abdominal wall*—suggests peritoneal inflammation.

- *Guarding* if the patient flinches, grimaces, or reports pain during palpation.

- *Rebound tenderness* from peritoneal inflammation; pain is greater when you withdraw your hand than when you press down. Press slowly on a tender area, then quickly "let go."

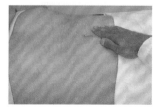

- Deeply for masses or tenderness

Tumors, a distended viscus

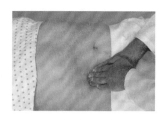

THE LIVER

Percuss span of liver dullness in the midclavicular line (MCL).

Hepatomegaly

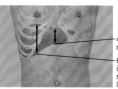

4–8 cm in midsternal line
6–12 cm in right midclavicular line
} Normal liver spans

Feel the liver edge, if possible, as patient breathes in.

Firm edge of cirrhosis

| EXAMINATION TECHNIQUES | POSSIBLE FINDINGS |

Measure its distance from the costal margin in the MCL.

Increased in hepatomegaly—may be missed (as below) by starting palpation too high in the RUQ

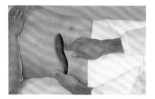

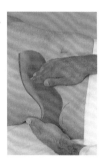

Note any tenderness or masses.

Tender liver of hepatitis or heart failure; tumor mass

THE SPLEEN

Percuss across left lower anterior chest, noting change from tympany to dullness.

Try to feel spleen with the patient:

Splenomegaly

- Supine

- Lying on the right side with legs flexed at hips and knees

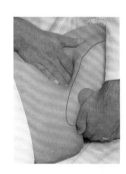

| EXAMINATION TECHNIQUES | POSSIBLE FINDINGS |

THE KIDNEYS

○— Try to palpate each kidney.

Enlargement from cysts, cancer, hydronephrosis

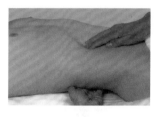

Check for costovertebral angle (CVA) tenderness.

Tender in *pyelonephritis*

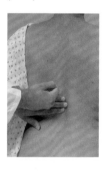

THE AORTA

○— Palpate the aorta's pulsations. In older people, estimate its width.

Periumbilical mass with expansile pulsations ≥3 cm in diameter in *abdominal aortic aneurysm*. Assess further due to risk of rupture.

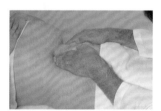

Chapter 11 | The Abdomen

EXAMINATION TECHNIQUES	POSSIBLE FINDINGS

ASSESSING ASCITES

○—/○— Palpate for shifting dullness. Map areas of tympany and dullness with patient supine, then lying on side (see below).

Ascitic fluid usually shifts to dependent side, changing the margin of dullness (see below)

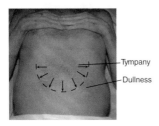

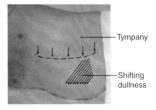

○— Check for a fluid wave. Ask patient or an assistant to press edges of both hands into midline of abdomen. Tap one side and feel for a wave transmitted to the other side.

A palpable wave suggests but does not prove ascites.

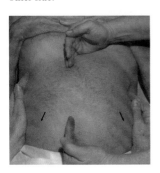

EXAMINATION TECHNIQUES	POSSIBLE FINDINGS
○— Ballotte an organ or mass in an ascitic abdomen. Place your stiffened and straightened fingers on the abdomen, briefly jab them toward the structure, and try to touch its surface.	Your hand, quickly displacing the fluid, stops abruptly as it touches the solid surface.

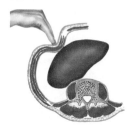

ASSESSING POSSIBLE APPENDICITIS

Ask:	In *classic appendicitis*:
"Where did the pain begin?"	Near the umbilicus
"Where is it now?"	Right lower quadrant (RLQ)
Ask patient to cough. "Where does it hurt?"	RLQ at "McBurney's point"
Palpate for local tenderness.	RLQ tenderness
Palpate for muscular rigidity.	RLQ rigidity
Perform a rectal examination and, in women, a pelvic examination (see Chapters 14 and 15).	Local tenderness, especially if appendix is retrocecal
• *Rovsing's sign:* Press deeply and evenly in the *left* lower quadrant. Then quickly withdraw your fingers.	Pain in the *right* lower quadrant during *left*-sided pressure suggests appendicitis (a *positive* Rovsing's sign).
• *Psoas sign:* Place your hand just above the patient's right knee. Ask the patient to raise that thigh against your hand. Or, ask the patient to turn onto the left side. Then extend the patient's right leg at the hip to stretch the psoas muscle.	Pain from irritation of the psoas muscle suggests an inflamed appendix (a *positive* psoas sign).

EXAMINATION TECHNIQUES

| | POSSIBLE FINDINGS |

- *Obturator sign:* Flex the patient's right thigh at the hip, with the knee bent, and rotate the leg internally at the hip, which stretches the internal obturator muscle.

Right hypogastric pain in a *positive* obturator sign, suggesting irritation of the obturator muscle by an inflamed appendix.

ASSESSING POSSIBLE ACUTE CHOLECYSTITIS

Auscultate, percuss, and palpate the abdomen for tenderness.

Bowel sounds may be active or decreased; tympany may increase with an ileus: Assess any RUQ tenderness.

Assess for *Murphy's sign.* Hook your thumb under the right costal margin at edge of rectus muscle, and ask patient to take a deep breath.

Sharp tenderness and a sudden stop in inspiratory effort constitute a *positive* Murphy's sign.

Recording Your Findings

Recording the Physical Examination—The Abdomen

"Abdomen is protuberant with active bowel sounds. It is soft and nontender; no palpable masses or hepatosplenomegaly. Liver span is 7 cm and in the right MCL; edge is smooth and palpable 1 cm below the right costal margin. Spleen and kidneys not felt. No CVA tenderness."
OR
"Abdomen is flat. No bowel sounds heard. It is firm and boardlike, with increased tenderness, guarding, and rebound in the right midquadrant. Liver percusses to 7 cm in the MCL; edge not felt. Spleen and kidneys not felt. No palpable mass. No CVA tenderness." *(Suggests peritonitis from possible appendicitis; see pp. 192–193.)*

Aids to Interpretation

Table 11-1 Diarrhea

Problem/Process	Characteristics of Stool
Acute Diarrhea	
Secretory Infections (noninflammatory)	
Infection by viruses; preformed bacterial toxins such as *Staphylococcus aureus, Clostridium perfringens,* toxigenic *Escherichia coli; Vibrio cholerae, Cryptosporidium, Giardia lamblia*	Watery, without blood, pus, or mucus
Inflammatory Infections	
Colonization or invasion of intestinal mucosa as in nontyphoid *Salmonella, Shigella, Yersinia, Campylobacter,* enteropathic *E. coli, Entamoeba histolytica*	Loose to watery, often with blood, pus, or mucus
Drug-Induced Diarrhea	
Action of many drugs, such as magnesium-containing antacids, antibiotics, antineoplastic agents, and laxatives	Loose to watery
Chronic Diarrhea (≥30 days)	
Diarrheal Syndromes	
• *Irritable bowel syndrome:* A disorder of bowel motility with alternating diarrhea and constipation	Loose; may show mucus but no blood. Small, hard stools with constipation
• *Cancer of the sigmoid colon:* Partial obstruction by a malignant neoplasm	May be blood-streaked

Table 11-1 Diarrhea (continued)

Problem/Process	Characteristics of Stool
Inflammatory Bowel Disease	
• *Ulcerative colitis:* inflammation and ulceration of the mucosa and submucosa of the rectum and colon	Soft to watery, often containing blood
• *Crohn's disease* of the small bowel (regional enteritis) or colon (granulomatous colitis): chronic inflammation of the bowel wall, typically involving the terminal ileum, proximal colon, or both	Small, soft to loose or watery, usually free of gross blood (enteritis) or with less bleeding than ulcerative colitis (colitis)
Voluminous Diarrheas	
• *Malabsorption syndrome:* Defective absorption of fat, including fat-soluble vitamins, with steatorrhea (excessive excretion of fat) as in pancreatic insufficiency, bile salt deficiency, bacterial overgrowth	Typically bulky, soft, light yellow to gray, mushy, greasy or oily, and sometimes frothy; particularly foul-smelling; usually floats in the toilet
• *Osmotic diarrheas*	
• Lactose intolerance: Deficiency in intestinal lactase	Watery diarrhea of large volume
• Abuse of osmotic purgatives: Laxative habit, often surreptitious	Watery diarrhea of large volume
• *Secretory diarrheas* from bacterial infection, secreting villous adenoma, fat or bile salt malabsorption, hormone-mediated conditions (gastrin in Zollinger–Ellison syndrome, vasoactive intestinal peptide): Process is variable.	Watery diarrhea of large volume

Table 11-2	Urinary Incontinence
Problem	**Mechanisms**
Stress Incontinence: Urethral sphincter weakened. Transient increases in intra-abdominal pressure raise bladder pressure to levels exceeding urethral resistance. Leads to voiding *small amounts* during laughing, coughing, and sneezing.	• In women, weakness of the pelvic floor with inadequate muscular support of the bladder and proximal urethra and a change in the angle between the bladder and the urethra from childbirth, surgery, and local conditions affecting the internal urethral sphincter, such as postmenopausal atrophy of the mucosa and urethral infection • In men, prostatic surgery
Urge Incontinence: Detrusor contractions are stronger than normal and overcome normal urethral resistance. Bladder is typically small. Results in voiding *moderate amounts,* urgency, frequency, and nocturia.	• Decreased cortical inhibition of detrusor contractions, as in stroke, brain tumor, dementia, and lesions of the spinal cord above the sacral level • Hyperexcitability of sensory pathways, as in bladder infection, tumor, and fecal impaction • Deconditioning of voiding reflexes, caused by frequent voluntary voiding at low bladder volumes
Overflow Incontinence: Detrusor contractions are insufficient to overcome urethral resistance. Bladder is typically large, even after an effort to void, leading to *continuous dribbling.*	• Obstruction of the bladder outlet, as by benign prostatic hyperplasia or tumor • Weakness of detrusor muscle associated with peripheral nerve disease at the sacral level • Impaired bladder sensation that interrupts the reflex arc, as in diabetic neuropathy

Table 11-2 Urinary Incontinence (continued)

Problem	Mechanisms
Functional Incontinence: Inability to get to the toilet in time because of impaired health or environmental conditions	• Problems in mobility from weakness, arthritis, poor vision, other conditions; environmental factors such as unfamiliar setting, distant bathroom facilities, bed rails, physical restraints
Incontinence Secondary to Medications: Drugs may contribute to any type of incontinence listed.	• Sedatives, tranquilizers, anticholinergics, sympathetic blockers, potent diuretics

Table 11-3 Abdominal Tenderness

Visceral Tenderness

Peritoneal Tenderness

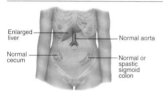
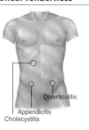

Tenderness From Disease in the Chest and Pelvis

Acute Pleurisy

Acute Salpingitis

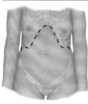

Unilateral or bilateral, upper or lower abdomen

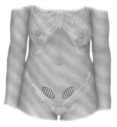

CHAPTER 12

The Peripheral Vascular System

The Health History

Common or Concerning Symptoms

- Abdominal, flank, or back pain
- Pain in the arms or legs
- Intermittent claudication
- Cold, numbness, pallor in the legs; hair loss
- Color change in fingertips or toes in cold weather
- Swelling in calves, legs, or feet
- Swelling with redness or tenderness

Ask about abdominal, flank, or back pain, especially in older male smokers.

An expanding abdominal aortic aneurysm (AAA) may compress arteries or ureters.

Ask about any *pain in the arms and legs*.

Is there *intermittent claudication*, exercise-induced pain that is absent at rest, makes the patient stop exertion, and abates within about 10 minutes? Ask "Have you ever had any pain or cramping in your legs when you walk or exercise?" "How far can you walk without stopping to rest?" and "Does pain improve with rest?"

Peripheral arterial disease (PAD) can cause symptomatic limb ischemia with exertion; distinguish this from *spinal stenosis*, which produces leg pain with exertion often reduced by leaning forward (stretching the spinal cord in the narrowed vertebral canal) and less readily relieved by rest.

Ask also about *coldness, numbness*, or *pallor* in legs or feet or *hair loss* over the anterior tibial surfaces.

Hair loss over the anterior tibiae in PAD. "Dry" or brown–black ulcers from gangrene may ensue.

199

Because patients have few symptoms, identify risk factors—tobacco abuse, hypertension, diabetes, hyperlipidemia, and history of myocardial infarction or stroke.	Only approximately 10% to 30% of affected patients have the classic symptoms of exertional calf pain relieved by rest.
"Do your fingertips or toes ever change color in cold weather or when you handle cold objects?"	Digital ischemic changes from arterial spasm cause blanching, followed by cyanosis and then rubor with cold exposure and rewarming in *Raynaud's phenomenon* or *disease*
Ask about *swelling of feet and legs,* or any ulcers on lower legs, often near the ankles from peripheral vascular disease.	Calf swelling in deep venous thrombosis; hyperpigmentation, edema, and possible cyanosis, especially when legs are dependent, in *venous stasis ulcers;* swelling with redness and tenderness in *cellulitis*

Health Promotion and Counseling: Evidence and Recommendations

Important Topics for Health Promotion and Counseling

- Screening for peripheral arterial disease (PAD); the ankle–brachial index
- Screening for renal artery disease
- Screening for abdominal aortic aneurysm

Screening for Peripheral Arterial Disease (PAD). PAD involves the femoral and popliteal arteries most commonly, followed by the tibial and peroneal arteries. PAD affects from 12% to 29% of community populations; despite significant association with cardiovascular and cerebrovascular disease, PAD often is underdiagnosed in office practices. Most patients with PAD have either no symptoms or a range of *nonspecific leg symptoms,* such as *aching, cramping, numbness,* or *fatigue.*

Screen patients for PAD risk factors, such as tobacco abuse, elevated cholesterol, diabetes, age older than 70 years, hypertension, or atherosclerotic coronary, carotid, or renal artery disease. Pursue aggressive risk factor intervention. Consider use of the ankle–brachial index (ABI), a highly accurate test for detecting stenoses of 50% or more in major vessels of the legs (see pp. 209–210).

A wide range of interventions reduces both onset and progression of PAD, including meticulous foot care and well-fitting shoes, tobacco cessation, treatment of hyperlipidemia, optimal control and treatment of diabetes and hypertension, use of antiplatelet agents, graded exercise, and surgical revascularization. Patients with ABIs in the lowest category have a 20% to 25% annual risk of death.

Screening for Renal Artery Disease. The American College of Cardiology and the American Heart Association recommend diagnostic studies for renal artery disease, usually beginning with ultrasound, in patients with hypertension before age 30 years; severe hypertension (see p. 56) after age 55 years; accelerated, resistant, or malignant hypertension; new worsening of renal function or worsening after use of an angiotensin-converting enzyme inhibitor or an angiotensin-receptor blocking agent; an unexplained small kidney; or sudden unexplained pulmonary edema, especially in the setting of worsening renal function. Symptoms arise from these conditions rather than directly from atherosclerotic changes in the renal artery.

Screening for Abdominal Aortic Aneurysm (AAA). An AAA is present when the infrarenal aortic diameter exceeds 3.0 cm. Rupture and mortality rates dramatically increase for AAAs exceeding 5.5 cm in diameter. The strongest risk factor for rupture is excess aortic diameter. Additional risk factors are smoking, age older than 65 years, family history, coronary artery disease, PAD, hypertension, and elevated cholesterol level. Because symptoms are rare, and screening is now shown to reduce mortality by approximately 40%, the U.S. Preventive Services Task Force recommends one-time screening by ultrasound in men between 65 and 75 years of age with a history of "ever smoking," defined as more than 100 cigarettes in a lifetime.

Techniques of Examination

| EXAMINATION TECHNIQUES | POSSIBLE FINDINGS |

ARMS

Inspect for:

- Size and symmetry, any swelling — Lymphedema, venous obstruction

- Venous pattern — Venous obstruction

- Color and texture of skin and nails — *Raynaud's disease*

Palpate and grade the pulses:

Grading Arterial Pulses

3+	Bounding
2+	Brisk, expected (normal)
1+	Diminished, weaker than expected
0	Absent, unable to palpate

- Radial

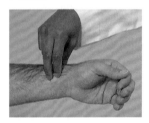

Bounding radial, carotid, and femoral pulses in *aortic regurgitation*

Lost in *thromboangiitis obliterans* or *acute arterial occlusion*

- Brachial

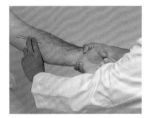

EXAMINATION TECHNIQUES	POSSIBLE FINDINGS
Feel for the epitrochlear nodes.	Lymphadenopathy from local cut, infection

ABDOMEN

Palpate and estimate the width of the abdominal aorta between your two fingers. (See p. 190)	Pulsatile mass, AAA if width ≥4 cm.

LEGS

Inspect for:	See Table 12-1, Chronic Insufficiency of Arteries and Veins, p. 207, and Table 12-2, Common Ulcers of the Feet and Ankles, p. 208.
• Size and symmetry, any swelling in thigh or calf	Venous insufficiency, lymphedema; deep venous thrombosis
• Venous pattern	Varicose veins
• Color and texture of skin	Pallor, rubor, cyanosis; erythema, warmth in *cellulitis, thrombophlebitis*
• Hair distribution, temperature	Loss hair and coldness in arterial insufficiency
Palpate the inguinal lymph nodes:	Lymphadenopathy in genital infections, lymphoma, AIDs
• Horizontal group	
• Vertical group	

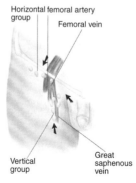

| EXAMINATION TECHNIQUES | POSSIBLE FINDINGS |

Palpate and grade the pulses:

Loss of pulses in acute arterial occlusion and arteriosclerosis obliterans

- Femoral

- Popliteal

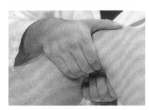

- Dorsalis pedis

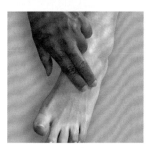

- Posterior tibial

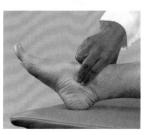

See Table 12-3, Using the Ankle-Brachial Index, p. 209–210.

Check for pitting edema.

Dependent edema, heart failure, hypoalbuminemia, nephrotic syndrome

Palpate the calves.

Tenderness in deep venous thrombosis (though tenderness often not present)

Ask patient to stand, and reinspect the venous pattern.

Varicose veins

| EXAMINATION TECHNIQUES | POSSIBLE FINDINGS |

SPECIAL TECHNIQUES

EVALUATING ARTERIAL SUPPLY TO THE HAND

Feel ulnar pulse, if possible. Perform an **Allen test**.

Persisting pallor of palm indicates occlusion of the released artery or its distal branches.

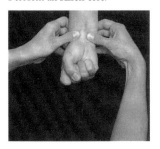

1. Ask the patient to make a tight fist, palm up. Occlude both radial and ulnar arteries with your thumb.

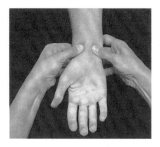

2. Ask the patient to open hand into a relaxed, slightly flexed position.

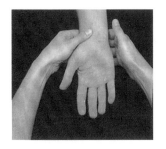

3. Release your pressure over one artery. Palm should flush within 3 to 5 seconds.

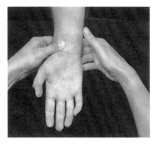

4. Repeat, releasing other artery.

EXAMINATION TECHNIQUES

POSTURAL COLOR CHANGES OF CHRONIC ARTERIAL INSUFFICIENCY

Raise both legs to 60 degrees for about 1 minute. Then ask patient to sit up with legs dangling down. Note time required for (1) return of pinkness (normally 10 seconds) and (2) filling of veins on feet and ankles (normally about 15 seconds).

POSSIBLE FINDINGS

Marked pallor of feet on elevation, delayed color return and venous filling, and rubor of dependent feet suggest arterial insufficiency.

Recording Your Findings

Recording the Physical Examination—The Peripheral Vascular System

"Extremities are warm and without edema. No varicosities or stasis changes. Calves are supple and nontender. No femoral or abdominal bruits. Brachial, radial, femoral, popliteal, dorsalis pedis (DP), and posterior tibial (PT) pulses are 2+ and symmetric."

OR

"Extremities are pale below the midcalf, with notable hair loss. Rubor noted when legs dependent but no edema or ulceration. Bilateral femoral bruits; no abdominal bruits heard. Brachial and radial pulses 2+; femoral, popliteal, DP, and PT pulses 1+." (Alternatively, pulses can be recorded as below.) *Suggests atherosclerotic PAD.*

	Radial	Brachial	Femoral	Popliteal	Dorsalis Pedis	Posterior Tibial
RT	2+	2+	1+	1+	1+	1+
LT	2+	2+	1+	1+	1+	1+

Aids to Interpretation

Table 12-1 Chronic Insufficiency of Arteries and Veins

Condition	Characteristics
Chronic Arterial Insufficiency 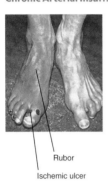 Rubor / Ischemic ulcer	Intermittent claudication progressing to pain at rest. Decreased or absent pulses. Pale, especially on elevation; dusky red on dependency. Cool. Absent or mild edema, which may develop on lowering the leg to relieve pain. Thin, shiny, atrophic skin; hair loss over foot and toes; thickened, ridged nails. Possible ulceration on toes or points of trauma on feet. Potential gangrene.
Chronic Venous Insufficiency 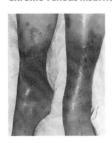	No pain to aching pain on dependency. Normal pulses, though may be hard to feel because of edema. Color normal or cyanotic on dependency; petechiae or brown pigment may develop. Often marked edema. Stasis dermatitis, possible thickening of skin, and narrowing of leg as scarring develops. Potential ulceration at sides of ankles. No gangrene.

Table 12-2 Common Ulcers of the Feet and Ankles

Ulcer	Characteristics
Arterial Insufficiency 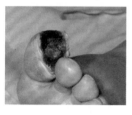	Located on toes, feet, or possible areas of trauma. No callus or excess pigment. May be atrophic. Pain often severe, unless masked by neuropathy. Possible gangrene. Decreased pulses, trophic changes, pallor of foot on elevation, dusky rubor on dependency.
Chronic Venous Insufficiency 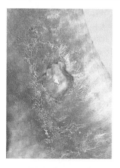	Located on inner or outer ankle. Pigmented, sometimes fibrotic. Pain not severe. No gangrene. Edema, pigmentation, stasis dermatitis, and possibly cyanosis of feet on dependency.
Neuropathic Ulcer 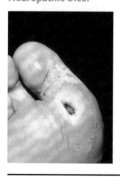	Located on pressure points in areas with diminished sensation, as in diabetic neuropathy. Skin calloused. No pain (which may cause ulcer to go unnoticed). Usually no gangrene. Decreased sensation, absent ankle jerks.

Table 12-3 Using the Ankle–Brachial Index

Instructions for Measuring the Ankle–Brachial Index (ABI)

1. Patient should rest supine in a warm room for at least 10 minutes before testing.

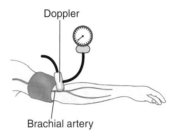

2. Place blood pressure cuffs on both arms and ankles as illustrated, then apply ultrasound gel over brachial, dorsalis pedis, and posterior tibial arteries.
3. Measure systolic pressures in the arms
   - Use vascular Doppler to locate brachial pulse
   - Inflate cuff 20 mm Hg above last audible pulse
   - Deflate cuff slowly and record pressure at which pulse becomes audible
   - Obtain 2 measures in each arm and record the average as the brachial pressure in that arm

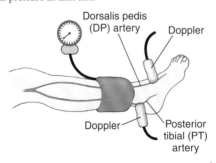

(continued)

Table 12-3 Using the Ankle–Brachial Index (continued)

4. Measure systolic pressures in ankles
   - Use vascular Doppler to locate dorsalis pedis pulse
   - Inflate cuff 20 mm Hg above last audible pulse
   - Deflate cuff slowly and record pressure at which pulse becomes audible
   - Obtain 2 measures in each ankle and record the average as the dorsalis pedis pressure in that leg
   - Repeat above steps for posterior tibial arteries
5. Calculate ABI

$$\text{Right ABI} = \frac{\text{highest right average ankle pressure (DP or PT)}}{\text{highest average arm pressure (right or left)}}$$

$$\text{Left ABI} = \frac{\text{highest left average ankle pressure (DP or PT)}}{\text{highest average arm pressure (right or left)}}$$

Interpretation of Ankle–Brachial Index

Ankle–Brachial Index Result	Clinical Interpretation
>0.90 (with a range of 0.90 to 1.30)	Normal lower extremity blood flow
<0.89 to >0.60	Mild PAD
<0.59 to >0.40	Moderate PAD
<0.39	Severe PAD

Source: Wilson JF, Laine C, Goldman D. In the clinic: peripheral arterial disease. Ann Int Med 2007;146(5):ITC3-1.

CHAPTER 13

Male Genitalia and Hernias

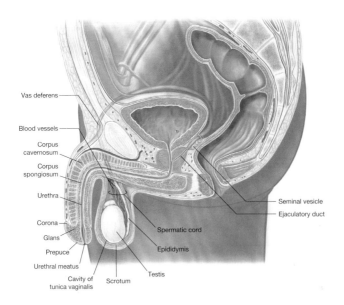

The Health History

Common or Concerning Symptoms

- Sexual orientation and sexual response
- Penile discharge or lesions
- Scrotal pain, swelling, or lesions
- Sexually transmitted infections (STIs)

Explain your concern for the patient's sexual health. Pose questions in a neutral and nonjudgmental way.

- "What is your relationship status? Tell me about your sexual preference."

- "How is sexual function for you?" "Are you satisfied with your sexual life?" "What about your ability to perform sexually?"

To assess *libido*, or desire: "Have you maintained an interest in sex?"

Decreased libido from depression, endocrine dysfunction, or side effects of medications

For the *arousal* phase: "Can you achieve and maintain an erection?"

Erectile dysfunction from psychogenic causes, especially if early morning erection is preserved; also from decreased testosterone, decreased blood flow in hypogastric arterial system, impaired neural innervation, diabetes

If *ejaculation* is premature or early: "About how long does intercourse last?" "Do you climax too soon?" For reduced or absent ejaculation: "Do you find that you cannot have orgasm even though you can have an erection?" "Does the problem involve the pleasurable sensation of *orgasm*, the ejaculation of seminal fluid, or both?"

Premature ejaculation is common, especially in young men. Less common is reduced or absent ejaculation affecting middle-aged or older men. Consider medications, surgery, neurologic deficits, or lack of androgen. Lack of orgasm with intact ejaculation is usually psychogenic.

To assess possible infection from sexually transmitted infections (STIs), ask about any *discharge from the penis.*

Penile discharge in *gonococcal* (usually yellow) and *nongonococcal* (clear or white) *urethritis*

Inquire about *sores or growths on the penis* and any *pain or swelling in the scrotum.*

See Table 13-1, Abnormalities of the Penis and Scrotum, p. 218, and Table 13-2, Sexually Transmitted Infections of Male Genitalia, pp. 219–220.

STIs may involve other parts of the body. Ask about practices of oral and anal sex and any related sore throat, oral itching or pain, diarrhea, or rectal bleeding.

Rash in disseminated gonococcal infection

Health Promotion and Counseling: Evidence and Recommendations

Important Topics for Health Promotion and Counseling

- Prevention of STIs and HIV
- Screening for testicular cancer; testicular self-examination

Prevention of STIs and HIV Infection. Focus on patient education about STIs and HIV, early detection of infection during history taking and physical examination, and identification and treatment of infected partners. Identify the patient's sexual orientation, the number of sexual partners in the past month, and any history of STIs. Also query use of alcohol and drugs, particularly injection drugs. Counsel patients at risk about limiting the number of partners, using condoms, and establishing regular medical care for treatment of STIs and HIV infection.

Counseling and testing for HIV are recommended for: all people at increased risk for infection with HIV, STIs, or both; men with male partners; past or present injection drug users; men and women having unprotected sex with multiple partners; sex workers; any past or present partners of people with HIV infection, bisexual practices, or injection drug use; and patients with a history of transfusion between 1978 and 1985.

Testicular Self-Examination. Encourage men, especially those between 15 and 35 years of age, to perform monthly testicular self-examinations. Testicular cancer strikes men ages 15 to 34, especially those with a positive family history or cyptorchidism (see p. 221).

Techniques of Examination

EXAMINATION TECHNIQUES	POSSIBLE FINDINGS

MALE GENITALIA

Wear gloves. The patient may be standing or supine.

THE PENIS

Inspect the:

- Development of the penis and the skin and hair at its base

  Sexual maturation, lice

- Prepuce

  Phimosis

- Glans

  Balanitis, chancre, herpes, warts, cancer

- Urethral meatus

  Hypospadias, discharge of *urethritis*

Palpate:

- Any visible lesions

  Chancre, cancer

- The shaft

  Urethral stricture or cancer

| EXAMINATION TECHNIQUES | POSSIBLE FINDINGS |

THE SCROTUM AND ITS CONTENTS

Inspect:

- Contours of scrotum — Hernia, *hydrocele*, *cryptorchidism*

- Skin of scrotum — Rashes

Palpate each:

- Testis, noting any: — See Table 13-3, Abnormalities of the Testis, p. 221.

  - Lumps — Testicular carcinoma

  - Tenderness — Orchitis, torsion of the spermatic cord, strangulated inguinal hernia

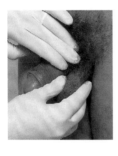

- Epididymis — Epididymitis, cyst

- Spermatic cord and adjacent areas — Varicocele if multiple tortuous veins; cystic structure may be a hydrocele

See Table 13-4, Abnormalities of the Epididymis and Spermatic Cord, p. 222.

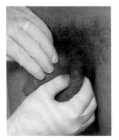

| EXAMINATION TECHNIQUES | POSSIBLE FINDINGS |

HERNIAS

Patient is usually standing.

See Table 13-5, Hernias in the Groin, p. 223.

Inspect inguinal and femoral areas as patient strains down.

Inguinal and femoral hernias

Palpate external inguinal ring through scrotal skin and ask patient to strain down.

Indirect and direct inguinal hernias

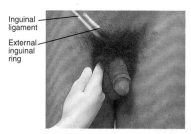

SPECIAL TECHNIQUE

Patient Instructions for the Testicular Self-Examination

This examination is best performed after a warm bath or shower. The heat relaxes the scrotum and makes it easier to find anything unusual.

- Standing in front of a mirror, check for any swelling on the skin of the scrotum.
- With the penis out of the way, examine each testicle separately.
- Cup the testicle between your thumbs and forefingers with both hands and roll it gently between the thumbs and fingers. One testicle may be larger than the other; that's normal, but be concerned about any lump or area of pain.

(continued)

EXAMINATION TECHNIQUES

Patient Instructions for the Testicular Self-Examination (continued)

- Find the epididymis. This is a soft, tubelike structure at the back of the testicle that collects and carries sperm, not an abnormal lump.

- If you find any lump, don't wait. See your doctor. The lump may just be an infection, but if it is cancer, it will spread unless stopped by treatment.

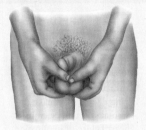

Source: Medline Plus. U.S. National Library of Medicine and National Institutes of Health. Medical Encyclopedia—Testicular self-examination. Available at www.nlm.nih.gov/medlineplus/ency/article/003909.htm. Accessed December 19, 2010.

Recording Your Findings

Recording the Physical Examination—Male Genitalia and Hernias

"Circumcised male. No penile discharge or lesions. No scrotal swelling or discoloration. Testes descended bilaterally, smooth, without masses. Epididymis nontender. No inguinal or femoral hernias."

OR

"Uncircumcised male; prepuce easily retractible. No penile discharge or lesions. No scrotal swelling or discoloration. Testes descended bilaterally; right testicle smooth; 1 × 1 cm firm nodule on left lateral testicle. It is fixed and nontender. Epididymis nontender. No inguinal or femoral hernias." (*Suspicious for testicular carcinoma, the most common form of cancer in men between 15 and 35 years of age.*)

Aids to Interpretation

Table 13-1   Abnormalities of the Penis and Scrotum

Hypospadias
A congenital displacement of the urethral meatus to the inferior surface of the penis. A groove extends from the actual urethral meatus to its normal location on the tip of the glans.

Scrotal Edema
Pitting edema may make the scrotal skin taut; seen in heart failure or nephrotic syndrome.

Peyronie's Disease
Palpable, nontender, hard plaques are found just beneath the skin, usually along the dorsum of the penis. The patient complains of crooked, painful erections.

Fingers can get above mass

Hydrocele
A nontender, fluid-filled mass within the tunica vaginalis. It transilluminates, and the examining fingers can get above the mass within the scrotum.

Carcinoma of the Penis
An indurated nodule or ulcer that is usually nontender. Limited almost completely to men who are not circumcised, it may be masked by the prepuce. Any persistent penile sore is suspicious.

Fingers cannot get above mass

Scrotal Hernia
Usually an *indirect inguinal hernia* that comes through the external inguinal ring, so the examining fingers cannot get above it within the scrotum.

Table 13-2: Sexually Transmitted Infections of Male Genitalia

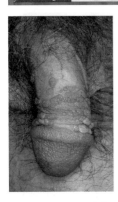

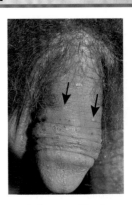

Genital Warts (condylomata acuminata)
- *Appearance:* Single or multiple papules or plaques of variable shapes; may be round, acuminate (or pointed), or thin and slender. May be raised, flat, or cauliflowerlike (verrucous).
- *Causative organism: Human papillomavirus (HPV),* usually from subtypes 6, 11; carcinogenic subtypes rare, approximately 5% to 10% of all anogenital warts.
- *Incubation:* weeks to months; infected contact may have no visible warts.
- Can arise on penis, scrotum, groin, thighs, anus; usually asymptomatic, occasionally cause itching and pain.
- May disappear without treatment.

Genital Herpes Simplex
- *Appearance:* Small scattered or grouped vesicles, 1 to 3 mm in size, on glans or shaft of penis. Appear as erosions if vesicular membrane breaks.
- *Causative organism:* Usually *Herpes simplex virus 2* (90%), a double-stranded DNA virus. *Incubation:* 2 to 7 days after exposure.
- Primary episode may be asymptomatic; recurrence usually less painful, of shorter duration.
- Associated with fever, malaise, headache, arthralgias; local pain and edema, lymphadenopathy.
- Need to distinguish from genital herpes zoster (usually in older patients with dermatomal distribution); candidiasis.

(continued)

Table 13-2	**Sexually Transmitted Infections of Male Genitalia** (*continued*)

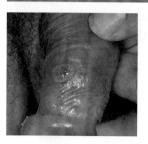 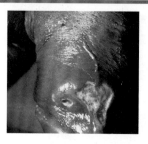

Primary Syphilis
- *Appearance:* Small red papule that becomes a *chancre*, or *painless* erosion up to 2 cm in diameter. Base of chancre is clean, red, smooth, and glistening; borders are raised and indurated. Chancre heals within 3 to 8 weeks.
- *Causative organism: Treponema pallidum*, a spirochete.
- *Incubation:* 9 to 90 days after exposure.
- May develop inguinal lymphadenopathy within 7 days; lymph nodes are rubbery, nontender, mobile.
- 20% to 30% of patients develop secondary syphilis while chancre still present (suggests coinfection with HIV).
- Distinguish from: genital herpes simplex, chancroid, granuloma inguinale from *Klebsiella granulomatis* (rare in the United States; 4 variants, so difficult to identify).

Chancroid
- *Appearance:* Red papule or pustule initially, then forms a *painful* deep ulcer with ragged nonindurated margins; contains necrotic exudate, has a friable base.
- *Causative organism: Haemophilus ducreyi,* an anaerobic bacillus.
- *Incubation:* 3 to 7 days after exposure.
- Painful inguinal adenopathy; suppurative bobos in 25% of patients.
- Need to distinguish from: primary syphilis; genital herpes simplex; lymphomogranuloma venereum, granuloma inguinale from *Klebsiella granulomatis* (both rare in the United States).

Table 13-3 Abnormalities of the Testes

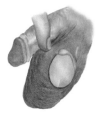

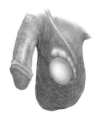

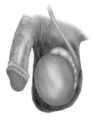

Cryptorchidism
Testis is atrophied and may lie in the inguinal canal or the abdomen, resulting in an unfilled scrotum. As above, there is no palpable left testis or epididymis. Cryptorchidism markedly raises the risk for testicular cancer.

Small Testis
In adults, testicular length is usually ≤3.5 cm. Small, firm testes seen in *Klinefelter's syndrome*, usually ≤2 cm. Small, soft testes suggesting atrophy seen in cirrhosis, myotonic dystrophy, use of estrogens, and hypopituitarism; may also follow orchitis.

Acute Orchitis
The testis is acutely inflamed, painful, tender, and swollen. It may be difficult to distinguish from the epididymis. The scrotum may be reddened. Seen in mumps and other viral infections; usually unilateral.

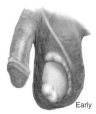
Early

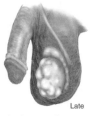
Late

Tumor of the Testis
Usually appears as a painless nodule. Any nodule within the testis warrants investigation for malignancy.

As a testicular neoplasm grows and spreads, it may seem to replace the entire organ. The testicle characteristically feels heavier than normal.

| | Table 13-4 | **Abnormalities of the Epididymis and Spermatic Cord** |

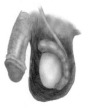 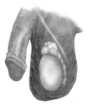

Acute Epididymitis
An acutely inflamed epididymis is tender and swollen and may be difficult to distinguish from the testis. The scrotum may be reddened and the vas deferens inflamed. It occurs chiefly in adults. Coexisting urinary tract infection or prostatitis supports the diagnosis.

Spermatocele and Cyst of the Epididymis
A painless, movable cystic mass just above the testis suggests a spermatocele or an epididymal cyst. Both transilluminate. The former contains sperm, and the latter does not, but they are clinically indistinguishable.

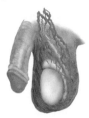 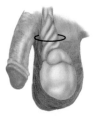

Varicocele of the Spermatic Cord
Varicocele refers to varicose veins of the spermatic cord, usually found on the left. It feels like a soft "bag of worms" separate from the testis, and slowly collapses when the scrotum is elevated in the supine patient.

Torsion of the Spermatic Cord
Twisting of the testicle on its spermatic cord produces an acutely painful and swollen organ that is retracted upward in the scrotum, which becomes red and edematous. There is no associated urinary infection. It is a surgical emergency because of obstructed circulation.

Table 13-5 Hernias in the Groin

Indirect Inguinal

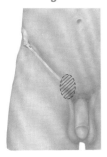

Most common hernia at all ages, both sexes. Originates above inguinal ligament and often passes into scrotum. *May touch examiner's fingertip in inguinal canal.*

Direct Inguinal

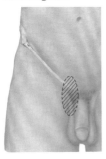

Less common than indirect hernia, usually occurs in men older than 40 years. Originates above inguinal ligament near external inguinal ring and *rarely enters scrotum. May bulge anteriorly, touching side of examiner's finger.*

Femoral

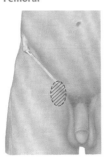

Least common hernia, more common in women than in men. Originates below inguinal ligament, more lateral than inguinal hernia. *Never enters scrotum.*

CHAPTER 14

Female Genitalia

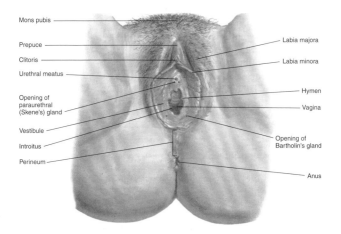

The Health History

Common Concerns

- Menarche, menstruation, menopause, postmenopausal bleeding
- Pregnancy
- Vulvovaginal symptoms
- Sexual preference and sexual response
- Pelvic pain—acute and chronic
- Sexually transmitted infections (STIs)

For the *menstrual history*, ask when menstrual periods began (age at menarche).	Changes in the interval between periods can signal possible pregnancy or menstrual irregularities.

When did her last menstrual period (LMP) start, and the one prior menstrual period (PMP)? What is the interval between periods, from the first day of one to the first day of the next? Are menses regular or irregular? How long do they last? How heavy is the flow?

In amenorrhea from *pregnancy*, common early symptoms are tenderness, tingling, or increased size of breasts; urinary frequency; nausea and vomiting; easy fatigability; and feelings that the baby is moving (usually noted at about 20 weeks).

Amenorrhea followed by heavy bleeding in threatened abortion or dysfunctional uterine bleeding

Dysmenorrhea, or painful menses, is common.

Primary dysmenorrhea from increased prostaglandin production; secondary dysmenorrhea from *endometriosis, pelvic inflammatory disease,* and endometrial polyps

Amenorrhea is the absence of periods. Failure to begin periods is *primary amenorrhea*, whereas cessation of established periods is *secondary amenorrhea*.

Secondary amenorrhea from low body weight is seen in malnutrition, *anorexia nervosa,* stress, chronic illness, and hypothalamic–pituitary–ovarian dysfunction.

Menopause, the absence of menses for 12 consecutive months, usually occurs between 48 and 55 years. Associated symptoms include hot flashes, flushing, sweating, and sleep disturbances.

Postmenopausal bleeding, or bleeding occurring 6 months after menses have stopped, suggests endometrial cancer, hormone replacement therapy, or uterine or cervical polyps.

For *vaginal discharge* and local *itching*, inquire about amount, color, consistency, and odor of discharge.

See Table 14-1, Lesions of the Vulva, pp. 233–234; and Table 14-2, Vaginal Discharge, p. 235.

Ask, "Tell me about your sexual preferences. Are your partners men, women or do you have partners of both sexes?"

To assess sexual function, start with general nonjudgmental questions like "How is sex for you?" or "Are you having any problems with sex?"

Direct questions help you assess each phase of the sexual response: desire, arousal, and orgasm.

Ask also about *dyspareunia*, or discomfort or pain during intercourse.

Superficial pain suggests local inflammation, atrophic vaginitis, or inadequate lubrication; deeper pain may result from pelvic disorders or pressure on a normal ovary.

For *sexually transmitted infections (STIs)* and diseases, identify sexual preference (male, female, or both) and the number of sexual partners in the previous month. Ask if the patient has concerns about HIV infection, desires HIV testing, or has current or past partners at risk.

In women, some STIs do not produce symptoms, but do increase the risk of infertility.

Health Promotion and Counseling: Evidence and Recommendations

Important Topics for Health Promotion and Counseling

- Cervical cancer screening; Pap smear and HPV infection
- Ovarian cancer: symptoms and risk factors
- STIs and HIV
- Options for family planning
- Menopause and hormone replacement therapy

New Pap Smear Screening Guidelines. Observe the new Pap smear guidelines from the American College of Obstetricians and Gynecologists (ACOG) in 2012 based on scientific advances related to the biology of human papillomavirus (HPV) infection.

- **First screening:** Begin screening at age 21

- **Women ages 21–29:**
  - Screen every 3 years if normal pap smears
  - Screen more frequently in patients with positive Pap or at high risk of positive HPV test; HIV infection; immunosuppression; DES exposure in utero; prior history of cervical cancer

- **Women ages 30–65:** Screen every 3 years with cytology if 3 consecutive normal Pap smears, no history of CIN 2 or CIN 3, and no high-risk factors; or with cytology and HPV testing every 5 years.

- **Women with hysterectomy:** Discontinue routine screening **if** hysterectomy for benign indications and no history of high-grade CIN. If hysterectomy for CIN 2, CIN 3, or cancer and cervix removed, screen annually for 20 years

- **Women ages >65:** Discontinue screening if ≥3 negative pap smears in a row and no abnormal Pap smears for 20 years

The most important risk factor for cervical cancer is HPV infection from HPV strains 16, 18, 6, or 11. The HPV vaccine prevents HPV infection from the strains when given *before* sexual exposure at age 11.

Ovarian Cancer. There are no effective screening tests to date. Risk factors include family history of breast or ovarian cancer and BRCA1 or BRCA2 mutation.

STIs and HIV Infection. *For STIs and HIV*, assess risk factors by taking a careful sexual history and counseling patients about spread of disease and ways to reduce high-risk practices. Test women younger than 26 years and pregnant women for *Chlamydia*; in women at increased risk and pregnant women, test for *gonorrhea, syphilis,* and *HIV.* In 2006, the CDC recommended universal screening for HIV for those ages 13 to 64 because infection occurs in many without known risk factors.

Options for Family Planning. More than half of U.S. pregnancies are unintended. Counsel women, particularly adolescents, about the *timing of ovulation*, which occurs midway in the regular menstrual cycle. Discuss methods for contraception and their effectiveness: natural (periodic abstinence, withdrawal, lactation); barrier (condom, diaphragm, cervical cap); implantable (intrauterine device, subdermal implant); pharmacologic (spermicide, oral contraceptives, subdermal implant of levonorgestrel, estrogen/progesterone injectables and patch, vaginal ring); and surgical (tubal ligation, transcervical sterilization).

Menopause and Hormone Replacement Therapy (HRT). Be familiar with the psychological and physiologic changes of *menopause*. Help the patient to weigh the risks of hormone replacement therapy (HRT), including increased risk of stroke, pulmonary embolism, and breast cancer. One to 2 years of HRT may be indicated for menopausal symptoms.

Techniques of Examination

Tips for the Successful Pelvic Examination

The Patient	The Examiner
▸ Avoids intercourse, douching, or use of vaginal suppositories for 24 to 48 hours before examination ▸ Empties bladder before examination ▸ Lies supine, with head and shoulders elevated, arms at sides or folded across chest to enhance eye contact and reduce tightening of abdominal muscles	▸ Obtains permission; selects chaperone ▸ Explains each step of the examination in advance ▸ Drapes patient from midabdomen to knees; depresses drape between knees to provide eye contact with patient ▸ Avoids unexpected or sudden movements ▸ Chooses a speculum that is the correct size ▸ Warms speculum with tap water ▸ Monitors comfort of the examination by watching the patient's face ▸ Uses excellent but gentle technique, especially when inserting the speculum

Male examiners should be accompanied by female chaperones. Female examiners should be assisted whenever possible.

| EXAMINATION TECHNIQUES | POSSIBLE FINDINGS |

EXTERNAL GENITALIA

Observe pubic hair to assess sexual maturity.

Normal or *delayed puberty*

Examine the external genitalia.

- Labia minora

  Ulceration in *herpes simplex, syphilitic chancre;* inflammation in Bartholin's cyst

- Clitoris

  Enlarged in masculinization

- Urethral orifice

  Urethral caruncle or *prolapse;* tenderness in *interstitial cystitis*

- Introitus

  Imperforate hymen

Milk the urethra for discharge, if indicated.

Discharge of urethritis

INTERNAL GENITALIA AND PAP SMEAR

Locate the cervix with a gloved and water-lubricated index finger.

Assess support of vaginal outlet by asking patient to strain down.

Cystocele, *cystourethrocele, rectocele*

Enlarge the introitus by pressing its posterior margin downward.

Insert a water-lubricated speculum of suitable size. Start with speculum held obliquely, then rotate to horizontal position for full insertion.

ENTRY ANGLE

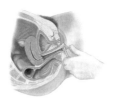

ANGLE AT FULL INSERTION

Chapter 14 | Female Genitalia

| EXAMINATION TECHNIQUES | POSSIBLE FINDINGS |

Open the speculum and inspect cervix.

See Table 14-3, Shapes of the Cervical Os, p. 236, and Table 14-4, Abnormalities of the Cervix, p. 237.

Observe:

- Position

  Cervix faces forward if uterus is retroverted.

- Color

  Purplish in pregnancy

- Epithelial surface

  Squamous and columnar epithelium

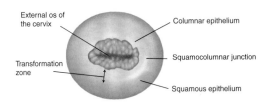

- Any discharge or bleeding

  Discharge from os in mucopurulent cervicitis from *Chlamydia* or *gonorrhea*

- Any ulcers, nodules, or masses

  Herpes, polyp, cancer

Obtain specimens for cytology (Pap smears) with:

Early cancer before it is clinically evident

- An endocervical broom or brush with scraper (except in pregnant women), to collect both squamous and columnar cells

- Or, if the woman is pregnant, use a cotton-tipped applicator moistened with water

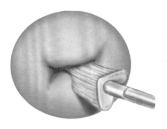

Inspect the vaginal mucosa as you withdraw the speculum.

Bluish color and deep rugae in pregnancy; vaginal cancer

| EXAMINATION TECHNIQUES | POSSIBLE FINDINGS |

Palpate, by means of a bimanual examination:

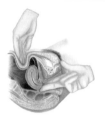

- The cervix and fornices

    Pain on moving cervix in *pelvic inflammatory disease*

- The uterus

    Pregnancy, myomas; soft isthmus in early pregnancy

- Right and left adnexa (ovaries)

    Ovarian cysts or masses, salpingitis, PID, tubal pregnancy

Assess strength of pelvic muscles. With your vaginal fingers clear of the cervix, ask patient to tighten her muscles around your fingers as hard and long as she can.

A firm squeeze that compresses your fingers, moves them up and inward, and lasts more than 3 seconds is full strength.

 Perform a rectovaginal examination to palpate a retroverted uterus, uterosacral ligaments, cul-de-sac, and adnexa or screen for colorectal cancer in women 50 years or older (see p. 245).

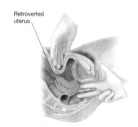

SPECIAL TECHNIQUE

HERNIAS

Ask the woman to strain down, as you palpate for a bulge in:

- The femoral canal

    Femoral hernia

- The *labia majora* up to just lateral to the pubic tubercle

    Indirect inguinal hernia

Chapter 14 | Female Genitalia

EXAMINATION TECHNIQUES

Recording Your Findings

Recording the Physical Examination—Female Genitalia

> "No inguinal adenopathy. External genitalia without erythema, lesions, or masses. Vaginal mucosa pink. Cervix parous, pink, and without discharge. Uterus anterior, midline, smooth, and not enlarged. No adnexal tenderness. Pap smear obtained. Rectovaginal wall intact. Rectal vault without masses. Stool brown and Hemoccult negative."
>
> OR
>
> "Bilateral shotty inguinal adenopathy. External genitalia without erythema or lesions. Vaginal mucosa and cervix coated with thin, white homogenous discharge with mild fishy odor. After swabbing cervix, no discharge visible in cervical os. Uterus midline; no adnexal masses. Rectal vault without masses. Stool brown and Hemoccult negative." (*Suggests bacterial vaginosis.*)

Aids to Interpretation

Table 14-1　Lesions of the Vulva

Epidermoid Cyst

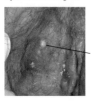

Cystic nodule in skin

A small, firm, round cystic nodule in the labia suggests *epidermoid cyst*. They are yellowish in color. Look for the dark punctum marking the blocked opening of the gland.

Venereal Wart
(Condyloma Acuminatum)

Warts

Warty lesions on the labia and within the vestibule suggest *condylomata acuminata* from infection with human papillomavirus.

(continued)

Table 14-1 Lesions of the Vulva (continued)

Genital Herpes

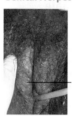

Shallow ulcers on red bases

Shallow, small, painful ulcers on red bases suggest a herpes infection. Initial infection may be extensive, as illustrated here. Recurrent infections are usually confined to a small local patch.

Syphilitic Chancre

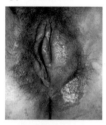

A firm, painless ulcer suggests the chancre of *primary syphilis*. Because most chancres in women develop internally, they often go undetected.

Secondary Syphilis (*Condyloma Latum*)

Flat, gray papules

Slightly raised, round or oval flat-topped papules covered by a gray exudate suggest *condylomata lata*, a manifestation of *secondary syphilis*. They are contagious.

Carcinoma of the Vulva

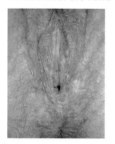

An ulcerated or raised red vulvar lesion in an elderly woman may indicate vulvar carcinoma.

Table 14-2 Vaginal Discharge

Note: Accurate diagnosis depends on laboratory assessment and cultures.

Trichomonas vaginitis

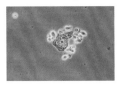

Discharge: Yellowish green, often profuse, may be malodorous
Other Symptoms: Itching, vaginal soreness, dyspareunia
Vulva: May be red
Vagina: May be normal or red, with red spots, petechiae
Laboratory Assessment: Saline wet mount for trichomonads

Candida vaginitis

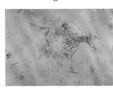

Discharge: White, curdy, often thick, not malodorous
Other Symptoms: Itching, vaginal soreness, external dysuria, dyspareunia
Vulva: Often red and swollen
Vagina: Often red with white patches of discharge
Laboratory Assessment: KOH preparation for branching hyphae

Bacterial vaginosis

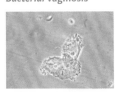

Discharge: Gray or white, thin, homogeneous, scant, malodorous
Other Symptoms: Fishy genital odor
Vulva: Usually normal
Vagina: Usually normal
Laboratory Assessment: Saline wet mount for "clue cells," "whiff test" with KOH for fishy odor

Table 14-3	**Shapes of the Cervical Os**

Normal Variations

Oval

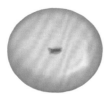

Slitlike

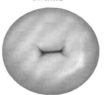

Lacerations

Unilateral Transverse

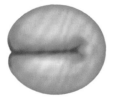

Bilateral Transverse

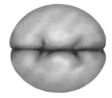

Stellate

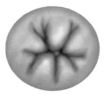

Table 14-4 Abnormalities of the Cervix

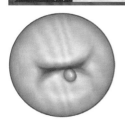

Endocervical polyp. A bright red, smooth mass that protrudes from the os suggests a polyp. It bleeds easily.

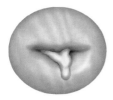

Mucopurulent cervicitis. A yellowish exudate emerging from the cervical os suggests infection from *Chlamydia*, *gonorrhea* (often asymptomatic), or *herpes*.

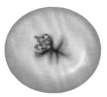

Carcinoma of the cervix. An irregular, hard mass suggests cancer. Early lesions are best detected by colposcopy following abnormal Pap smear from of high risk of HPV.

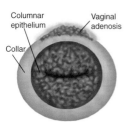

Fetal exposure to diethylstilbestrol (DES). Several changes may occur: a collar of tissue around the cervix, columnar epithelium that covers the cervix or extends to the vaginal wall (then termed *vaginal adenosis*), and, rarely, carcinoma of the vagina.

Table 14-5 Relaxations of the Pelvic Floor

When the pelvic floor is weakened, various structures may become displaced. These displacements are seen best when the patient strains down.

A **cystocele** is a bulge of the anterior wall of the upper part of the vagina, together with the urinary bladder above it.

A **cystourethrocele** involves both the bladder and the urethra as they bulge into the anterior vaginal wall throughout most of its extent.

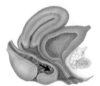

A **rectocele** is a bulge of the posterior vaginal wall, together with a portion of the rectum.

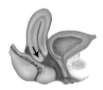

A **prolapsed uterus** has descended down the vaginal canal. There are three degrees of severity: first, still within the vagina (as illustrated); second, with the cervix at the introitus; and third, with the cervix outside the introitus.

Table 14-6 — Positions of the Uterus and Uterine Myomas

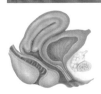

An anteverted uterus lies in a forward position at roughly a right angle to the vagina. This is the most common position. *Anteflexion*—a forward flexion of the uterine body in relation to the cervix—often coexists.

A retroverted uterus is tilted posteriorly with its cervix facing anteriorly.

A retroflexed uterus has a posterior tilt that involves the uterine body but not the cervix. A uterus that is retroflexed or retroverted may be felt only through the rectal wall; some cannot be felt at all.

A myoma of the uterus is a very common benign tumor that feels firm and often irregular. There may be more than one. A myoma on the posterior surface of the uterus may be mistaken for a retrodisplaced uterus; one on the anterior surface may be mistaken for an anteverted uterus.

CHAPTER

15

The Anus, Rectum, and Prostate

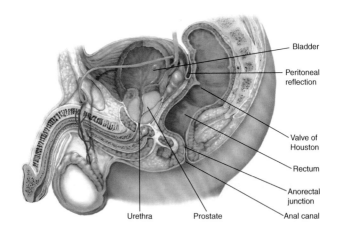

The Health History

Common or Concerning Symptoms

- Change in bowel habits
- Blood in the stool
- Pain with defecation; rectal bleeding or tenderness
- Anal warts or fissures
- Weak stream of urine
- Burning with urination

241

Ask about any change in bowel habits, diarrhea, or constipation. Is there any blood in the stool, or dark tarry stools?	Pencil-like stool or blood in stool in *colon cancer;* dark tarry stools in *gastrointestinal bleeding*
Any pain with defecation, or rectal bleeding or tenderness?	Hemorrhoids; proctitis from STIs
Any anal warts or fissures?	*Human papillomavirus* (HPV), *condylomata lata* in secondary syphilis; fissures in proctitis, *Crohn's disease*
In men, is there difficulty starting the urine stream or holding back urine? Is the flow weak? What about frequent urination, especially at night? Or pain or burning when passing urine? Any blood in the urine or semen or pain with ejaculation? Is there frequent pain or stiffness in the lower back, hips, or upper thighs?	These symptoms suggest urethral obstruction from *benign prostatic hyperplasia* (BPH) or *prostate cancer*, especially in men age ≥70. The American Urological Association (AUA) Symptom Index helps quantify BPH severity (see Table 15-1, BPH Score Index: American Urological Association (AUA), pp. 246–247).

Health Promotion and Counseling: Evidence and Recommendations

Important Topics for Health Promotion and Counseling

- Screening for prostate cancer
- Screening for colorectal cancer
- Counseling for sexually transmitted infections (STIs)

Screening for Prostate Cancer. Prostate cancer is the leading cancer diagnosed in U.S. men and the second leading cause of death. Risk factors are age, family history of prostate cancer, and African American ethnicity.

Screening methods such as the digital rectal examination (DRE) and the prostate-specific antigen (PSA) test are not highly accurate, which complicates decisions about screening men *without symptoms*.

- The *DRE* reaches only the posterior and lateral surfaces of the prostate, missing 25% to 35% of tumors in other areas. Sensitivity of the

DRE for prostate cancer is low, 59%, and the rate of false positives is high.

- *The PSA.* PSA testing is controversial. The PSA can be elevated in benign conditions like hyperplasia, prostatitis, ejaculation, and urinary retention. Its detection rate for prostate cancer is about 28% to 35% in asymptomatic men. It does not distinguish small-volume indolent cancers from aggressive life-threatening disease. Discussion and shared decision making are warranted. Several groups recommend annual combined screening with PSA and DRE for men older than 50 years and for African Americans and men older than 40 years with a positive family history. Studies of baseline PSA testing at age 40, and reducing the threshold for biopsy from 4.0 ng/mL to 2.5 ng/mL are inconclusive.

For *symptomatic prostate disorders*, the clinician's role is more straightforward. Men with incomplete emptying of the bladder, urinary frequency or urgency, weak or intermittent stream or straining to initiate flow, hematuria, nocturia, or even bony pains in the pelvis should be encouraged to seek evaluation and treatment early.

Screening for Colorectal Cancer. In 2008, screening recommendations were revised to promote more aggressive surveillance:

- Clinicians should first identify whether patients are at average or increased risk, ideally by age 20 years, but earlier if the patient has inflammatory bowel disease or a family history of familial adenomatous polyposis.

- Average-risk patients 50 years or older should be offered a range of screening options to increase compliance: annual screening with high-sensitivity fecal occult blood tests (FOBTs); flexible sigmoidoscopy every 5 years, with annual high-sensitivity FOBT every 3 years; or colonoscopy every 10 years.

- People at increased risk should undergo colonoscopy at intervals ranging from 3 to 5 years.

Clinicians should also use the 6-sample fecal occult blood test. Avoid single-sample FOBT and DRE, which have inadequate detection rates.

Counseling for STIs. Anal intercourse increases risk for HIV and STIs. Promote abstinence, use of condoms, and good hygiene.

Techniques of Examination

EXAMINATION TECHNIQUES	POSSIBLE FINDINGS

○— Wear gloves.

MALE

Position the patient on his side, or standing leaning forward over the examining table and hips flexed.

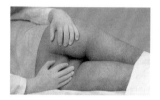

Inspect the:

- Sacrococcygeal area

  Pilonidal cyst or sinus

- Perianal area

  Hemorrhoids, warts, herpes, chancre, cancer, fissures from *proctitis* or *Crohn's disease*

Palpate the anal canal and rectum with a lubricated and gloved finger. Feel the:

Lax sphincter tone in some neurologic disorders; tightness in proctitis

- Walls of the rectum

  Cancer of the rectum, polyps

- Prostate gland, as shown below, including median sulcus

  Prostate nodule or cancer; BPH; tenderness in prostatitis

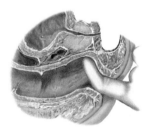

Chapter 15 | The Anus, Rectum, and Prostate

EXAMINATION TECHNIQUES	POSSIBLE FINDINGS
Try to feel above the prostate for irregularities or tenderness, if indicated.	See Table 15-2, Abnormalities on Rectal Examination, pp. 248–249.

♀ FEMALE

The patient is usually in the lithotomy position or lying on her side.	Rectal shelf of peritoneal metastases; tenderness of inflammation
Inspect the anus.	Hemorrhoids
Palpate the anal canal and rectum.	Rectal cancer, normal uterine cervix or tampon (felt through the rectal wall)

Recording Your Findings

Recording the Physical Examination—The Anus, Rectum, and Prostate

> "No perirectal lesions or fissures. External sphincter tone intact. Rectal vault without masses. Prostate smooth and nontender with palpable median sulcus. (Or in a female, uterine cervix nontender.) Stool brown and Hemoccult negative."
>
> **OR**
>
> "Perirectal area inflamed; no ulcerations, warts, or discharge. Cannot examine external sphincter, rectal vault, or prostate because of spasm of external sphincter and marked inflammation and tenderness of anal canal." (*Raises concern of proctitis from infectious cause.*)
>
> **OR**
>
> "No perirectal lesions or fissures. External sphincter tone intact. Rectal vault without masses. Left lateral prostate lobe with 1 × 1 cm firm hard nodule; right lateral lobe smooth; medial sulcus is obscured. Stool brown and Hemoccult negative." (*Raises concern of prostate cancer.*)

Aids to Interpretation

Table 15-1	BPH Symptom Score Index: American Urological Association (AUA)

Score or ask the patient to score each of the questions below on a scale of 1 to 5.

0 = Not at all

1 = Less than 1 time in 5

2 = Less than half the time

3 = About half the time

4 = More than half the time

5 = Almost always

Higher scores (maximum 35) indicate more severe symptoms; scores ≤7 are considered mild and generally do not warrant treatment.

PART A	Score
1. **Incomplete emptying:** Over the past month, how often have you had a sensation of not emptying your bladder completely after you finished urinating?	_____
2. **Frequency:** Over the past month, how often have you had to urinate again <2 hours after you finished urinating?	_____
3. **Inter-mittency:** Over the past month, how often have you stopped and started again several times when you urinated?	_____
4. **Urgency:** Over the past month, how often have you found it difficult to postpone urination?	_____
5. **Weak stream:** Over the past month, how often have you had a weak urinary stream?	_____
6. **Straining:** Over the past month, how often have you had to push or strain to begin urination?	_____
PART A TOTAL SCORE	_____

Table 15-1: BPH Symptom Score Index: American Urological Association (AUA) *(continued)*

Score or ask the patient to score each of the questions below on a scale of 1 to 5.

0 = Not at all

1 = Less than 1 time in 5

2 = Less than half the time

3 = About half the time

4 = More than half the time

5 = Almost always

Higher scores (maximum 35) indicate more severe symptoms; scores ≤7 are considered mild and generally do not warrant treatment.

PART B	Score
7. **Nocturia:** Over the past month, how many times did you most typically get up to urinate from the time you went to bed at night until the time you got up in the morning? (Score 0 to 5 times on night)	_____
TOTAL PARTS A and B (maximum 35)	_____

Adapted from: Madsen FA, Burskewitz RC. Clinical Manifestations of benign prostatic hyperplasia. Urol Clin North Am 1995;22:291–298.

Table 15-2 — Abnormalities on Rectal Examination

External Hemorrhoids (*Thrombosed*).
Dilated hemorrhoidal veins that originate below the pectinate line, covered with skin; a tender, swollen, bluish ovoid mass is visible at the anal margin

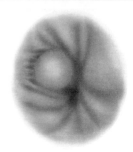

Polyps of the Rectum. A soft mass that may or may not be on a stalk; may not be palpable

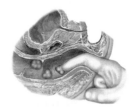

Benign Prostatic Hyperplasia. An enlarged, nontender, smooth, firm but slightly elastic prostate gland; can cause symptoms without palpable enlargement

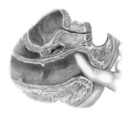

Acute Prostatitis. A prostate that is very tender, swollen, and firm because of acute infection

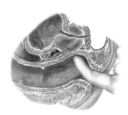

Table 15-2 Abnormalities on Rectal Examination (continued)

Cancer of the Prostate. A hard area in the prostate that may or may not feel nodular

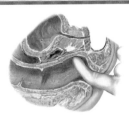

Cancer of the Rectum. Firm, nodular, rolled edge of an ulcerated cancer

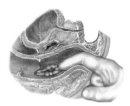

The Musculoskeletal System

CHAPTER 16

Fundamentals for Assessing Joints

Assessing joints requires knowledge of their structure and function. Learn the surface landmarks and underlying anatomy of each major joint. Be familiar with the following terms:

- *Articular structures* include the joint capsule and articular cartilage, synovium and synovial fluid, intra-articular ligaments, and juxta-articular bone.

- *Extra-articular structures* include periarticular ligaments, tendons, bursae, muscle, fascia, bone, nerve, and overlying skin.

  - *Ligaments* are the ropelike bundles of collagen fibrils that connect bone to bone.

  - *Tendons* are collagen fibers that connect muscle to bone.

  - *Bursae* are pouches of synovial fluid that cushion the movement of tendons and muscles over bone or other joint structures.

Review the three primary types of joint articulation—synovial, cartilaginous, and fibrous—and the varying degrees of movement each type allows.

Joints

Synovial Joints

- Freely movable within limits of surrounding ligaments
- Separated by *articular cartilage* and a *synovial cavity*
- Lubricated by synovial fluid
- Surrounded by a joint capsule
- *Example:* knee, shoulder

SYNOVIAL

Cartilaginous Joints

- Slightly movable
- Contain fibrocartilaginous discs that separate the bony surfaces
- Have a central *nucleus pulposus* of discs that cushions bony contact
- *Example:* vertebral bodies

CARTILAGINOUS

Fibrous Joints

- No appreciable movement
- Consist of fibrous tissue or cartilage
- Lack a joint cavity
- *Example:* skull sutures

FIBROUS

Review the types of synovial joints and their associated features as well.

Note that joint structure determines joint function and range of motion.

Synovial Joints

Type of Joint	Articular Shape	Movement	Example
Spheroidal (ball and socket)	Convex surface in concave cavity	Wide-ranging flexion, extension, abduction, adduction, rotation, circumduction	Shoulder, hip
Hinge	Flat, planar	Motion in one plane; flexion, extension	Interphalangeal joints of hand and foot; elbow
Condylar	Convex or concave	Movement of two articulating surfaces, not dissociable	Knee; temporomandibular joint

The Health History

Common or Concerning Symptoms

- Low back pain
- Neck pain
- Monoarticular or polyarticular joint pain
- Inflammatory or infectious joint pain
- Joint pain with systemic features such as fever, chills, rash, anorexia, weight loss, and weakness
- Joint pain with symptoms from other organ systems

Assess the seven features of any joint pain (see p. 38).

> **Tips for Assessing Joint Pain**
>
> - Ask the patient to *"point to the pain."* This may save considerable time, because the patient's verbal description is often imprecise.
> - Clarify and record the onset of pain and the *mechanism of injury*, particularly if there is a history of trauma.
> - Determine whether the pain is *localized* or *diffuse*, *acute* or *chronic*, *inflammatory* or *noninflammatory*.

Low Back Pain. Ask, "Any pains in your back?" *Low back pain* is the second most common reason for office visits. Ask if the pain is in the midline over the vertebrae, or off midline. If the pain radiates into the legs, ask about any associated numbness, tingling, or weakness. Ask about history of trauma.

See Table 16-1, Low Back Pain, pp. 277–278. Causes of *midline back pain* include vertebral collapse, disc herniation, epidural abscess, spinal cord compression, or spinal cord metastases. *Pain off the midline* in muscle strain, sacroiliitis, trochanteric bursitis, sciatica, hip arthritis, renal conditions such as *pyelonephritis* or renal stones

Check for bladder or bowel dysfunction.

Present in *cauda equine syndrome* from S2–4 tumor or disc herniation, especially if "saddle anesthesia" from perianal numbness

Neck Pain. Ask about location, radiation into the shoulders or arms, arm or leg weakness, bladder or bowel dysfunction.

C7 or C6 spinal nerve compression from foraminal impingement more common than disc herniation. See Table 16-2, Pains in the Neck, pp. 279–280.

Joint Pain. Proceed with "Do you have any pain in your joints?"

See Table 16-3, Patterns of Pain in and Around the Joints, p. 281.

Ask the patient to *point to the pain*. If *localized* and involving only one joint, it is *monoarticular*.

Consider trauma, monoarticular arthritis, tendonitis, or bursitis. Hip pain near the greater trochanter suggests trochanteric bursitis.

If *polyarticular*, does it migrate from joint to joint, or steadily spread from one joint to multiple joint involvement? Is the involvement symmetric?

Migratory pattern in *rheumatic fever* or *gonococcal arthritis;* progressive and symmetric pattern in *rheumatoid arthritis*

Ask if pain is extra-articular (bones, muscles, and tissues around the joint, such as the tendons, bursae, or even overlying skin). Are there generalized "aches and pains" (*myalgia* if in muscles, *arthralgia* if in joints with no evidence of arthritis)?	*Bursitis* if inflammation of bursae; *tendonitis* if in tendons, and *tenosynovitis* if in tendon sheaths; also *sprains* from stretching or tearing of ligaments
Assess the timing, quality, and severity of joint symptoms. If from trauma, what was the *mechanism of injury* or series of events that caused the joint pain? Furthermore, what aggravates or relieves the pain? What are the effects of exercise, rest, and treatment?	Severe pain of rapid onset in a red, swollen joint in *acute septic arthritis* or *gout*
Is the problem *inflammatory* or *noninflammatory*? Is there *tenderness, warmth,* or *redness*?	Fever, chills, warmth, redness in *septic arthritis*; also consider *gout* or *rheumatic fever*
Is the pain *articular* in origin, with *swelling, stiffness,* or *decreased range of motion*?	Pain, swelling, loss of active and passive motion, "locking," deformity in *articular joint pain*; loss of active but not passive motion, tenderness outside the joint, no deformity in *nonarticular pain*
Assess any *limitations of motion*.	Transient stiffness after limited activity in *degenerative arthritis*; prolonged stiffness in *rheumatoid arthritis, fibromyalgia, polymyalgia rheumatica*
Ask about any *systemic* symptoms such as fever, chills, rash, anorexia, weight loss, and weakness.	Common in *rheumatoid arthritis, systemic lupus erythematosus, polymyalgia rheumatica,* and other inflammatory arthritides. High fever and chills suggest an infectious cause.

Health Promotion and Counseling: Evidence and Recommendations

Important Topics for Health Promotion and Counseling

- Nutrition, weight, and physical activity
- Profiling low back pain
- Osteoporosis: screening and prevention
- Preventing falls

Nutrition, Weight, and Physical Activity. Advise patients that a healthy lifestyle conveys direct benefits to the skeleton. Good nutrition supplies the calcium needed for bone mineralization and bone density. Optimal weight reduces excess mechanical stress on weight-bearing joints like the hips and knees. Exercise helps maintain bone mass and improves outlook and stress management.

Profiling Low Back Pain. The low back is especially vulnerable, most notably at L5–S1, where the sacral vertebrae make a sharp posterior angle. Approximately 60% to 80% of the population experiences low back pain at least once. Current evidence supports active exercise with minimal bed rest and delay of back-specific exercise while pain is acute; cognitive-behavioral counseling; and occupational interventions targeting graded exercise and early return to modified work. *Depression* is a major predictor of new low back pain, warranting prompt treatment of psychiatric comorbidities.

Osteoporosis Screening and Prevention. Osteoporosis is a major public health threat for postmenopausal women and some men. The U.S. Preventive Services Task Force recommends routine bone density screening for women 65 years or older and earlier for those with the risk factors on next page.

Risk Factors for Osteoporosis and Fracture

- Prior fragility fracture
- Postmenopausal status in white women
- Age ≥50 years
- Weight ≤70 kg (154 lb)
- Lower dietary calcium
- Vitamin D deficiency
- Tobacco and alcohol use
- Family history of fracture in a first-degree relative
- Use of corticosteroids
- Medical conditions such as thyrotoxicosis, celiac sprue, chronic renal disease, organ transplantation, diabetes, HIV, primary or secondary hypogonadism, multiple myeloma, and anorexia nervosa
- Medications such as aromatase inhibitors for breast cancer, methotrexate, selected antiseizure medications, immunosuppressive agents, and anti-gonadal therapy
- Inflammatory disorders of the musculoskeletal, pulmonary, or gastrointestinal systems, including rheumatoid arthritis

Use the country-specific FRAX calculator to assess fracture risk. If risk is >9.3% for any fracture and >3% for hip fracture, bone density screening is warranted. The Web site for the FRAX Calculator for Assessing Fracture Risk for the United States is http://www.shef.ac.uk/FRAX/tool.jsp?country=9.

Use the World Health Organization scoring criteria to determine bone density. A 10% drop in bone density, equivalent to 1.0 standard deviation, is associated with a 20% increase in risk of fracture.

World Health Organization Bone Density Criteria

Osteoporosis: T score <-2.5 (>2.5 standard deviations below the mean for young adult white women)
Osteopenia: T score -2.5 to 1.5 (1.0 to 2.5 standard deviations below the mean for young adult white women)

Several agents inhibit bone resorption: calcium, vitamin D, and antiresorptive agents such as bisphosphonates, selective estrogen-receptor modulators (SERMs), and calcitonin. Learn the therapeutic uses of these agents and exercise.

Recommended Dietary Intakes of Calcium and Vitamin D for Adults (Institute of Medicine 2010)

Age Group	Calcium (elemental) mg/day	Vitamin D IU/day
19–50	1,000	600
50–71		
Women	1,200	600
Men	1,000	600
≥71	1,200	800

Source: Ross AC, Manson JE, Abrams SA, et al. The 2011 report on dietary reference intakes for calcium and vitamin D from the Institute of Medicine: what clinicians need to know. J Endocrinol Metab 2011;96:53–58.

Preventing Falls. Falls are the leading cause of nonfatal injuries and account for a dramatic rise in death rates after 65 years of age. Risk factors include unstable gait, imbalanced posture, reduced strength, cognitive loss and dementia, deficits in vision and proprioception, and osteoporosis. Urge patients to correct poor lighting, dark or steep stairs, chairs at awkward heights, slippery or irregular surfaces, and ill-fitting shoes. Scrutinize any medications affecting balance, especially benzodiazepines, vasodilators, and diuretics.

Techniques of Examination

Approach to Individual Joint Examination

Inspect the joints and surrounding tissues as you do the various regional examinations.

Identify joints with changes in structure and function, carefully assessing for:

- Symmetry of involvement—one or both sides of the body; one joint or several
- Deformity or malalignment of bones
- Changes in surrounding soft tissue—skin changes, subcutaneous nodules, muscle atrophy, crepitus
- Limitations in range of motion and maneuvers, ligamentous laxity
- Changes in muscle strength

Note signs of inflammation and arthritis: swelling, warmth, tenderness, redness.

| EXAMINATION TECHNIQUES | POSSIBLE FINDINGS |

TEMPOROMANDIBULAR JOINT (TMJ)

Inspect the TMJ for swelling or redness.

Palpate the TMJ as the patient opens and closes the mouth.

Palpate the muscles of mastication: the *masseters*, *temporal muscles*, and *pterygoid muscles*.

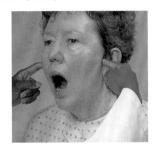

SHOULDERS

Inspect the contour of the shoulders and shoulder girdles from front and back.

Muscle atrophy; anterior or posterior dislocation of humeral head; scoliosis if shoulder heights asymmetric

See Table 16-4, Painful Shoulders, p. 282.

Palpate:
- The clavicle from the sternoclavicular joint to the acromioclavicular joint

"Step-offs" if fracture from trauma

- The bicipital tendon

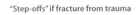

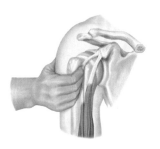

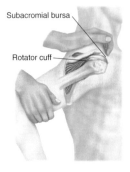

- The subacromial and subdeltoid bursae after lifting arm posteriorly

Subacromial or subdeltoid bursitis

| EXAMINATION TECHNIQUES | POSSIBLE FINDINGS |

Assess range of motion.

- Flexion—"Raise your arm in front of you and overhead."

  Intact glenohumeral motion if patient raises arms to shoulder level, palms facing *down*

- Extension—"Move your arms behind you."

  Intact scapulothoracic motion if patient raises arms an additional 60 degrees, palms facing *up*

- Abduction—"Raise your arms out to the side and overhead."

- Adduction—"Cross your arm in front of your body, keeping the arm straight."

  Acromioclavicular joint arthritis

- External and internal rotation

  Shoulder arthritis

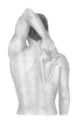
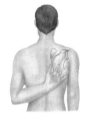

| TESTS ABDUCTION AND EXTERNAL ROTATION | TESTS ADDUCTION AND INTERNAL ROTATION |

Perform maneuvers to assess the "SITS" muscles and tendons of the *rotator cuff*—supraspinatus, infraspinatus, teres minor, subscapularis, and the bicipital tendon.

- "Empty can test" for supraspinatus strength

  Weakness in *rotator cuff tear*

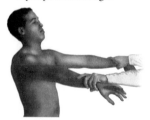

EXAMINATION TECHNIQUES

POSSIBLE FINDINGS

- Infraspinatus strength

Weakness in *rotator cuff tear* or *bicipital tendonitis*

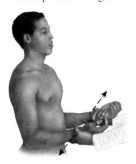

- Forearm supination

Pain in *rotator cuff tear*

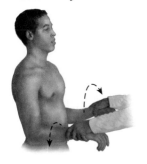

- "Drop arm" test

If patient cannot hold arm fully abducted at shoulder level, possible *rotator cuff tear*

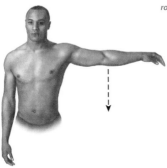

| EXAMINATION TECHNIQUES | POSSIBLE FINDINGS |

ELBOWS

Inspect and palpate:

- Olecranon process

    Olecranon bursitis; posterior dislocation from direct trauma or supracondylar fracture

- Medial and lateral epicondyles

    Tenderness distal to epicondyle in epicondylitis (medial → "tennis elbow"; lateral → "pitcher's elbow")

- Extensor surface of the ulna

    Rheumatoid nodules

- Grooves between the epicondyles and the olecranon

    Tender in arthritis

Ask patient to:

- Flex and extend elbows
- Turn palms up and down (supination and pronation)

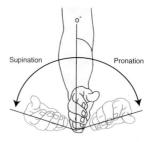

WRISTS AND HANDS

Inspect:

- Movement of the wrist (flexion, extension, ulnar and medial deviation), hands, and fingers

    Guarded movement in injury

- Contours of wrists, hands, and fingers

    Deformities in *rheumatoid* and *degenerative arthritis;* swelling in arthritis, ganglia; impaired alignment of fingers in flexor tendon damage; flexion contractures in Dupuytren's contractures

- Contours of palms

    Thenar atrophy in median nerve compression (*carpal tunnel syndrome*); hypothenar atrophy in ulnar nerve compression

Chapter 16 | The Musculoskeletal System

| EXAMINATION TECHNIQUES | POSSIBLE FINDINGS |

Palpate:

- Wrist joints

Swelling and tenderness in *rheumatoid arthritis*, *gonococcal infection* of joint or extensor tendon sheaths

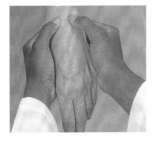

- Distal radius and ulna

Tenderness over ulnar styloid in *Colles' fracture*

- "Anatomic snuffbox," the hollow space distal to the radial styloid bone; thumb extensor and abductor tendons.

Tenderness suggests *scaphoid fracture*. Tenderness over extensor and abductor tendons in de Quervain's tenosynovitis.

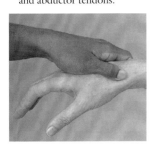

- Metacarpophalangeal joint

Swelling in *rheumatoid arthritis*

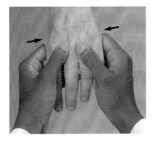

EXAMINATION TECHNIQUES

- Proximal and distal interphalangeal joint

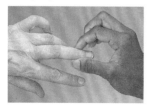

POSSIBLE FINDINGS

Proximal nodules in rheumatoid arthritis (*Bouchard's nodes*), distal nodules in osteoarthritis (*Heberden's nodes*)

Assess range of motion:

- Wrists: Flexion, extension, adduction (radial deviation), abduction (lateral deviation)

Arthritis, tenosynovitis

- Fingers: Flexions, extension, abduction/adduction (spread fingers apart and back)

Trigger finger, Dupuytren's contracture

- Thumbs

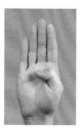

FLEXION

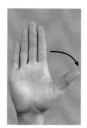

EXTENSION

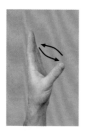

ABDUCTION AND ADDUCTION

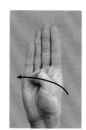

OPPOSITION

Chapter 16 | The Musculoskeletal System

EXAMINATION TECHNIQUES

POSSIBLE FINDINGS

Perform selected maneuvers.

- Hand grip strength

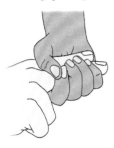

Decreased grip strength if weakness of finger flexors or intrinsic hand muscles

- Thumb movement

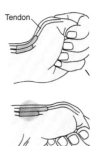

Pain if de Quervain's tenosynovitis

- Carpal tunnel testing

  - *Thumb adduction*

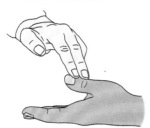

Weakness of abductor pollicis longus is specific to median nerve.

  - *Tinel's sign:* Tap lightly over median nerve at volar wrist

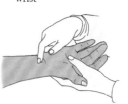

Aching, tingling, and numbness in second, third, and fourth fingers is a positive Tinel's sign.

EXAMINATION TECHNIQUES	POSSIBLE FINDINGS
• *Phalen's sign:* Patient flexes wrists for 60 seconds	Aching, tingling, and numbness in second, third, and fourth volar fingers is a *positive Phalen's sign*.

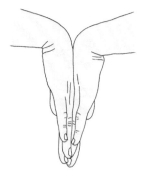

SPINE

Inspect spine from the side and back, noting any abnormal curvatures.	Kyphosis, scoliosis, lordosis, gibbus, list curvatures
Look for asymmetric heights of shoulders, iliac crests, or buttocks.	Scoliosis, pelvic tilt, unequal leg length

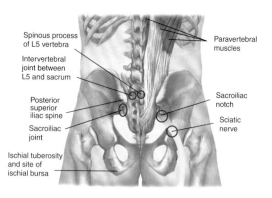

| EXAMINATION TECHNIQUES | POSSIBLE FINDINGS |

Identify and palpate:

- Spinous processes of each vertebra

  Tender if trauma, infection; "step-offs" in spondylolisthesis, fracture

- Sacroiliac joints

  Sacroiliitis, ankylosing spondylitis

- Paravertebral muscles, if painful

  Paravertebral muscle spasm in abnormal posture, degenerative and inflammatory muscle disorders, overuse

- Sciatic nerve (midway between greater trochanter and ischial tuberosity)

  Herniated disc or nerve root compression

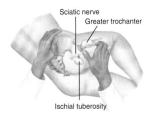

Test the range of motion in the neck and spine in: flexion, extension, rotation, and lateral bending.

Decreased mobility in arthritis

HIPS

Inspect gait for:

- *Stance* (see below) and *swing* (foot moves forward, does not bear weight)

  Most problems arise during the weight-bearing stance phase.

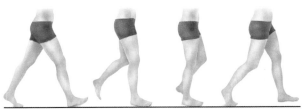

Heelstrike Foot flat Midstance Push-off

PHASES OF GAIT: STANCE (RIGHT LEG) AND SWING (LEFT LEG)

EXAMINATION TECHNIQUES	POSSIBLE FINDINGS
• *Width of base* (usually 2 to 4 inches from heel to heel), shift of pelvis, flexion of knee	Cerebellar disease or foot problems if wide base; impaired shift of pelvis in arthritis, hip dislocation, abductor weakness; disrupted gait if poor knee flexion

Palpate:

• Along the inguinal ligament	Bulges in inguinal hernia, aneurysm
• The *trochanteric bursa*, on the greater trochanter of the femur	Focal tenderness in *trochanteric bursitis*, often described by patients as "low back pain"
• The *ischiogluteal bursa*, superficial to the ischial tuberosity	Tender in bursitis ("weaver's bottom") from prolonged sitting

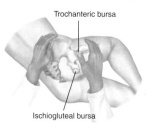

TROCHANTERIC AND ISCHIOGLUTEAL BURSA

Check range of motion, including:

• Flexion—"Bend your knee and pull it against your abdomen."	Flexion of opposite leg suggests deformity of that hip.

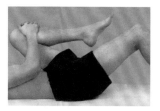

| EXAMINATION TECHNIQUES | POSSIBLE FINDINGS |

- Extension

Painful in iliopsoas abscess

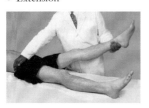

- Abduction and adduction

Restricted in hip arthritis

- Internal and external rotation

Restricted in hip arthritis

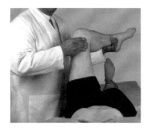

KNEES

Review the structures of the knee.

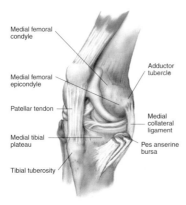

EXAMINATION TECHNIQUES	POSSIBLE FINDINGS

Inspect:

- Gait for knee extension at heel strike, flexion during all other phases of swing and stance

    Stumbling or "giving way" during heel strike in *quadriceps weakness* or abnormal patellar tracking

- Alignment of knees

    Bowlegs, knock-knees; flexion contractures in limb paralysis or hamstring tightness

- Contours of knees, including any atrophy of the quadriceps muscles

    Quadriceps atrophy with *patellofemoral disorder*

Inspect and palpate:

See Table 16-5, Painful Knees, pp. 283–284.

- The tibiofemoral joint—with knees flexed, including:

    - Joint line—place thumbs on either side of the patellar tendon.

        Irregular, bony ridges in osteoarthritis.

    - Medial and lateral meniscus

        Tenderness if meniscus tear

    - Medial and lateral collateral ligaments

        Tenderness if MCL tear (LCL injuries less common)

- The patellofemoral compartment:

    - Patella

        Swelling over the patella in prepatellar bursitis ("housemaid's knee")

    - Palpate the patellar tendon and ask patient to extend the leg.

        Tenderness or inability to extend the leg in partial or complete tear of the patellar tendon

    - Press the patella against the underlying femur.

        Pain, crepitus, and a history of knee pain in *patellofemoral disorder*

    - Push patella distally and ask patient to tighten knee against table.

        Pain during contraction of quadriceps in *chondromalacia*

Chapter 16 | The Musculoskeletal System

EXAMINATION TECHNIQUES	POSSIBLE FINDINGS

- Also:

  - Suprapatellar pouch — Swelling in synovitis and arthritis

  - Infrapatellar spaces (hollow areas adjacent to patella) — Swelling in arthritis

  - Medial tibial condyle — Swelling in *pes anserine* bursitis

  - Popliteal surface — Popliteal or Baker's cyst

Assess any effusions.

- *Bulge sign* (minor effusions): Compress the suprapatellar pouch, stroke downward on medial surface, apply pressure to force fluid to lateral surface, and then tap knee behind lateral margin of patella.

  A fluid wave returning to the medial surface after a lateral tap confirms an effusion—a positive "bulge sign."

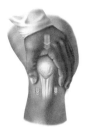

Milk downward

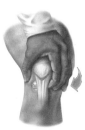

Apply medial pressure

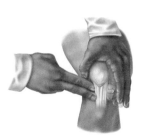

Tap and watch for fluid wave

| EXAMINATION TECHNIQUES | POSSIBLE FINDINGS |

- *Balloon sign* (major effusions): Compress suprapatellar pouch with one hand; with thumb and finger of other hand, feel for fluid entering the spaces next to the patella.

A palpable fluid wave is a positive sign.

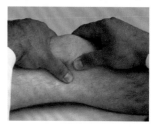

- *Ballotte the patella* (major effusion): Push the patella sharply against the femur; watch for fluid returning to the suprapatellar space.

Visible wave is a positive sign.

Assess range of motion: flexion, extension, internal and external rotation.

Use maneuvers to assess menisci and ligaments.

- *Medial meniscus and lateral meniscus—McMurray test:* With the patient supine, grasp the heel and flex the knee. Cup your other hand over the knee joint with fingers and thumb along the medial joint line. From the heel, externally rotate the lower leg, then push on the lateral side to apply a valgus stress on the medial side of the joint. Slowly extend the lower leg in external rotation.

Click or pop along the medial joint with valgus stress, external rotation, and leg extension in tear of posterior medial meniscus.

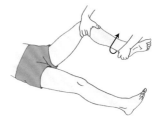

The same maneuver with internal rotation stresses the lateral meniscus.

Chapter 16 | The Musculoskeletal System

EXAMINATION TECHNIQUES

- *Medial collateral ligament:* With knee slightly flexed, push medially against lateral surface of knee with one hand and pull laterally at the ankle with the other hand (*abduction* or *valgus stress*).

- *Lateral collateral ligament (LCL):* With knee slightly flexed, push laterally along medial surface of knee with one hand and pull medially at the ankle with the other hand (an *adduction* or *varus stress*).

- *Anterior cruciate ligament (ACL):* (1) With knee flexed, place thumbs on medial and lateral joint line and place fingers on hamstring insertions. Pull tibia forward, observe if tibia slides forward "like a drawer." Compare to opposite knee.

(2) *Lachman test:* Grasp the distal femur with one hand and the proximal tibia with the other (place the thumb on the joint line). Move the femur forward and the tibia back.

POSSIBLE FINDINGS

Pain or a gap in the medial joint line points to a partial or complete MCL tear.

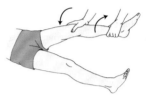

Pain or a gap in the lateral joint line points to a partial or complete LCL tear.

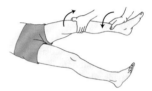

Forward slide of proximal tibia is a positive *anterior drawer sign* in ACL laxity or tear.

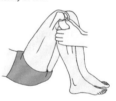

Significant forward excursion of tibia in ACL tear

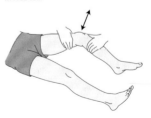

| EXAMINATION TECHNIQUES | POSSIBLE FINDINGS |

- *Posterior cruciate ligament (PCL): Posterior drawer sign:* Position patient and hands as in the ACL test. Push the tibia posteriorly and observe for posterior movement, like a drawer sliding posteriorly.

Isolated PCL tears are rare.

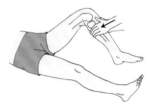

ANKLES AND FEET

Inspect ankles and feet.

Hallux valgus, corns, calluses

Palpate:

- Ankle joint

Tender joint in arthritis

- Ankle ligaments: medial-deltoid; lateral-anterior and posterior talofibular, calcaneofibular

Tenderness in sprain: lateral ligaments weaker, inversion injuries (ankle bows outward) more common

- Achilles tendon

Rheumatoid nodules, tenderness in tendonitis

- Compress the metatarsophalangeal joints; then palpate each joint between the thumb and forefinger.

Tenderness in arthritis, Morton's neuroma third and fourth MTP joints; inflammation of first MTP joint in gout

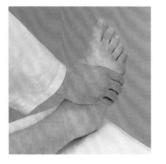

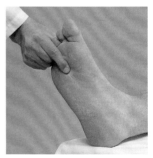

Chapter 16 | The Musculoskeletal System

EXAMINATION TECHNIQUES	POSSIBLE FINDINGS

Assess range of motion.

- Dorsiflex and plantar flex the ankle (*tibiotalar joint*).

  Arthritic joint often painful when moved in any direction; sprain, when injured ligament is stretched

- Stabilize the ankle and invert and evert the heel (*subtalar* or *talocalcaneal joint*).

  Ankle sprain

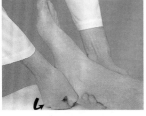

INVERSION

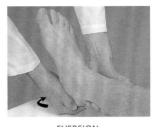

EVERSION

- Stabilize the heel and invert and evert the forefoot (*transverse tarsal joints*).

  Trauma, arthritis

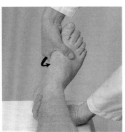

INVERSION

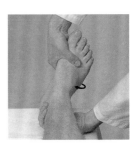

EVERSION

- Move proximal phalanx of each toe up and down (metatarsophalangeal joints).

SPECIAL TECHNIQUES

EXAMINATION TECHNIQUES

Measuring Leg Length. Patient's legs should be aligned symmetrically. With a tape, measure distance from anterior superior iliac spine to medial malleolus. Tape should cross knee medially.

Measuring Range of Motion. To measure range of motion precisely, a simple pocket goniometer is needed. Estimates may be made visually. Movement in the elbow at the right is limited to range indicated by red lines.

POSSIBLE FINDINGS

Unequal leg length may be the cause of *scoliosis*.

A flexion deformity of 45 degrees and further flexion to 90 degrees (45 degrees → 90 degrees)

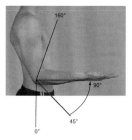

Recording Your Findings

Recording the Physical Examination—The Musculoskeletal System

"Full range of motion in all joints. No evidence of swelling or deformity."
OR
"Full range of motion in all joints. Hand with degenerative changes of Heberden's nodes at the distal interphalangeal joints, Bouchard's nodes at proximal interphalangeal joints. Mild pain with flexion, extension, and rotation of both hips. Full range of motion in the knees, with moderate crepitus; no effusion but boggy synovium and osteophytes along the tibiofemoral joint line bilaterally. Both feet with hallux valgus at the first metatarsophalangeal joints." (*Suggests osteoarthritis.*)

Aids to Interpretation

Table 16-1 Low Back Pain

Patterns	Physical Signs
Mechanical Low Back Pain Aching pain in lumbosacral area; may radiate into lower leg, along L5 or S1 dermatomes. Usually acute, work related, in age group 30 to 50 years; no underlying pathology	Paraspinal muscle or facet tenderness, muscle spasm or pain with back movement, loss of normal lumbar lordosis but no motor or sensory loss or reflex abnormalities. In osteoporosis, check for thoracic kyphosis, percussion tenderness over a spinous process, or fractures in the thoracic spine or hip.
Sciatica (Radicular Low Back Pain) Usually from disc herniation; more rarely from nerve root compression, primary or metastatic tumor	Disc herniation most likely if calf wasting, weak ankle dorsiflexion, absent ankle jerk, positive *crossed straight-leg raise* (pain in affected leg when healthy leg tested); negative straight-leg raise makes diagnosis highly unlikely.
Lumbar Spinal Stenosis Pseudoclaudication pain in the back or legs that improves with rest, forward lumbar flexion. Pain vague but usually bilateral, with paresthesias in one or both legs; usually from arthritic narrowing of spinal canal	Posture may be flexed forward with lower extremity weakness and hyporeflexia; straight-leg raise usually negative

(continued)

Table 16-1	Low Back Pain *(continued)*
Patterns	**Physical Signs**
Chronic Back Stiffness Consider ankylosing spondylitis in inflammatory polyarthritis, most common in men younger than 40 years. Diffuse idiopathic skeletal hyperostosis (DISH) affects men more than women, usually age older than 50 years.	Loss of the normal lumbar lordosis, muscle spasm, limited anterior and lateral flexion; improves with exercise. Lateral immobility of the spine, especially thoracic segment
Nocturnal Back Pain, Unrelieved by Rest Consider metastasis to spine from cancer of the prostate, breast, lung, thyroid, and kidney, and multiple myeloma.	Findings vary with the source. Local vertebral tenderness may be present.
Pain Referred from the Abdomen or Pelvis Usually a deep, aching pain, the level of which varies with the source (~2% of low back pain)	Spinal movements are not painful and range of motion is not affected. Look for signs of the primary disorder, such as peptic ulcer, pancreatitis, dissecting aortic aneurysm.

Table 16-2	Pains in the Neck
Patterns	**Physical Signs**
Mechanical Neck Pain Aching pain in the cervical paraspinal muscles and ligaments with associated muscle spasm, stiffness, and tightness in the upper back and shoulder, lasting up to 6 weeks. No associated radiation, paresthesias, or weakness. Headache may be present.	Local muscle tenderness, pain on movement. No neurologic deficits. Possible trigger points in *fibromyalgia*. *Torticollis* if prolonged abnormal neck posture and muscle spasm.
Mechanical Neck Pain—Whiplash Also mechanical neck pain with aching paracervical pain and stiffness, often beginning the day after injury. Occipital headache, dizziness, malaise, and fatigue may be present. Chronic whiplash syndrome if symptoms last more than 6 months, present in 20% to 40% of injuries.	Localized paracervical tenderness, decreased neck range of motion, perceived weakness of the upper extremities. Causes of cervical cord compression such as fracture, herniation, head injury, or altered consciousness are excluded.
Cervical Radiculopathy—from nerve root compression Sharp burning or tingling pain in the neck and one arm, with associated paresthesias and weakness. Sensory symptoms often in myotomal pattern, deep in muscle, rather than dermatomal pattern.	C7 nerve root affected most often (45%–60%), with weakness in triceps and finger flexors and extensors. C6 nerve root involvement also common, with weakness in biceps, brachioradialis, wrist extensors.

(continued)

Table 16-2	Pains in the Neck (continued)
Patterns	**Physical Signs**
Cervical Myelopathy—from cervical cord compression Neck pain with bilateral weakness and paresthesias in both upper and lower extremities, often with urinary frequency. Hand clumsiness, palmar paresthesias, and gait changes may be subtle. Neck flexion often exacerbates symptoms.	Hyperreflexia; clonus at the wrist, knee, or ankle; extensor plantar reflexes (positive Babinski signs); and gait disturbances. May also see *Lhermitte's sign:* neck flexion with resulting sensation of electrical shock radiating down the spine. Confirmation of cervical myelopathy warrants neck immobilization and neurosurgical evaluation.

Table 16-3   Patterns of Pain in and Around the Joints

	Rheumatoid Arthritis	Osteoarthritis (Degenerative Joint Disease, or DJD)
Process	Chronic inflammation of synovial membranes with secondary erosion of adjacent cartilage and bone, damage to ligaments and tendons	Degeneration and progressive loss of cartilage within joints, damage to underlying bone, formation of new bone at margins of cartilage
Common Locations	Hands (proximal interphalangeal and metacarpophalangeal joints), feet (metatarsophalangeal joints), wrists, knees, elbows, ankles	Knees, hips, hands (distal, sometimes proximal interphalangeal joints), cervical and lumbar spine, and wrists (first carpometacarpal joint); also joints previously injured or diseased
Pattern of Spread	Symmetrically additive: progresses to other joints; persists in initial ones	Additive; however, sometimes only one joint affected
Onset	Usually insidious	Usually insidious
Progression and Duration	Often chronic, with remissions and exacerbations	Slowly progressive, with exacerbations after overuse
Associated Symptoms	Frequent swelling of synovial tissue in joints or tendon sheaths; also subcutaneous nodules Tender, often warm but seldom red Prominent stiffness, often for >1 hour in mornings	Small joint effusions may be present, especially in knees; also bony enlargement Tender, seldom warm or red Frequent but brief stiffness in the morning

| Table 16-4 | **Painful Shoulders** |

Acromioclavicular Arthritis

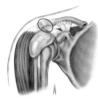

Tenderness over the acromioclavicular joint, especially with adduction of the arm across the chest. Pain often increases with shrugging the shoulders, due to movement of scapula.

Subacromial and Subdeltoid Bursitis

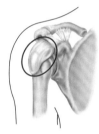

Pain over anterior superior aspect of shoulder, particularly when raising the arm overhead. Tenderness common anterolateral to the acromion, in hollow recess formed by the acromiohumeral sulcus. Often seen in overuse syndromes.

Rotator Cuff Tendinitis

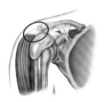

Tenderness over the rotator cuff, when elbow passively lifted posteriorly or with "drop-arm" maneuver.

Bicipital Tendinitis

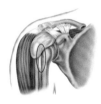

Tenderness over the long head of the biceps when rolled in the bicipital groove or when flexed arm is supinated against resistance suggests *bicipital tendinitis*.

Table 16-5 Painful Knees

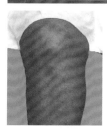

Arthritis. *Degenerative arthritis* usually occurs after age 50; associated with obesity. Often with medial joint line tenderness, palpable osteophytes, bowleg appearance, suprapatellar bursae and joint effusion. Systemic involvement, swelling, and subcutaneous nodules in *rheumatoid arthritis*.

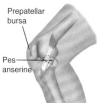

Bursitis. Inflammation and thickening of bursa seen in repetitive motion and overuse syndromes. Can involve *prepatellar bursa* ("housemaid's knee"), *pes anserine* bursa medially (runners, osteoarthritis), *iliotibial band* laterally (over lateral femoral condyle), especially in runners.

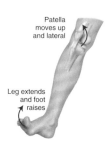

Patellofemoral instability. During flexion and extension of knee, due to subluxation and/or malalignment, patella tracks laterally instead of centrally in trochlear groove of femoral condyle. Inspect or palpate for lateral motion with leg extension. May lead to chondromalacia, osteoarthritis.

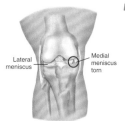

Meniscal tear. Commonly arises from twisting injury of knee; in older patients may be degenerative, often with clicking, popping, or locking sensation. Check for tenderness along joint line over medial or lateral meniscus and for effusion. May have associated tears of medial collateral of anterior cruciate ligaments.

(continued)

Table 16-5 Painful Knees (continued)

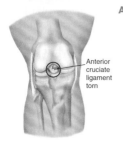

Anterior cruciate tear or sprain. In twisting injuries of the knee, often with popping sensation, immediate swelling, pain with flexion/extension, difficulty walking, and sensation of knee "giving way." Check for anterior drawer sign, swelling of hemarthrosis, injuries to medial meniscus or medial collateral ligament. Consider evaluation by an orthopedic surgeon.

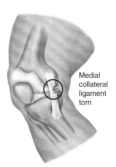

Collateral ligament sprain or tear. From force applied to medial or lateral surface of knee (valgus or varus stress), producing localized swelling, pain, stiffness. Patients able to walk but may develop an effusion. Check for tenderness over affected ligament and ligamentous laxity during valgus or varus stress.

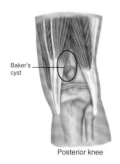

Posterior knee

Baker's cyst. Cystic swelling palpable on the medial surface of the popliteal fossa, prompting complaints of aching or fullness behind the knee. Inspect, palpate for swelling adjacent to medial hamstring tendons. If present, suggests involvement of posterior horn of medial meniscus. In rheumatoid arthritis, cyst may expand into calf or ankle.

CHAPTER 17

The Nervous System

Fundamentals for Assessing the Nervous System

The *central nervous system* (CNS) consists of the brain and spinal cord. The *peripheral nervous system* consists of the 12 pairs of cranial nerves and the spinal and peripheral nerves. Most peripheral nerves contain both motor and sensory fibers.

CENTRAL NERVOUS SYSTEM

The Brain

- *Gray matter*, or aggregations of neuronal cell bodies; rims the surfaces of the cerebral hemispheres, forming the cerebral cortex

- *White matter*, or neuronal axons coated with myelin, allowing nerve impulses to travel more rapidly

- *Basal ganglia*, which affect movement

- *Thalamus*, which processes and relays sensory impulses to the cerebral cortex

- *Hypothalamus*, which maintains homeostasis and regulates temperature, heart rate, and blood pressure; affects endocrine system, and governs emotional behaviors such as anger and sex drive; and contains hormones that act directly on the pituitary gland

- *Brainstem*, which connects the upper part of the brain with the spinal cord and has three sections: midbrain, pons, and medulla

- *Reticular activating (arousal) system,* in the diencephalon and upper brainstem; activation linked to consciousness

- *Cerebellum,* at the base of the brain, which coordinates all movement and helps maintain the body upright in space

The Spinal Cord

- A cylindrical mass of nerve tissue encased within the bony vertebral column, extending from medulla to first or second lumbar vertebra

- Contains important motor and sensory nerve pathways that exit and enter the cord via anterior and posterior nerve roots and spinal and peripheral nerves

- Mediates reflex activity of the deep tendon (or spinal nerve) reflexes

- Divided into five segments: cervical (C1–8), thoracic (T1–12), lumbar (L1–5), sacral (S1–5), and coccygeal

- Roots fan out like a horse's tail at L1–2, the *cauda equina*

 PERIPHERAL NERVOUS SYSTEM

The Cranial Nerves

- Cranial nerves I and II are actually fiber tracts emerging from the brain.

- Cranial nerves III through XII arise from the diencephalon and brainstem.

The Peripheral Nerves

- Thirty-one pairs of nerves carry impulses to and from the cord: 8 cervical, 12 thoracic, 5 lumbar, 5 sacral, and 1 coccygeal.

- Each nerve has an anterior (ventral) root containing motor fibers, and a posterior (dorsal) root containing sensory fibers.

- These merge to form a short (<5 mm) *spinal nerve*.

- Spinal nerve fibers commingle with similar fibers in plexuses outside the cord—from these emerge *peripheral nerves*.

The Health History

Common or Concerning Symptoms

- Headache
- Dizziness or vertigo
- Generalized, proximal, or distal weakness
- Numbness, abnormal or lost sensations
- Loss of consciousness, syncope, or near-syncope
- Seizures
- Tremors or involuntary movements

Headache: ask about location, severity, duration, and any associated symptoms, such as visual changes, weakness, or loss of sensation. Ask if coughing, sneezing, or sudden movements of the head affect the headache.

See Table 7-1, Primary Headaches, p. 111, and Table 7-2, Secondary Headaches, pp. 112–113. *Subarachnoid hemorrhage* may evoke "the worst headache of my life." Dull headache affected by maneuvers, especially on awakening and in the same location are seen in mass lesions such as brain tumors

Dizziness can have many meanings. Is the patient lightheaded or feeling faint (*presyncope*)? Is there unsteady gait from disequilibrium or ataxia, or true *vertigo*, a perception that the room is spinning or rotating?

Lightheadedness in palpitations; near-syncope from vasovagal stimulation, low blood pressure, febrile illness, and others; vertigo in benign positional vertigo, Ménière's disease, brainstem tumor

Are any medications contributing to dizziness?

Are associated symptoms present, such as double vision (*diplopia*), difficulty forming words (*dysarthria*), or difficulty with gait or balance (*ataxia*)? Is there any weakness?

Diplopia, dysarthria, ataxia in vertebrobasilar *transient ischemic attack (TIA)* or *stroke*

See Table 17-1, Types of Stroke, pp. 308–311

Weakness or paralysis in *TIA* or *stroke*

Distinguish *proximal* from *distal* **weakness**. For *proximal weakness*, ask about combing hair, reaching for things on a high shelf, difficulty getting out of a chair or taking a high step up. For *distal weakness*, ask about hand movements such as opening a jar or can or using hand tools (e.g., scissors, pliers, screwdriver). Ask about frequent tripping.

Bilateral proximal weakness in *myopathy*; bilateral, predominantly distal weakness in *polyneuropathy*; weakness worsened by repeated effort and improved by rest in *myasthenia gravis*

Is there any **loss of sensation**, difficulty moving a limb, or altered sensation such as tingling or pins and needles? Peculiar sensations without an obvious stimulus (*paresthesias*)? *Dysesthesias*, or disordered sensations in response to a stimulus, may last longer than the stimulus itself.

Loss of sensation, paresthesias, and dysesthesias in brain and spinal cord lesions; also in disorders of peripheral sensory roots and nerves; paresthesias in hands and around mouth in hyperventilation

Synope: "Have you ever fainted or passed out?" leads to discussion of any *loss of consciousness (syncope)*.

Syncope if sudden but temporary loss of consciousness from decreased cerebral blood flow, commonly called *fainting*.

Get a complete description of the event. What brought on the episode? Were there any warning symptoms? Was the patient standing, sitting, or lying down when it began? How long did it last? Could voices be heard while passing out and coming to? How rapid was recovery? Were onset and offset slow or fast?

Young people with emotional stress and warning symptoms of flushing, warmth, or nausea may have *vasodepressor (or vasovagal) syncope* of slow onset, slow offset. *Cardiac syncope* from dysrhythmias, more common in older patients, often with sudden onset, sudden offset.

Also ask if anyone observed the episode. What did the patient look like before, during, and after the episode? Was there any seizurelike movement of the arms or legs? Any incontinence of the bladder or bowel?

Tonic–clonic motor activity, incontinence, and *postictal state* in generalized *seizures*. Unlike syncope, injury such as tongue biting or bruising of limbs may occur.

A **seizure** is a paroxysmal disorder caused by sudden excessive electrical discharge in the cerebral cortex or its underlying structures.

Depending on the type of seizure, there may be loss of consciousness or abnormal feelings, thought processes, and sensations, including smells, as well as abnormal movements.

Health Promotion and Counseling: Evidence and Recommendations

Important Topics for Health Promotion and Counseling

- Preventing stroke or transient ischemic attack (TIA)
- Preventing risk of peripheral neuropathy
- Preventing the "three Ds": delirium, dementia, and depression

Preventing Stroke or TIA. Cerebrovascular disease is the third leading cause of death in the United States. Decreased vascular perfusion results in sudden focal but transient brain dysfunction in *TIA*, or in permanent neurological deficits in *stroke*, as determined by neurodiagnostic imaging.

Counsel patients about the *warning signs of stroke:* sudden numbness or weakness of the face, arm, or leg; sudden confusion or trouble speaking or understanding; sudden difficulty walking, dizziness, or loss of balance or coordination; sudden trouble seeing in one or both eyes; or sudden severe headache. Detecting TIAs is important—in the first 3 months after a TIA, subsequent stroke occurs in approximately 15% of patients.

Primary prevention of stroke requires aggressive management of risk factors and patient education. Risk factors include smoking, excess weight, hypertension, dyslipidemia, heavy alcohol use, physical inactivity, obesity, and diabetes. Blood pressure should be ≤140/90 mm Hg and ≤130/80 mm Hg for those with diabetes or renal disease with proteinuria. Lipid-lowering agents may reduce risk of stroke. Urge patients to replace saturated and transunsaturated fats, found in dairy products, meat, and stick margarine, with polyunsaturated and unhydrogenated monosaturated fats, found in soybeans, liquid margarine, and fish oils. Or recommend increased intake of fruits, vegetables, and fiber. Encourage regular exercise, optimal body weight, and moderate intake of alcohol. Aim for optimal blood glucose levels, approximately 100 mg/dL for patients with diabetes.

Preventing Risk of Peripheral Neuropathy. In diabetics, promote optimal glucose control to reduce risk of sensorimotor polyneuropathy, autonomic dysfunction, mononeuritis multiplex, or diabetic neuropathy.

Preventing the "Three Ds": Delirium, Dementia, and Depression

Delirium is an acute confusional state marked by sudden onset, fluctuating course, inattention and changes in the level of consciousness; it is often undetected. Learn to use the Confusional Assessment Method (CAM) algorithm.

Dementia is best assessed by the Mini-Mental State examination and the Mini-Cog, but may be difficult to distinguish from *benign forgetfulness* and *mild cognitive impairment.*

Depression is common in individuals with significant medical conditions. See screening questions on p. 45, Chapter 3. See also Chapter 20, The Older Adult, pp. 378–379, and Table 20-2, Delirium and Dementia, pp. 391–392, and Table 20-3, Screening for Dementia: The Mini-Cog, p. 393.

Techniques of Examination

Cranial Nerves and Function

No.	Cranial Nerve	Function
I	Olfactory	Sense of smell
II	Optic	Vision
III	Oculomotor	Pupillary constriction, opening the eye (lid elevation), and most extraocular movements
IV	Trochlear	Downward, internal rotation of the eye
V	Trigeminal	*Motor*—temporal and masseter muscles (jaw clenching), also lateral pterygoid's (lateral jaw movement)
		Sensory—facial. The nerve has three divisions: (1) ophthalmic, (2) maxillary, and (3) mandibular.
VI	Abducens	Lateral deviation of the eye
VII	Facial	*Motor*—facial movements, including those of facial expression, closing the eye, and closing the mouth
		Sensory—taste for salty, sweet, sour, and bitter substances on the anterior two-thirds of the tongue
VIII	Acoustic	Hearing (cochlear division) and balance (vestibular division)
IX	Glossopharyngeal	*Motor*—pharynx
		Sensory—posterior portions of the eardrum and ear canal, the pharynx, and the posterior tongue, including taste (salty, sweet, sour, bitter)
X	Vagus	*Motor*—palate, pharynx, and larynx
		Sensory—pharynx and larynx
XI	Spinal accessory	*Motor*—the sternomastoid and upper portion of the trapezius
XII	Hypoglossal	*Motor*—tongue

| EXAMINATION TECHNIQUES | POSSIBLE FINDINGS |

CRANIAL NERVES

CN I (OLFACTORY)

Test sense of smell on each side. — Loss in frontal lobe lesions

CN II (OPTIC)

Assess visual acuity. — Blindness

Check visual fields. — Hemianopsia

Inspect optic discs. — Papilledema, optic atrophy

CN II, III (OPTIC AND OCULOMOTOR)

Test pupillary reactions to light. If abnormal, test reactions to near effort. — Blindness, CN III paralysis, tonic pupils; Horner's syndrome may affect light reactions

CN III, IV, VI (OCULOMOTOR, TROCHLEAR, AND ABDUCENS)

Assess extraocular movements. — Strabismus from paralysis of CN III, IV, or VI; nystagmus, intranuclear opthalmoplegia

CN V (TRIGEMINAL)

Test pain and light touch sensations on face in (1) ophthalmic, (2) maxillary and (3) mandibular zones.

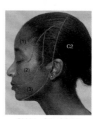

CN V—SENSORY

EXAMINATION TECHNIQUES	POSSIBLE FINDINGS
Feel the contractions of temporal and masseter muscles.	Motor or sensory loss from lesions of CN V or its higher motor pathways

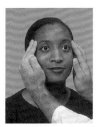

TEMPORAL MUSCLES

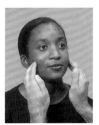

MASSETER MUSCLES

Check corneal reflexes.

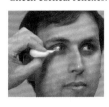

CN VII (FACIAL)

Ask patient to raise both eyebrows, frown, close eyes tightly, show teeth, smile, and puff out cheeks.

Weakness from lesion of peripheral nerve, as in Bell's palsy, or of CNS, as in a stroke. See Table 17-2, Facial Paralysis, p. 312.

CN VIII (ACOUSTIC)

Assess hearing of whispered voice. If decreased:

- Test for lateralization (*Weber test*).

Sensorineural loss causes lateralization to affected ear where AC > BC. Conduction loss causes lateralization to affected ear and BC > AC. See p. 108.

- Compare air and bone conduction (*Rinne test*).

See p. 108.

EXAMINATION TECHNIQUES	POSSIBLE FINDINGS

CN IX, X (GLOSSOPHARYNGEAL AND VAGUS)

Observe any difficulty swallowing.	A weakened palate or pharynx impairs swallowing.
Listen to the voice.	Hoarseness or nasality
Watch soft palate rise with "ah."	Palatal paralysis in CVA
Test gag reflex on each side.	Absent reflex is often normal.

CN XI (SPINAL ACCESSORY)

Trapezius Muscles. Assess muscles for bulk, involuntary movements, and strength of shoulder shrug.	Atrophy, fasciculations, weakness

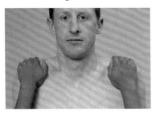

Sternomastoid Muscles. Assess strength as head turns against your hand.	Weakness of sternomastoid muscle when head turns to *opposite* side

CN XII (HYPOGLOSSAL)

Listen to patient's articulation.	Dysarthria from damage to CN X or CN XII
Inspect the resting tongue.	Atrophy, fasciculations in ALS, polio
Inspect the protruded tongue.	Deviation to weak side in contralateral CVA

THE MOTOR SYSTEM

See Table 17-3, Motor Disorders, p. 313.

BODY POSITION

Observe the patient's body position during movement and at rest.	Hemiplegia in stroke

EXAMINATION TECHNIQUES

INVOLUNTARY MOVEMENTS

If present, observe location, quality, rate, rhythm, amplitude, and setting.

MUSCLE BULK AND TONE

Inspect muscle contours.

Assess resistance to passive stretch of arms and legs.

MUSCLE STRENGTH

Test and grade the major muscle groups, with the examiner providing resistance.

POSSIBLE FINDINGS

Tremors, fasciculations, tics, chorea, athetosis, oral–facial dyskinesias. See Table 17-4, Involuntary Movements, pp. 314–315.

Atrophy of bulk. See Table 17-5, Disorders of Muscle Tone, p. 316.

Spasticity, rigidity, flaccidity of tone

Grading Muscle Strength

Grade	Description
0	No muscular contraction detected
1	A barely detectable trace of contraction
2	Active movement with gravity eliminated
3	Active movement against gravity
4	Active movement against gravity and some resistance
5	Active movement against full resistance (normal)

Look for a pattern if any detectable *weakness*. It may suggest a lower motor neuron lesion affecting a peripheral nerve or nerve root. Weakness of one side of body suggests an upper motor neuron lesion. A *polyneuropathy* causes symmetric distal weakness, and a *myopathy* usually causes proximal weakness. Weakness that worsens with repeated effort and improves with rest suggests *myasthenia gravis*.

| EXAMINATION TECHNIQUES | POSSIBLE FINDINGS |

- Elbow flexion (C5, C6)—biceps

- Elbow extension (C6, C7, C8)—triceps

- Wrist extension (C6, C7, C8)—radial nerve

    Peripheral radial nerve damage; central *stroke* or *multiple sclerosis* if hemiplegia

- Grip (C7, C8, T1)

    Weak grip in *cervical radiculopathy, de Quervain's tenosynovitis, carpal tunnel syndrome*

- Finger abduction (C8, T1)—ulnar nerve

    Weak in ulnar nerve disorders

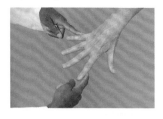

- Thumb opposition (C8, T1)—median nerve

    Weak in *Carpal tunnel syndrome*

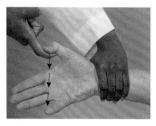

- Trunk—flexion extension, lateral bending

- Hip flexion (L2, L3, L4)—iliopsoas

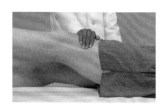

Chapter 17 | The Nervous System

| EXAMINATION TECHNIQUES | POSSIBLE FINDINGS |

- Hip extension (S1)—gluteus maximus

- Hip adduction (L2, L3, L4)—adductors

- Hip abduction (L4, L5, S1)—gluteus medius and minimus

- Knee extension (L2, L3, L4)—quadriceps

- Knee flexion (L4, L5, S1, S2)—hamstrings

- Ankle dorsiflexion (L4, L5)

- Ankle plantar flexion (S1)

COORDINATION

Check *rapid alternating movements* in arms and legs (tap foot)

Clumsy, slow movements in cerebellar disease

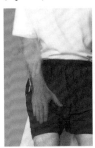

Point-to-point movements in arms and legs–finger to nose, heel to shin

Clumsy, unsteady movements in cerebellar disease

Gait. Ask patient to:

- Walk away, turn, and come back

CVA, cerebellar ataxia, parkinsonism, or loss of position sense may affect performance.

| EXAMINATION TECHNIQUES | POSSIBLE FINDINGS |

- Walk heel to toe

Ataxia

- Walk on toes, then on heels

Corticospinal tract injury

- Hop in place on each foot; do one-legged shallow knee bends. Substitute rising from a chair and climbing on a stool for hops and bends as indicated.

Proximal hip girdle weakness increases risk of falls.

Stance

- Do a *Romberg test* (a sensory test of stance). Ask patient to stand with feet together and eyes open, then closed for 20 to 30 seconds. Mild swaying may occur. Stand close by to prevent falls.

Loss of balance when eyes are closed is a *positive* Romberg test, suggesting poor position sense.

- Look for a *pronator drift* as patient holds arms forward, with eyes closed, for 20 to 30 seconds.

Flexion and pronation at elbow and downward drift of arm from *contralateral corticospinal tract lesion*

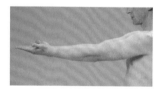
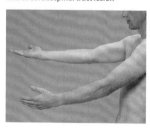

Ask patient to keep arms up and tap them downward. A smooth return to position is normal.

Weakness, incoordination, poor position sense

THE SENSORY SYSTEM

Use an object like a broken cotton swab to test sharp and dull sensation; compare **symmetric areas on the two sides of the body.** Do not reuse the object on another patient.

A hemisensory loss pattern suggests a contralateral cortical lesion.

EXAMINATION TECHNIQUES	POSSIBLE FINDINGS

Compare proximal and distal areas of arms and legs for *pain, temperature,* and *touch sensation.* Scatter stimuli to sample most dermatomes and major peripheral nerves.

"Glove-and-stocking" loss of peripheral neuropathy, often seen in alcoholism and diabetes

See Table 17-6, Dermatones, pp. 317–318.

Map any area of abnormal response, including dermatomes, if present.

Dermatomal sensory loss in *herpes zoster, nerve root compression.*

Assess response to the following stimuli, with the patient's eyes closed.

- *Pain.* Use the sharp end of a pin or other suitable tool. The dull end serves as a control.

Analgesia, hypalgesia, hyperalgesia

- *Temperature* (if indicated). Use test tubes with hot and cold water, or other objects of suitable temperature.

Temperature and pain sensation usually correlate.

- *Light touch.* Use a fine wisp of cotton.

Anesthesia, hyperesthesia

Check for *vibration and position senses.* If responses are abnormal, test more proximally

Loss of vibration and position senses in peripheral neuropathy from diabetes or alcoholism and in posterior column disease from syphilis or vitamin B_{12} deficiency

- *Vibration and position.* Vibration: Use a 128-Hz tuning fork, held on a *bony* prominence. Vibration and position senses, both carried in the posterior columns, often correlate.

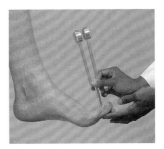

EXAMINATION TECHNIQUES

- *Position.* Holding patient's finger or big toe by its sides, move it up or down.

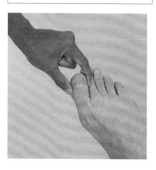

POSSIBLE FINDINGS

Assess *discriminative* sensations:

- *Stereognosis.* Ask for identification of a common object placed in patient's hand.

Lesions in the posterior columns or sensory cortex impair stereognosis, number identification, and two-point discrimination.

- *Number identification (graphesthesia).* Draw a number on patient's palm with blunt end of a pen and ask the patient to identify the number.

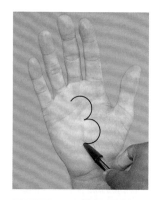

- *Two-point discrimination.* Use two pins of the sides of a paper clip to find minimal distance on pad of patient's finger at which two points can be distinguished (normally <5 mm).

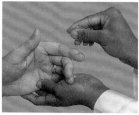

Chapter 17 | The Nervous System

EXAMINATION TECHNIQUES

POSSIBLE FINDINGS

- *Point localization.* Touch skin briefly, and ask patient to open both eyes and identify the place touched.

  A lesion in the sensory cortex may impair point localization on the contralateral side and cause extinction of the touch sensation.

- *Extinction.* Simultaneously touch opposite, corresponding areas of the body; ask whether the patient feels one touch or two.

REFLEXES

Grading Reflexes

Grade	Description
4+	Hyperactive (clonus must be present)
3+	Brisker than average, not necessarily abnormal
2+	Average, normal
1+	Diminished, low normal
0	No response

Biceps (C5, C6)

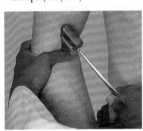

Triceps (C6, C7)

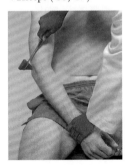

Hyperactive deep tendon reflexes, absent abdominal reflexes, and a positive Babinski response in *upper motor neuron lesions*

EXAMINATION TECHNIQUES	POSSIBLE FINDINGS

Supinator (brachioradialis) (C5, C6)

Knee (L2, L3, L4)

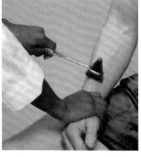
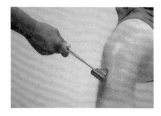

Ankle (S1)

Check for clonus if reflexes seem hyperactive.

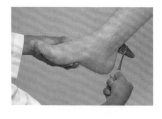
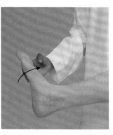

Ankle jerks symmetrically, decreased or absent in peripheral polyneuropathy; slowed ankle jerk in hypothyroidism.

CUTANEOUS STIMULATION REFLEXES

Abdominal reflexes (upper T8, T9, T10; lower T10, T11, T12)

May be absent with upper or lower neuron lesions

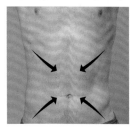

| EXAMINATION TECHNIQUES | POSSIBLE FINDINGS |

Plantar response (L5, S1), normally flexor

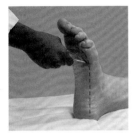

Babinski extensor response (big toe fans up) from corticospinal tract lesion

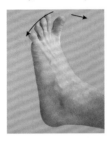

Anal Reflex. With a dull object, stroke outward from anus in four quadrants. Watch for anal contraction.

Loss of reflex suggests cauda equina lesion at the S2–3–4 level.

SPECIAL TECHNIQUES

Meningeal Signs. With patient supine, flex head and neck toward chest. Note resistance or pain, and watch for flexion of hips and knees (*Brudzinski's sign*).

Meningeal irritation in the subarachnoid space may cause resistance or pain on flexion during both maneuvers.

Flex one of patient's legs at hip and knee, then straighten knee. Note resistance or pain (*Kernig's sign*).

A compressed lumbosacral nerve root also causes pain on straightening the knee of the raised leg.

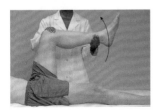

| EXAMINATION TECHNIQUES | POSSIBLE FINDINGS |

Lumbosacral Radiculopathy: Straight-Leg Raise.

With patient supine, raise relaxed and straightened leg, flexing the leg at the hip. Then dorsiflex the foot.

Pain and muscle weakness if herniated disc; ipsilateral calf wasting and weak ankle dorsiflexion may also be present.

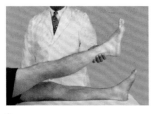

Asterixis. Ask patient to hold both arms forward, with hands cocked up and fingers spread. Watch for 1 to 2 minutes.

Sudden brief flexions in liver disease, uremia and hypercapnia.

Winging of the Scapula. Ask patient to push against the wall of your hand with a partially straightened arm. Inspect scapula. It should stay close to the chest wall.

Winging of scapula away from chest wall suggests weakness of the serratus anterior muscle, seen in muscular dystrophy or injury to long thoracic nerve.

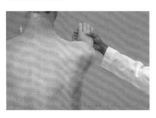 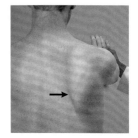

The Stuporous or Comatose Patient.

Assess ABCs (airway, breathing, and circulation).

See Table 17-7, Metabolic and Structural Coma, p. 319, Table 17-8, Glascow Coma Scale, p. 320, and Table 17-9, Pupils in Comatose Patients, p. 321.

Chapter 17 | The Nervous System

EXAMINATION TECHNIQUES	POSSIBLE FINDINGS

- Take pulse, blood pressure, and rectal temperature.

- Establish level of consciousness with escalating stimuli.
  Lethargy, obtundation, stupor, coma

However, don't dilate pupils, and **don't flex patient's neck** if any suspicion of cervical cord injury.

Levels of Consciousness

Alertness	Patient is awake and aware of self and environment. When spoken to in a normal voice, patient looks at you and responds fully and appropriately to stimuli.
Lethargy	When spoken to in a loud voice, patient appears drowsy but opens eyes and looks at you, responds to questions, and then falls asleep.
Obtundation	When shaken gently, patient opens eyes and looks at you but responds slowly and is somewhat confused. Alertness and interest in environment are decreased.
Stupor	Patient arouses from sleep only after painful stimuli. Verbal responses are slow or absent. Patient lapses into unresponsiveness when stimulus stops. Patient has minimal awareness of self or environment.
Coma	Despite repeated painful stimuli, patient remains unarousable with eyes closed. No evident response to inner need or external stimuli is shown.

- Conduct neurological examination, looking for asymmetric findings.

NEUROLOGIC EXAMINATION

Observe:

- Breathing pattern — Cheyne-Stokes, ataxic breathing

- Pupils — Asymmetric if structural lesions or brain herniation

- Ocular movements — Deviation to affected side in hemispheric stroke

EXAMINATION TECHNIQUES	POSSIBLE FINDINGS

Check for the *oculocephalic reflex (doll's eye movements).* Holding upper eyelids open, turn head quickly to each side, and then flex and extend patient's neck. This patient's head will be turned to her right.

In a comatose patient with an **intact brainstem,** the eyes move in the opposite direction, in this case to her left (doll's eye movements) as below.

Very deep coma or a lesion in the midbrain or pons abolishes this reflex, so eyes *do not move.*

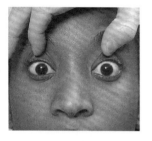

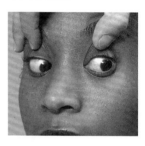

Note posture of body.

Decorticate rigidity, decerebrate rigidity, flaccid hemiplegia

Test for flaccid paralysis.

- Hold forearms vertically; note wrist positions.

A flaccid hand droops to the horizontal.

- From 12 to 18 inches above bed, drop each arm.

A flaccid arm drops more rapidly.

- Support both knees in a somewhat flexed position, and then extend each knee and let leg drop to the bed.

The flaccid leg drops more rapidly.

- From a similar starting position, release both legs.

A flaccid leg falls into extension and external rotation.

Complete the neurologic and general physical examination.

EXAMINATION TECHNIQUES

Recording Your Findings

Recording the Examination—The Nervous System

> "*Mental Status:* Alert, relaxed, and cooperative. Thought process coherent. Oriented to person, place, and time. Detailed cognitive testing deferred. *Cranial Nerves:* I—not tested; II through XII intact. *Motor:* Good muscle bulk and tone. Strength 5/5 throughout. *Cerebellar:* Rapid alternating movements (RAMs), finger-to-nose (F→N), heel-to-shin (H→S) intact. Gait with normal base. Romberg—maintains balance with eyes closed. No pronator drift. *Sensory:* Pinprick, light touch, position, and vibration intact. *Reflexes:* 2+ and symmetric with plantar reflexes downgoing."
>
> OR
>
> "*Mental Status:* The patient is alert and tries to answer questions but has difficulty finding words. *Cranial Nerves:* I—not tested; II—visual acuity intact; visual fields full; III, IV, VI—extraocular movements intact; V motor—temporal and masseter strength intact, sensory corneal reflexes present; VII motor—prominent right facial droop and flattening of right nasolabial fold, left facial movements intact, sensory—taste not tested; VIII—hearing intact bilaterally to whispered voice; IX, X—gag intact; XI—strength of sternomastoid and trapezius muscles 5/5; XII—tongue midline. *Motor:* strength in right biceps, triceps, iliopsoas, gluteals, quadriceps, hamstring, and ankle flexor and extensor muscles 3/5 with good bulk but increased tone and spasticity; strength in comparable muscle groups on the left 5/5 with good bulk and tone. Gait—unable to test. Cerebellar—unable to test on right due to right arm and leg weakness; RAMs, F→N, H→S intact on left. Romberg—unable to test due to right leg weakness. Right pronator drift present. *Sensory:* decreased sensation to pinprick over right face, arm, and leg; intact on the left. Stereognosis and two-point discrimination not tested. *Reflexes* (can record in two ways):
>
> Suggests left hemispheric CVA in distribution of the left middle cerebral artery, with right sided hemiparesis.

	Biceps	Triceps	Brach	Knee	Ankle	Pl
RT	2+	2+	2+	2+	2+	↓
LT	2+	2+	2+	2+	1+	↓

OR

(stick figure diagram with H markings at reflex points; arrows showing plantar response; labeled R and L)

Aids to Interpretation

Table 17-1 Types of Stroke

Assessing patients with stroke involves three fundamental questions:

- *What brain area and related vascular territory explain the patient's findings?*
- *Is the stroke ischemic or hemorrhagic?*
- *If ischemic, is the mechanism thrombus or embolus?*

Stroke is a medical emergency, and timing is of the essence. Answers to these questions are critical to patient outcomes and use of antithrombotic therapies.

In *acute ischemic stroke*, ischemic brain injury begins with a central core of very low perfusion and often irreversible cell death. This core is surrounded by an *ischemic penumbra* of metabolically disturbed cells that are still potentially viable, depending on restoration of blood flow and duration of ischemia. Because most irreversible damage occurs in the first 3 to 6 hours after onset of symptoms, therapies targeted to the initial 3-hour window achieve the best outcomes, with recovery in up to 50% of patients in some studies.

Understanding the pathophysiology of stroke takes dedication, expert supervision to improve techniques of neurological examination, and perseverance. *This brief overview is intended to prompt further study and practice.*

Table 17-1 Types of Stroke (continued)

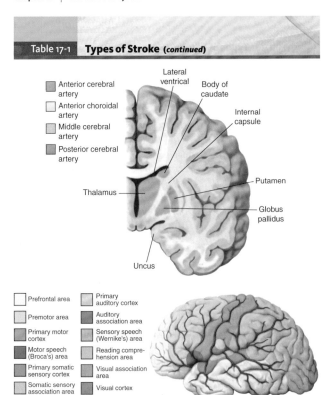

(continued)

Table 17-1 Types of Stroke *(continued)*

Clinical Features and Vascular Territories of Stroke

Major Clinical Features	Vascular Territory
Contralateral leg weakness	*Anterior circulation*—anterior cerebral artery (ACA) Includes stem of circle of Willis connecting internal carotid artery to ACA, and the segment distal to ACA and its anterior choroidal branch
Contralateral face, arm > leg weakness, sensory loss, field cut, aphasia (left MCA) or neglect, apraxia (right MCA)	*Anterior circulation*—middle cerebral artery (MCA) Largest vascular bed for stroke
Contralateral motor or sensory deficit without cortical signs	*Subcortical circulation*—lenticulostriate deep penetrating branches of MCA Small vessel subcortical *lacunar infarcts* in internal capsule, thalamus, or brainstem. Four common syndromes: pure motor hemiparesis; pure sensory hemianesthesia; ataxic hemiparesis; clumsy hand—dysarthria syndrome
Contralateral field cut	*Posterior circulation*—posterior cerebral artery (PCA) Includes paired vertebral arteries, the basilar artery, paired posterior cerebral arteries. Bilateral PCA infarction causes cortical blindness but preserved pupillary light reaction.

| Table 17-1 | Types of Stroke *(continued)* |

Clinical Features and Vascular Territories of Stroke *(continued)*

Major Clinical Features	Vascular Territory
Dysphagia, dysarthria, tongue/palate deviation and/or ataxia with crossed sensory/motor deficits (= ipsilateral face with contralateral body)	*Posterior circulation*—brainstem, vertebral, or basilar artery branches
Oculomotor deficits and/or ataxia with crossed sensory/motor deficits	*Posterior circulation*—basilar artery Complete basilar artery occlusion—"locked-in syndrome" with intact consciousness but inability to speak and quadriplegia

Source: Adapted from American College of Physicians. Stroke, in Neurology. Medical Knowledge Self-Assessment Program (MKSAP) 14. Philadelphia: American College of Physicians, 2006. pp. 52–68.

Table 17-2 Facial Paralysis

Distinguish peripheral from central lesions of CN VII by closely observing movements of the *upper face*. Because of innervation from both hemispheres, the movements are *preserved* in central lesions.

	Lesion of Peripheral Nervous System	Lesion of Central Nervous System
Side of face affected	**Same side as the lesion**	**Side opposite the lesion**
Upper face	Unable to wrinkle forehead, raise eyebrow, close eye	Movements normal or slightly weak
Lower face	Unable to smile, show teeth	Same

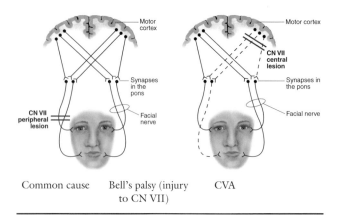

| Common cause | Bell's palsy (injury to CN VII) | CVA |

Table 17-3 Motor Disorders

	Peripheral Nervous System Disorder	Central Nervous System Disorder*	Parkinsonism (Basal Ganglia Disorder)	Cerebellar Disorder
Involuntary movements	Often fasciculations	No fasciculations	Resting tremors	Intention tremors
Muscle bulk	Atrophy	Normal or mild atrophy (disuse)	Normal	Normal
Muscle tone	Decreased or absent	Increased, spastic	Increased, rigid	Decreased
Muscle strength	Decreased or lost	Decreased or lost	Normal or slightly decreased	Normal or slightly decreased
Coordination	Unimpaired, though limited by weakness	Slowed and limited by weakness	Good, though slowed and often tremulous	Impaired, ataxic
Reflexes				
Deep tendon	Decreased or absent	Increased	Normal or decreased	Normal or decreased
Plantar	Flexor or absent	Extensor	Flexor	Flexor
Abdominals	Absent	Absent	Normal	Normal

*Upper motor neuron.

Table 17-4 Involuntary Movements

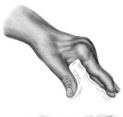

Resting static tremors. Fine, "pin-rolling" tremor seen at rest, usually disappear with movement; seen in basal ganglia disorders like Parkinson's disease.

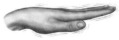

Postural tremor. Seen when maintaining active posture; in anxiety, hyperthyroidism; also familial. From basal ganglia disorder.

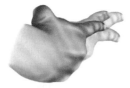

Intention tremor. Seen with intentional movement, absent at rest; in cerebellar disorders, including multiple sclerosis

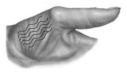

Fasciculations. Fine, rapid flickering of muscle bundles in lower motor neuron disorders.

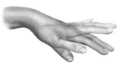

Chorea. Brief, rapid, irregular, jerky; face, head, arms, or hands (e.g., Huntington's disease)

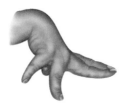

Athetosis. Slow, twisting, writhing; face, distal limbs, often with associated spasticity (e.g., cerebral palsy)

Table 17-4 Involuntary Movements (continued)

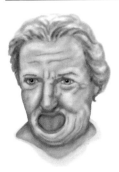

Oral-facial dyskinesias. Rhythmic, repetitive, bizarre movements of face, mouth. Tardive dyskinesias with prolonged use of psychotropic drugs such as phenothiazines

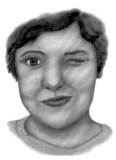

Tics. Brief, irregular, repetitive, coordinated movements (e.g., winking, shrugging); in Tourette's syndrome, users of phenothiazines, amphetamines

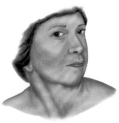

Dystonia. Grotesque, twisted postures, often in trunk or, as shown, in neck (*spasmodic torticollis*)

Table 17-5 Disorders of Muscle Tone

Spasticity	Rigidity
Location. Upper motor neuron or corticospinal tract systems.	**Location.** Basal ganglia system
Description. Increased muscle tone (*hypertonia*) that is rate-dependent. Tone is greater when passive movement is rapid, and less when passive movement is slow. Tone is also greater at the extremes of the movement arc. During rapid passive movement, initial hypertonia may give way suddenly as the limb relaxes. This spastic "catch" and relaxation is known as "clasp-knife" resistance.	**Description.** Increased resistance that persists throughout the movement arc, independent of rate of movement, is called *lead-pipe rigidity*. With flexion and extension of the wrist or forearm, a superimposed rachetlike jerkiness is called *cogwheel rigidity*.
Common Cause. Stroke, especially late or chronic stage	**Common Cause.** Parkinsonism

Flaccidity	Paratonia
Location. Lower motor neuron at any point from the anterior horn cell to the peripheral nerves	**Location.** Both hemispheres, usually in the frontal lobes
Description. Loss of muscle tone (*hypotonia*), causing the limb to be loose or floppy. The affected limbs may be hyperextensible or even flaillike.	**Description.** Sudden changes in tone with passive range of motion. Sudden loss of tone that increases the ease of motion is called *mitgehen* (moving with). Sudden increase in tone making motion more difficult is called *gegenhalten* (holding against).
Common Cause. Guillain–Barré syndrome; also initial phase of spinal cord injury (spinal shock) or stroke	**Common Cause.** Dementia

Chapter 17 | The Nervous System

Table 17-6 Dermatomes

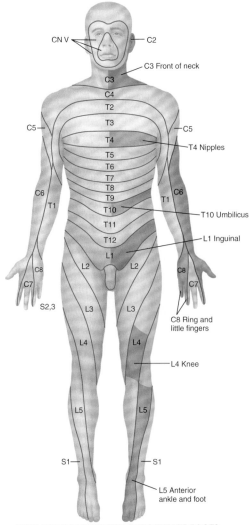

DERMATOMES INNERVATED BY POSTERIOR ROOTS

(continued)

Table 17-6 Dermatomes (continued)

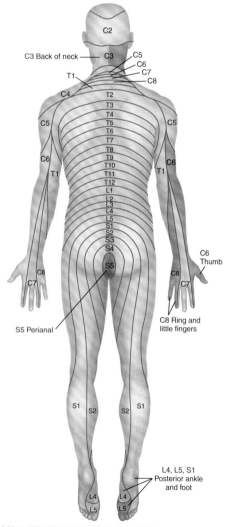

DERMATOMES INNERVATED BY POSTERIOR ROOTS

Table 17-7	**Metabolic and Structural Coma**
Toxic–Metabolic	**Structural**
Pathophysiology	
Arousal centers poisoned or critical substrates depleted	Lesion destroys or compresses brainstem arousal areas, either directly or secondary to more distant expanding mass lesions.
Clinical Features	
• Respiratory pattern. If regular, may be normal or hyperventilation. If irregular, usually Cheyne-Stokes	Respiratory pattern. Irregular, especially Cheyne-Stokes or ataxic breathing. Also with selected stereotypical patterns like "apneustic" respiration (peak inspiratory arrest) or central hyperventilation.
• Pupillary size and reaction. Equal, reactive to light. If *pinpoint* from opiates or cholinergics, you may need a magnifying glass to see the reaction. May be unreactive if *fixed and dilated* from anticholinergics or hypothermia	Pupillary size and reaction. Unequal or unreactive to light (fixed) *Midposition, fixed*—suggests midbrain compression *Dilated, fixed*—suggests compression of CN III from herniation
• Level of consciousness. Changes *after* pupils change	Level of consciousness. Changes *before* pupils change
Examples of Cause	**Examples of Cause**
Uremia, hyperglycemia	Epidural, subdural, or intracerebral hemorrhage
Alcohol, drugs, liver failure	Cerebral infarct or embolus
Hypothyroidism, hypoglycemia	Tumor, abscess
Anoxia, ischemia	
Meningitis, encephalitis	
	Brainstem infarct, tumor, or hemorrhage
Hyperthermia, hypothermia	Cerebellar infarct, hemorrhage, tumor, or abscess

Table 17-8: Glasgow Coma Scale

Activity	Score
Eye Opening	
None	1 = Even to supraorbital pressure
To pain	2 = Pain from sternum/limb/supraorbital pressure
To speech	3 = Nonspecific response, not necessarily to command
Spontaneous	4 = Eyes open, not necessarily aware _____
Motor Response	
None	1 = To any pain; limbs remain flaccid
Extension	2 = Shoulder adducted and shoulder and forearm internally rotated
Flexor response	3 = Withdrawal response or assumption of hemiplegic posture
Withdrawal	4 = Arm withdraws to pain, shoulder abducts
Localizes pain	5 = Arm attempts to remove supraorbital/chest pressure
Obeys commands	6 = Follows simple commands _____
Verbal Response	
None	1 = No verbalization of any type
Incomprehensible	2 = Moans/groans, no speech
Inappropriate	3 = Intelligible, no sustained sentences
Confused	4 = Converses but confused, disoriented
Oriented	5 = Converses and is oriented _____
	TOTAL (3–15)*

*Interpretation: Patients with scores of 3–8 usually are considered to be in a coma.
Source: Teasdale G, Jennett B. Assessment of coma and impaired consciousness. A practical scale. Lancet 1974;304(7872):81–84.

Table 17-9 Pupils in Comatose Patients

Small or Pinpoint Pupils

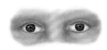

Bilaterally small pupils (1–2.5 mm) suggest (1) damage to the sympathetic pathways in the hypothalamus or (2) metabolic encephalopathy (a diffuse failure of cerebral function from drugs and other causes). Light reactions are usually normal.

Pinpoint pupils (<1 mm) suggest (1) a hemorrhage in the pons or (2) the effects of morphine, heroin, or other narcotics. Use a magnifying glass to see the light reactions.

Midposition Fixed Pupils

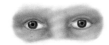

Midposition or *slightly dilated pupils* (4–6 mm) and *fixed to light* suggest damage in the midbrain.

Large Pupils

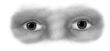

Bilaterally fixed and dilated pupils in severe anoxia with sympathomimetic effects, may be seen with cardiac arrest. They also result from atropinelike agents, phenothiazines, or tricyclic antidepressants.

One Large Pupil

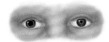

One fixed and dilated pupil warns of herniation of the temporal lobe, causing compression of the oculomotor nerve and midbrain. Also seen in diabetes with CN III infarction.

CHAPTER

18

Assessing Children: Infancy Through Adolescence

Child Development

Children display tremendous variations in physical, cognitive, and social development compared with adults.

Key Principles of Child Development

- Child development proceeds along a predictable pathway marked by developmental milestones.
- The range of normal development is wide. Children mature at different rates.
- Various physical, psychological, social, and environmental factors, as well as diseases, can affect child development and health. For example, chronic diseases, child abuse, and poverty can contribute to detectable physical abnormalities and influence the rate and course of developmental advancement.
- The child's developmental level affects how you conduct the medical history and physical examination.

The Health History

The child's history follows the same outline as the adult's history, with certain *additions* presented here.

Identifying Data. Record date and place of birth, nickname, and first names of parents (and last name of each, if different).

Chief Complaints. Determine if they are the concerns of the child, the parent(s), a schoolteacher, or some other person.

Present Illness. Determine how each family member responds to the child's symptoms, why he or she is concerned, and whether the illness may provide for the child any secondary gain.

History

Birth History. This is especially important when neurologic or developmental problems are present. Get hospital records if necessary.

- Prenatal—maternal health: medications; tobacco, drug, and alcohol use; weight gain; duration of pregnancy

- Natal—nature of labor and delivery, birth weight, Apgar scores at 1 and 5 minutes

- Neonatal—resuscitation efforts, cyanosis, jaundice, infections, bonding

Feeding History. This is particularly important with either undernutrition or obesity.

- Breast-feeding—frequency and duration of feeds, difficulties, timing and method of weaning

- Bottle-feeding—type; amount; frequency; vomiting; colic; diarrhea

- Vitamins, iron, and fluoride supplements; introduction of solid foods

- Eating habits—types and amounts of food eaten, parental attitudes and responses to feeding problems

Growth and Developmental History. This is particularly important with delayed growth or development and behavioral disturbances.

- Physical growth—weight and height at all ages; head circumference at birth and younger than 2 years; periods of slow or rapid growth

- Developmental milestones—ages child held head up, rolled over, sat, stood, walked, and talked

- Speech development, performance in preschool and school

- Social development—day and night sleeping patterns; toilet training; habitual behaviors; discipline problems; school behavior; relationships with family and peers

Current Health Status

Allergies. Pay particular attention to history of eczema, urticaria, perennial allergic rhinitis, asthma, food intolerance, insect hypersensitivity, and recurrent wheezing.

Immunizations. Include dates given and any untoward reactions.

Screening Tests. These are likely to vary according to the child's medical and social conditions. Include newborn screening results, anemia screening, blood lead, sickle cell disease, vision, hearing, developmental screening, and others (e.g., tuberculosis).

Health Promotion and Counseling: Evidence and Recommendations

1. Age-appropriate developmental achievement of the child
   - Physical (maturation, growth, puberty)
   - Motor (gross and fine motor skills)
   - Cognitive (milestones, language, school performance)
   - Emotional (self-efficacy, self-esteem, independence, morality)
   - Social (social competence, self-responsibility, integration with family and community)
2. Health supervision visits (per health supervision schedule)
   - Periodic assessment of medical and oral health
   - Adjustment of frequency for children or families with special needs
3. Integration of physical examination findings
4. Immunizations
5. Screening procedures
6. Anticipatory guidance
   - Healthy habits
   - Nutrition and healthy eating
   - Emotional and mental health
   - Oral health
   - Safety and prevention of injury
   - Sexual development and sexuality
   - Self-responsibility and efficacy
   - Family relationships (interactions, strengths, supports)
   - Prevention or recognition of illness
   - Prevention of risky behaviors and addictions
   - School and vocation
   - Peer relationships
   - Community interactions
7. Partnership between health provider, child, and family

Techniques of Examination

Sequence of Examination

The sequence of examination varies according to the child's age and comfort level.

- For infants and young children, *perform nondisturbing maneuvers early and potentially distressing maneuvers toward the end.* For example, palpate the head and neck and auscultate the heart and lungs early; examine the ears and mouth and palpate the abdomen near the end. If the child reports pain in an area, examine that part last.
- For older children and adolescents, use the same sequence as with adults, except examine the most painful areas last.

Assessing Newborns

| EXAMINATION TECHNIQUES | POSSIBLE FINDINGS |

IMMEDIATE ASSESSMENT AT BIRTH

Listen to the anterior thorax with your stethoscope. Palpate the abdomen. Inspect the head, face, oral cavity, extremities, genitalia, and perineum.

Apgar Score. Score each newborn according to the following table, at 1 and 5 minutes after birth, according to the 3-point scale (0, 1, or 2) for each component.

If the 5-minute score is 8 or more, proceed to a more complete examination.

Chapter 18 | Assessing Children: Infancy Through Adolescence

EXAMINATION TECHNIQUES | POSSIBLE FINDINGS

The Apgar Scoring System

Clinical Sign	Assigned Score		
	0	1	2
Heart rate	Absent	<100	>100
Respiratory effort	Absent	Slow and irregular	Good; strong
Muscle tone	Flaccid	Some flexion of the arms and legs	Active movement
Reflex irritability*	No responses	Grimace	Crying vigorously, sneeze, or cough
Color	Blue, pale	Pink body, blue extremities	Pink all over

1-Minute Apgar Score		5-Minute Apgar Score	
8–10	Normal	8–10	Normal
5–7	Some nervous system depression	0–7	High risk for subsequent central nervous system and other organ system dysfunction
0–4	Severe depression, requiring immediate resuscitation		

*Reaction to suction of nares with bulb syringe.

Gestational Age and Birth Weight.

Classify newborns according to their gestational age and birth weight.

Classification by Gestational Age and Birth Weight

Gestational Age

Classification	Gestational Age
▶ Preterm	<37 wks (<259th day)
▶ Term	37–42 wks
▶ Postterm	>42 wks (>294th day)

Birth Weight

Classification	Weight
▶ Extremely low birth weight	<1,000 g
▶ Very low birth weight	<1,500 g
▶ Low birth weight	<2,500 g
▶ Normal birth weight	≥2,500 g

| EXAMINATION TECHNIQUES | POSSIBLE FINDINGS |

Newborn Classifications

Category	Abbreviation	Percentile
Small for gestational age	SGA	<10th
Appropriate for gestational age	AGA	10–90th
Large for gestational age	LGA	>90th

Assessment Several Hours After Birth

During the first day of life, newborns should have a comprehensive examination following the technique outlined under "Infants." Wait until 1 or 2 hours after a feeding, when the newborn is more responsive. Ask parents to remain.

Observe the baby's color, size, body proportions, nutritional status, posture, respirations, and movements of the head and extremities.	Most newborns are *bowlegged*, reflecting their curled up intrauterine position.
Inspect the newborn's *umbilical cord* to detect abnormalities. Normally, there are two thick-walled umbilical arteries and one larger but thin-walled umbilical vein, which is usually located at the 12-o'clock position.	A *single umbilical artery* may be associated with congenital anomalies. *Umbilical hernias* in infants are from a defect in the abdominal wall.
The neurologic screening examination of all newborns should include assessment of mental status, gross and fine motor function, tone, cry, deep tendon reflexes, and primitive reflexes.	Signs of severe neurologic disease include *extreme irritability; persistent asymmetry of posture or extension of extremities; constant turning of head to one side; marked extension of head, neck, and extremities (opisthotonus); severe flaccidity;* and *limited pain response.*

Chapter 18 | Assessing Children: Infancy Through Adolescence 329

| EXAMINATION TECHNIQUES | POSSIBLE FINDINGS |

Assessing Infants

MENTAL AND PHYSICAL STATUS

Observe the parents' affect when talking about the baby and their manner of holding, moving, and dressing the baby. Observe a breast or bottle feeding. Determine attainment of developmental milestones, optimally using a standardized developmental screening test.

Common causes of *developmental delay* include abnormalities in embryonic development, hereditary and genetic disorders, environmental and social problems, other pregnancy or perinatal problems, childhood diseases such as infection (e.g., meningitis), trauma, and severe chronic disease.

GENERAL SURVEY

Growth, reflected in increases in height and weight within expected limits, is an excellent indicator of health during infancy and childhood. Deviations from normal may be early indications of an underlying problem. To assess growth, compare a child's parameters with respect to:

Failure to thrive is a condition reflecting significantly low weight gain (e.g., below 2nd percentile) for gestational-age corrected age and sex. Causes can be environmental or psychosocial, or various gastrointestinal, neurologic, cardiac, endocrine, renal, and other diseases.

- Normal values according to age and sex
- Prior readings to assess trends

Measures above the 97th or below the 3rd percentile, or recent rises or falls from prior levels, require investigation.

Height and Weight. Plot each child's height and weight on standard growth charts to determine progress.

Reduced growth in height may indicate *endocrine disease*, other *causes of short stature*, or, if weight is also low, other *chronic diseases*.

Head Circumference. Determine head circumference at every physical examination during the first 2 years.

Premature closure of the sutures or *microcephaly* may cause small head size. *Hydrocephalus, subdural hematoma,* or, rarely, *brain tumor* or *inherited syndromes* may cause an abnormally large head size.

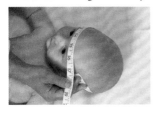

| EXAMINATION TECHNIQUES | POSSIBLE FINDINGS |

VITAL SIGNS

Blood Pressure. Measure blood pressure at least once during infancy. Although the hand-held method is shown here, the most easily used measure of systolic blood pressure in infants and young children is obtained with the *Doppler method*.

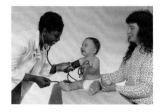

Causes of Sustained Hypertension in Children

Newborn	Middle Childhood
Renal artery disease (stenosis, thrombosis)	Primary hypertension
Congenital renal malformations	Renal parenchymal or arterial disease
Coarctation of the aorta	Coarctation of the aorta
Infancy and Early Childhood	**Adolescence**
Renal parenchymal or artery disease	Primary hypertension
Coarctation of the aorta	Renal parenchymal disease
	Drug induced

Pulse. The heart rate is quite variable and will increase markedly with excitement, crying, or anxiety. Therefore, measure the pulse when the infant or child is quiet.

Tachycardia (>180–200 beats per minute) usually indicates *paroxysmal supraventricular tachycardia*. Bradycardia may result from serious underlying disease.

Respiratory Rate. The respiratory rate has a very wide range and is more responsive to illness, exercise, and emotion than in adults.

Respiratory diseases such as *bronchiolitis* or *pneumonia* may cause rapid respirations (up to 80–90 breaths per minute), *and* increased work of breathing.

EXAMINATION TECHNIQUES | POSSIBLE FINDINGS

THE SKIN

Assess:

- Texture and appearance

  Cutis marmorata

- Vasomotor changes

  Acrocyanosis; cyanotic congenital heart disease

- Pigmentation (e.g., Mongolian spots)

  Café-au-lait spots

- Hair (e.g., lanugo)

  Midline hair tuft on back

- Common skin conditions (e.g., milia, erythema toxicum)

  Herpes simplex

- Color

  Jaundice can be from hemolytic disease.

- Turgor

  Dehydration

THE HEAD

Examine *sutures* and *fontanelles* carefully.

Anterior fontanelle
Posterior fontanelle
Lambdoidal suture
Sagittal suture
Coronal suture
Metopic suture

Head small with *microcephaly*, enlarged with *hydrocephaly*; fontanelles full and tense with *meningitis*, closed with *microcephaly*, separated with *increased intracranial pressure* (hydrocephaly, subdural hematoma, and brain tumor)

Swelling from subperiosteal hemorrhage (cephalohematoma) does not cross suture lines; swelling from bleeding associated with a fracture does.

Check the *face* for symmetry. Examine for an overall impression of the *facies*; comparing with the faces of the parents is helpful.

Abnormal facies occurs in a child with a constellation of facial features that appear abnormal. A variety of syndromes can cause abnormal facies (see table below for evaluation). Examples include *Down syndrome* and *fetal alcohol syndrome*.

| EXAMINATION TECHNIQUES | POSSIBLE FINDINGS |

Pearls to Evaluate Potentially Abnormal Facies

Carefully review the history, especially the *family history*, *pregnancy*, and *perinatal history*.

Note abnormalities, especially of *growth*, *development*, or *dysmorphic somatic features*.

Measure and plot percentiles, especially of *head circumference*, *height*, and *weight*.

Consider the three mechanisms of facial dysmorphogenesis:

- Deformations from intrauterine constraint
- Disruptions from amniotic bands or fetal tissue
- Malformations from an intrinsic abnormality (either face/head or brain)

Examine parents and siblings (similarity may be reassuring but might point to a familial disorder).

Determine whether facial features fit a recognizable syndrome. Compare against references, pictures, tables, and databases.

THE EYES

Newborns and young infants may look at your face and follow a bright light if you catch them while alert. *Normal visual milestones are as follows:*

Nystagmus, strabismus

Leukocoria is a white papillary reflex (instead of the normal red papillary reflex). It can be a sign of a rare tumor called *retinoblastoma*.

Visual Milestones of Infancy

Birth	Blinks, may regard face
1 month	Fixes on objects
1½–2 months	Coordinated eye movements
3 months	Eyes converge, baby reaches
12 months	Acuity around 20/50

THE EARS

Check *position*, *shape*, and *features*.

Small, deformed or low-set auricles may indicate associated *congenital defects*, especially renal disease.

EXAMINATION TECHNIQUES | POSSIBLE FINDINGS

Signs That an Infant Can Hear

Age	Signs
0–2 months	Startle response and blink to a sudden noise Calming down with soothing voice or music
2–3 months	Change in body movements in response to sound Change in facial expression to familiar sounds
3–4 months	Turning eyes and head to sound
6–7 months	Turning to listen to voices and conversation

THE NOSE

Test patency of the nasal passages by occluding alternately each nostril while holding the infant's mouth closed.

With *choanal atresia*, the baby cannot breathe if one nostril is occluded.

THE MOUTH AND PHARYNX

Inspect (with a tongue blade and flashlight) and palpate.

Supernumerary teeth, Epstein's pearls

You may see a whitish covering on the tongue. If this coating is from milk, you can easily remove it by scraping or wiping it away.

Oral candidiasis (thrush)

Vesicles in the mouth can be caused by *enteroviral infections* and *herpes simplex virus infections*.

THE NECK

Palpate the *lymph nodes*, and assess for any additional masses (e.g., *congenital cysts*).

Lymphadenopathy is usually from viral or bacterial infections.

Other neck masses include *malignancy*, *branchial cleft* or *thyroglossal duct cysts*, and *periauricular cysts and sinuses*.

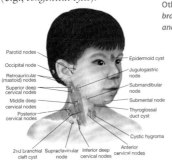

EXAMINATION TECHNIQUES	POSSIBLE FINDINGS

THE THORAX AND LUNGS

Carefully assess respirations and breathing pattern.

Apnea

Do not rush to the stethoscope, but observe the patient carefully first.

Upper respiratory infections may cause nasal flaring.

Examination of the Lungs in Infants—Before You Touch the Child!

Assessment	Possible Findings	Explanation
General appearance	Inability to feed or smile Lack of consolability	*Lower respiratory infections* below the vocal cords (e.g., *bronchiolitis, pneumonia*) are common in infants.
Respiratory rate	Tachypnea	Cardiac or respiratory disease
Color	Pallor or cyanosis	Cardiac or pulmonary disease
Nasal component of breathing	Nasal flaring (enlargement of both nasal openings during inspiration)	Upper or lower respiratory infection
Audible breath sounds	Grunting (repetitive, short expiratory sound) Wheezing (musical expiratory sound) Stridor (high-pitched, inspiratory noise) Obstruction (lack of breath sounds)	*Acute stridor* is a potentially serious condition with causes such as *laryngotracheobronchitis (croup), epiglottitis, bacterial tracheitis, foreign body, vascular ring*

Work of breathing	Nasal flaring
	Grunting
	Retractions (chest indrawing):
	  Supraclavicular (motion of soft tissue above clavicles)
	  Intercostal (indrawing of the skin between ribs)
	  Subcostal (just below the costal margin)
		In infants, abnormal work of breathing combined with abnormal findings on auscultation is the best finding for ruling in *pneumonia*.

| EXAMINATION TECHNIQUES | POSSIBLE FINDINGS |

Distinguishing Upper Airway From Lower Airway Sounds

Technique	Upper Airway	Lower Airway
Compare sounds from nose/stethoscope	Same sounds	Often different sounds
Listen to harshness of sounds	Harsh and loud	Variable
Note symmetry (left/right)	Symmetric	Often asymmetric
Compare sounds at different locations (higher or lower)	Sounds louder as stethoscope is moved up chest	Sounds louder lower in chest
Inspiratory vs. expiratory	Almost always inspiratory	Often has expiratory phase

THE HEART

Inspection. Observe carefully for any cyanosis. The best body part to assess cyanosis is the tongue or inside of the mouth.

At birth: *Transposition of the great arteries; pulmonary valve atresia or stenosis*

Within a few days of birth: The above; also *total anomalous pulmonary venous return, hypoplastic left heart*

Palpation. Palpate the *peripheral pulses*. The *point of maximal impulse (PMI)* is not always palpable in infants. *Thrills* are palpable when enough turbulence is within the heart or great vessels.

No or diminished femoral pulses suggest *coarctation of the aorta*. Weak or thready, difficult-to-feel pulses may reflect *myocardial dysfunction* and *heart failure*.

Auscultation. *Heart rhythm* is evaluated more easily in infants by listening to the heart than by feeling the peripheral pulses.

The most common dysrhythmia in children is *paroxysmal supraventricular tachycardia*.

Heart Sounds. Evaluate S_1 and S_2 carefully. They are normally crisp.

A louder-than-normal pulmonic component suggests *pulmonary hypertension*. Persistent splitting of S_2 may indicate *atrial septal defect*.

| EXAMINATION TECHNIQUES | POSSIBLE FINDINGS |

THE BREASTS

The breasts of males and females may be enlarged for months after birth as a result of maternal estrogen, and even engorged for 1 to 2 weeks with a white liquid.

THE ABDOMEN

You will find it easy to palpate an infant's abdomen, because infants like being touched. Palpate the liver and spleen and assess for hepatosplenomagaly.

Abnormal abdominal masses can be associated with kidney, bladder, or bowel tumors. In *pyloric stenosis*, deep palpation in the right upper quadrant or midline can reveal an "olive," or a 2-cm firm pyloric mass.

MALE GENITALIA

Inspect with the infant supine.

Common scrotal masses are *hydroceles* and *inguinal hernias*.

In 3% of infants, one or both testes cannot be felt in the scrotum or inguinal canal. Try to milk the testes into the scrotum.

Inability to palpate testes, even with maneuvers, indicates *undescended testicles*.

FEMALE GENITALIA

In females, genitalia may be prominent for several months after birth from the effects of maternal estrogen.

Ambiguous genitalia involves masculinization of the female external genitalia.

THE MUSCULOSKELETAL SYSTEM

Examine the extremities by inspection and palpation to detect congenital abnormalities, particularly in the hands, spine, hips, legs, and feet.

Skin tags, remnants of digits, *polydactyly* (extra fingers), or *syndactyly* (webbed fingers) are congenital defects. *Fracture of the clavicle* can occur during a difficult delivery.

| EXAMINATION TECHNIQUES | POSSIBLE FINDINGS |

Examine the *hips* carefully at each visit for signs of dislocation. There are two major techniques: one to test for a posteriorly dislocated hip (*Ortolani test*) and the other to test for the ability to sublux or dislocate an intact but unstable hip (*Barlow test*).

Congenital hip dysplasia may have a positive Ortolani or Barlow test, particularly during the first 3 months of age. With a *hip dysplasia*, you feel a "clunk."

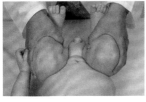
ORTOLANI TEST

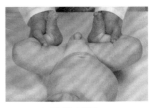
BARLOW TEST

Some normal infants exhibit twisting or *torsion of the tibia* inwardly or outwardly on its longitudinal axis.

Pathologic tibial torsion occurs only in association with *deformities of the feet or hips*.

THE NERVOUS SYSTEM

Evaluate the developing central nervous system by assessing *infantile automatisms*, called *primitive reflexes*.

Suspect a *neurologic* or *developmental abnormality* if primitive reflexes are absent at appropriate age, present longer than normal, asymmetric, or associated with posturing or twitching.

Neurologic and developmental abnormalities often co-exist. *Hypotonia* can be a sign of a variety of neurologic abnormalities.

| EXAMINATION TECHNIQUES | POSSIBLE FINDINGS |

Assessing Children (1 to 10 Years)

Tips for Interviewing Children

- **Establish rapport.** Refer to children by name and meet them on their own level. Maintain eye contact at their level (e.g., sit on the floor if needed). Participate in play and talk about their interests.
- **Work with families.** Ask simple, open-ended questions such as "Are you sick? Tell me about it," followed by more specific questions. Once the parent has started the conversation, direct questions back to the child. Also observe how parents interact with the child.
- **Identify multiple agendas.** Your job is to discover as many perspectives and agendas as possible.
- **Use the family as the key resource.** View parents as experts in the care of their child and you as their consultant.
- **Note hidden agendas.** As with adults, the chief complaint may not relate to the real reason the parent has brought the child to see you.

The following discussion focuses on those areas of the comprehensive physical examination that are different for children than for infants and for adults.

MENTAL AND PHYSICAL STATUS

In *children 1 to 5 years*, observe the degree of sickness or wellness, mood, nutritional state, speech, cry, facial expression, and developmental skills. Note parent–child interaction, including separation tolerance, affection, and response to discipline.	This overall examination can uncover evidence of *chronic disease, developmental delay, social or environmental disorders,* and *family problems*.
In *children 6 to 10 years*, determine orientation to time and place, factual knowledge, and language and number skills. Observe motor skills used in writing, tying laces, buttoning, cutting, and drawing.	Observing children performing tasks can reveal signs of inattentiveness or impulsivity, which may indicate *attention deficit disorder*.
Body Mass Index for Age. Age- and sex-specific charts are now available to assess body mass index (BMI) in children.	*Underweight* is <5th percentile, *at risk of overweight* is ≥85th percentile, and *overweight* is ≥95th percentile.

Chapter 18 | Assessing Children: Infancy Through Adolescence

| EXAMINATION TECHNIQUES | POSSIBLE FINDINGS |

BLOOD PRESSURE

Hypertension during childhood is more common than previously thought. Recognizing, confirming, and appropriately managing it is important. Blood pressure readings should be part of the physical examination of every child older than 2 years. *Proper cuff size is essential for accurate determination of blood pressure in children.*

The most frequent "cause" of elevated blood pressure in children is probably an *improperly performed examination*, often from an incorrect cuff size.

Causes of *sustained hypertension* in childhood include renal disease, coarctation of the aorta, and primary hypertension. Hypertension is often related to *childhood obesity*.

THE EYES

Test visual acuity in each eye and determine whether the gaze is conjugate or symmetric.

Strabismus can lead to *amblyopia*

Myopia or hyperopia often present in school-aged children.

SPECIAL TECHNIQUE

The corneal light reflex test (*left*) and the cover–uncover test (*right*) are particularly useful in young children.

Any difference in visual acuity between eyes is abnormal.

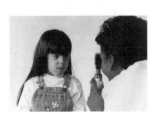
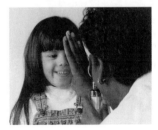

| EXAMINATION TECHNIQUES | POSSIBLE FINDINGS |

Visual Acuity

Age	Visual Acuity
3 months	Eyes converge, baby reaches
12 months	~20/200
Younger than 4 years	20/40
4 years and older	20/30

THE EARS

Examine the ear canal and drum. There are two positions for the child (lying down or sitting), and also two ways to hold the otoscope, as illustrated.

Pain on movement of the pinna occurs with *otitis externa.*

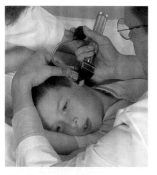
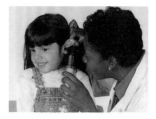

Pneumatic Otoscope. Learn to use a *pneumatic otoscope* to improve accuracy of diagnosis of otitis media.

- Insert the speculum, obtaining a proper seal.

Acute otitis media involves a red and bulging tympanic membrane.

| EXAMINATION TECHNIQUES | POSSIBLE FINDINGS |

- When air is introduced into the normal ear canal, the tympanic membrane and its light reflex move inward. When air is removed, the tympanic membrane moves outward toward you.

Diminished movement of tympanic membrane with *acute otitis media;* no movement with *otitis media with effusion.*

THE MOUTH AND PHARYNX

For anxious or young children, leave this examination toward the end. The best technique for a tongue blade is to push down and pull slightly forward toward you while the child says "ah." Do not place the blade too far posteriorly, eliciting a gag reflex.

A common cause of a strawberry tongue, red uvula, and pharyngeal exudate is *streptococcal pharyngitis.*

Examine the *teeth* for the timing and sequence of eruption, number, character, condition, and position.

Abnormalities of the enamel may reflect local or general disease.

Carefully inspect the inside of the upper teeth, as shown.

Nursing bottle caries; dental caries; staining of the teeth, which may be intrinsic or extrinsic

Dental caries are the most common health problem of children and are particularly prevalent in impoverished children.

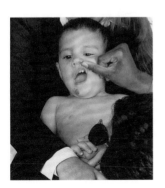

EXAMINATION TECHNIQUES	POSSIBLE FINDINGS

Look for abnormalities of tooth position.

Malocclusion

Note the size, position, symmetry, and appearance of the *tonsils*.

Peritonsillar abscess

THE HEART

A challenging aspect to cardiac examination of children is evaluation of *heart murmurs*, particularly distinguishing common benign murmurs from unusual or pathologic ones. Most children have one or more *functional*, or *benign*, *heart murmurs* at some point in time (see below).

See Table 18-4, Characteristics of Pathologic Heart Murmurs, pp. 351–352.

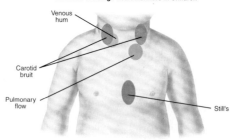

Location of Benign Heart Murmurs in Children

THE ABDOMEN

Most children are ticklish when you first place your hand on their abdomens for palpation. This reaction tends to disappear, particularly if you distract the child.

A pathologically enlarged liver in children usually is palpable more than 2 cm below the costal margin, has a round, firm edge, and often is tender.

| EXAMINATION TECHNIQUES | POSSIBLE FINDINGS |

MALE GENITALIA

There is an art to palpation of the young boy's scrotum and testes, because many have an active cremasteric reflex causing the testes to retract upward into the inguinal canal and appear undescended. A useful technique is to have the boy sit cross-legged on the examining table.

In *precocious puberty*, the penis and testes are enlarged, with signs of pubertal changes.

A painful testicle requires rapid treatment and may indicate *torsion*.

Inguinal hernias in older boys present as they do in adult men.

FEMALE GENITALIA

Use a calm, gentle approach, including a developmentally appropriate explanation.

Examine the genitalia in an efficient and systematic manner. The normal hymen can have various configurations.

Vaginal discharge in early childhood can result from *perineal irritation* (e.g., from bubble baths, soaps), *foreign body, vaginitis,* or *sexually transmitted infections* from sexual abuse. *Vaginal bleeding, abrasions,* or signs of trauma to the external genitalia can result from *sexual abuse.*

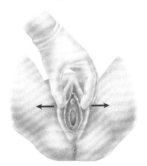

| EXAMINATION TECHNIQUES | POSSIBLE FINDINGS |

THE MUSCULOSKELETAL SYSTEM

Abnormalities of the upper extremities are rare in the absence of injury. To assess the lower extremities, observe the child standing and walking barefoot, and ask the child to touch the toes, rise from sitting, run a short distance, and pick up objects. You will detect most abnormalities by watching carefully.

A screening musculoskeletal examination for children participating in sports can detect injuries or abnormalities that may result in problems during athletics.

THE NERVOUS SYSTEM

Beyond infancy, the neurologic examination includes the components evaluated in adults. Again, combine the neurologic and developmental assessments. You can turn this into a game with the child to assess optimal development and neurologic performance.

Delayed language or cognitive skills can be due to neurologic disease as well as developmental disorders.

Soft neurological signs can suggest *minor developmental abnormalities.*

Assessing Adolescents

The key to successfully examining teens is a comfortable, confidential environment that makes the examination relaxed and informative. Adolescents are more likely to open up when the interview focuses on them rather than on their problems.

Consider the patient's cognitive and social development when deciding issues of privacy, parental involvement, and confidentiality. Explain to both teens and parents that the purpose of confidentiality is to improve health care, not keep secrets. Your goal is to help adolescents bring their concerns or questions to their parents. Never make confidentiality unlimited, however. Always state to teens explicitly that you may need to act on information that makes you concerned about safety.

EXAMINATION TECHNIQUES	POSSIBLE FINDINGS

The physical examination of the adolescent is similar to that of the adult. Keep in mind issues particularly relevant to teens, such as puberty, growth, development, family and peer relationships, sexuality, decision making, and risk behaviors. For more details on specific techniques of examination, the reader should refer to the corresponding chapter for the regional examination of interest or concern. Following are special areas to highlight when examining adolescents.

THE BREASTS

Assess normal maturational development.	See Table 18-5, Sex Maturity Ratings in Girls: Breasts, p. 353.

SPECIAL TECHNIQUE

Testing for Scoliosis. Inspect any child who can stand for *scoliosis*. Make sure the child bends forward with the knees straight (*Adams' bend test*). Evaluate any asymmetry in positioning or gait. If you detect scoliosis, use a *scoliometer* to test for the degree of scoliosis.

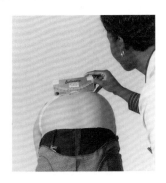

MALE AND FEMALE GENITALIA

An important goal when examining adolescent males and females is to assign a sexual maturity rating, regardless of chronologic age.	See Table 18-6, Sex Maturity Ratings in Boys, pp. 354–355, and Table 18-7, Sex Maturity Ratings in Girls: Pubic Hair, p. 356.

EXAMINATION TECHNIQUES

Recording Your Findings

The format of the pediatric medical record is the same as that of the adult. Thus, although the sequence of the physical examination may vary, convert your written findings back to the traditional format.

Recording the Physical Examination— The Pediatric Patient

Brian is a chubby, active, and energetic toddler. He plays with the reflex hammer, pretending it is a truck. He appears closely bonded with his mother, looking at her occasionally for comfort. She seems concerned that Brian will break something. His clothes are clean.

Vital Signs. Ht 90 cm (90th percentile). Wt 16 kg (>95th percentile). BMI 19.8 (>95th percentile). Head circumference 50 cm (75th percentile). BP 108/58. Heart rate 90 and regular. Respiratory rate 30; varies with activity. Temperature (ear) 37.5°C. Obviously no pain.

Skin. Normal except for bruises on legs, and patchy, dry skin over external surface of elbows.

HEENT. *Head:* Normocephalic; no lesions. *Eyes:* Difficult to examine because he won't sit still. Symmetric with normal extraocular movements. Pupils 4 to 5 mm constricting. Discs difficult to visualize; no hemorrhages noted. *Ears:* Normal pinna; no external abnormalities. Normal external canals and tympanic membranes (TMs). *Nose:* Normal nares; septum midline. *Mouth:* Several darkened teeth on inside surface of upper incisors. One clear cavity on upper right incisor. Tongue normal. Cobblestoning of posterior pharynx; no exudates. Tonsils large but adequate gap (1.5 cm) between them.

Neck. Supple, midline trachea, no thyroid palpable.

Lymph Nodes. Easily palpable (1.5 to 2 cm) tonsillar lymph nodes bilaterally. Small (0.5 cm) nodes in inguinal canal bilaterally. All lymph nodes mobile and nontender.

Lungs. Good expansion. No tachypnea or dyspnea. Congestion audible, but seems to be upper airway (louder near mouth, symmetric). No rhonchi, rales, or wheezes. Clear to auscultation.

Cardiovascular. PMI in 4th or 5th interspace and midsternal line. Normal S_1 and S_2. No murmurs or abnormal heart sounds. Normal femoral pulses; dorsalis pedis pulses palpable bilaterally.

(continued)

EXAMINATION TECHNIQUES

Breasts. Normal, with some fat under both.

Abdomen. Protuberant but soft; no masses or tenderness. Liver span 2 cm below right costal margin (RCM) and not tender. Spleen and kidneys not palpable.

Genitalia. Tanner I circumcised penis; no pubic hair, lesions, or discharge. Testes descended, difficult to palpate because of active cremasteric reflex. Normal scrotum both sides.

Musculoskeletal. Normal range of motion of upper and lower extremities and all joints. Spine straight. Gait normal.

Neurologic. *Mental Status:* Happy, cooperative child. *Developmental:* Gross motor—Jumps and throws objects. Fine motor—Imitates vertical line. Language—Does not combine words; single words only, three to four noted during examination. Personal–social—Washes face, brushes teeth, and puts on shirt. Overall—Normal, except for language, which appears delayed. *Cranial Nerves:* Intact, althwough several difficult to elicit. *Cerebellar:* Normal gait; good balance. *Deep tendon reflexes (DTRs):* Normal and symmetric throughout with downgoing toes. *Sensory:* Deferred.

Aids to Interpretation

Table 18-1   Classification of Newborn's Level of Maturity

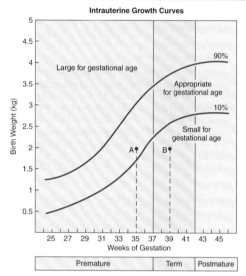

Weight Small for Gestational Age (SGA) = Birth weight <10th percentile on the intrauterine growth curve

Weight Appropriate for Gestational Age (AGA) = Birth weight within the 10th and 90th percentiles on the intrauterine growth curve

Weight Large for Gestational Age (LGA) = Birth weight >90th percentile on the intrauterine growth curve

---

Level of intrauterine growth based on birth weight and gestational age of liveborn, single, white infants. Point A represents a premature infant, while point B indicates an infant of similar birth weight who is mature but small for gestational age; the growth curves are representative of the 10th and 90th percentiles for all of the newborns in the sampling.

Adapted from Sweet YA. Classification of the low-birth-weight infant. In: Klaus MH, Fanaroff AA. Care of the High-Risk Neonate, 3rd ed. Philadelphia: WB Saunders, 1986. Reproduced with permission.

Table 18-2 Recommendations for Preventive Pediatric Health Care

Each child and family is unique; therefore, these recommendations are designed for the care of children who are receiving competent parenting, have no manifestation of any important health problems, and are growing and developing in satisfactory fashion. Additional visits may become necessary if circumstances suggest variation from normal.

AGE	INFANCY							EARLY CHILDHOOD					MIDDLE CHILDHOOD				ADOLESCENCE									
	2–4 days[1]	By 1 mo	2 mo	4 mo	6 mo	9 mo	12 mo	15 mo	18 mo	24 mo	3 y	4 y	5 y	6 y	8 y	10 y	11 y	12 y	13 y	14 y	15 y	16 y	17 y	18 y	19 y	20 y+
HISTORY Initial/Interval	•	•	•	•	•	•	•	•	•	•	•	•	•	•	•	•	•	•	•	•	•	•	•	•	•	•
MEASUREMENTS Height and Weight	•	•	•	•	•	•	•	•	•	•	•	•	•	•	•	•	•	•	•	•	•	•	•	•	•	•
Head Circumference	•	•	•	•	•	•	•	•	•	•																
Blood Pressure											•	•	•	•	•	•	•	•	•	•	•	•	•	•	•	•
SENSORY SCREENING Vision	S	S	S	S	S	S	S	S	S	S	O	O	O	O	O	O	S	O	S	S	S	O	S	S	S	S
Hearing	S	S	S	S	S	S	S	S	S	S	S	O	O	O	O	O	S	O	S	S	S	O	S	S	S	S
DEVELOPMENTAL/ BEHAVIORAL ASSESSMENT[2]	•	•	•	•	•	•	•	•	•	•	•	•	•	•	•	•	•	•	•	•	•	•	•	•	•	•
PHYSICAL EXAMINATION[3]	•	•	•	•	•	•	•	•	•	•	•	•	•	•	•	•	•	•	•	•	•	•	•	•	•	•

[1] For newborns discharged in <48 hours after delivery.
[2] By history and appropriate physical examination: if suspicious, by specific objective development testing.
[3] At each visit, a complete physical examination is essential, with infant totally unclothed, older child undressed and suitably draped.

Key: • = to be performed S = subjective, by history
O = objective, by a standard testing method

Adapted from Recommendations For Preventive Pediatric Health Care promulgated by the American Academy of Pediatrics Committee on Practice and Ambulatory Medicine, 1999.

Table 18-3   **Hypertension in Childhood**

Hypertension can start in childhood. Although young children with elevated blood pressure are more likely to have a renal, cardiac, or endocrine cause older children and adolescents with hypertension are most likely to have primary or essential hypertension. Hypertension is often related to obesity.

This child developed hypertension before adolescence, and it "tracked" into adulthood. Children tend to remain in the same percentile for blood pressure as they grow. This tracking of blood pressure continues into adulthood, supporting the concept that adult essential hypertension begins during childhood.

The consequences of untreated hypertension can be severe.

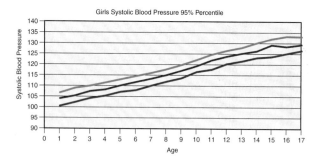

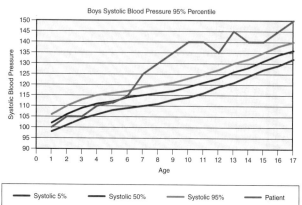

Table 18-4 — Characteristics of Pathologic Heart Murmurs

Congenital Defect	Characteristics of Murmur
Pulmonary Valve Stenosis *Mild* 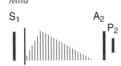 *Moderate* *Severe*	*Location.* Upper left sternal border *Radiation.* In mild degrees of stenosis, the murmur may be heard over the course of the pulmonary arteries in the lung fields. *Intensity.* Increases in intensity and duration as the degree of obstruction increases *Quality.* Ejection, peaking later in systole as the obstruction increases
Aortic Valve Stenosis 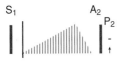	*Location.* Midsternum, upper right sternal border *Radiation.* To the carotid arteries and suprasternal notch; may also be a thrill *Intensity.* Varies, louder with increasingly severe obstruction *Quality.* An ejection, often harsh, systolic murmur
Tetralogy of Fallot *With Pulmonic Stenosis* 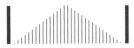	*General.* Variable cyanosis, increasing with activity *Location.* Mid to upper left sternal border. If pulmonary atresia, there is no systolic murmur but the continuous murmur of ductus arteriosus flow at upper left sternal border or in the back.

(continued)

Table 18-4	**Characteristics of Pathologic Heart Murmurs** (*continued*)
Congenital Defect	**Characteristics of Murmur**
With Pulmonic Atresia 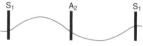	*Radiation.* Little, to upper left sternal border, occasionally to lung fields *Intensity.* Usually grade III–IV *Quality.* Midpeaking, systolic ejection murmur
Transposition of the Great Arteries	*General.* Intense generalized cyanosis *Location.* No characteristic murmur. If a murmur is present, it may reflect an associated defect such as VSD or patent ductus arteriosus. *Radiation.* Depends on associated abnormalities *Quality.* Depends on associated abnormalities
Ventricular Septal Defect	*Location.* Lower left sternal border
Small to Moderate	*Radiation.* Little *Intensity.* Variable, only partially determined by the size of the shunt. Small shunts with a high pressure gradient may have very loud murmurs. Large defects with elevated pulmonary vascular resistance may have no murmur. Grade II–IV/VI with a thrill if grade IV/VI or higher.

Table 18-5   Sex Maturity Ratings in Girls: Breasts

Stage 1

Preadolescent—elevation of nipple only

Stage 2

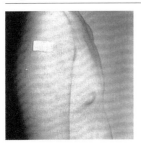

Breast bud stage. Elevation of breast and nipple as a small mound; enlargement of areolar diameter

Stage 3

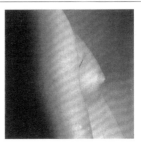

Further enlargement and elevation of breast and areola, with no separation of the contours

Stage 4

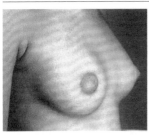

Projection of areola and nipple to form a secondary mound above the level of the breast

Stage 5

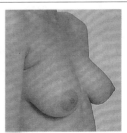

Mature stage; projection of nipple only. Areola has receded to general contour of the breast (although in some normal individuals areola continues to form a secondary mound).

Photos reprinted, with permission from the American Academy of Pediatrics, *Assessment of Sexual Maturity Stages in Girls*, 1995.

Table 18-6 Sex Maturity Ratings in Boys

In assigning SMRs in boys, observe each of the three characteristics separately. Record two separate ratings: pubic hair and genital. If the penis and testes differ in their stages, average the two into a single figure for the genital rating

---

Stage 1

Pubic Hair: Preadolescent—no pubic hair except for the fine body hair (vellus hair) similar to that on the abdomen

Genitalia

- **Penis:** Preadolescent—same size and proportions as in childhood

- **Testes and Scrotum:** Preadolescent—same size and proportions as in childhood

---

Stage 2

Pubic Hair: Sparse growth of long, slightly pigmented, downy hair, straight or only slightly curled, chiefly at the base of the penis

Genitalia

- **Penis:** Slight to no enlargement

- **Testes and Scrotum:** Testes larger; scrotum larger, somewhat reddened, and altered in texture

---

Stage 3

Pubic Hair: Darker, coarser, curlier hair spreading sparsely over the pubic symphysis

Genitalia
- **Penis:** Larger, especially in length

- **Testes and Scrotum:** Further enlarged

Table 18-6 Sex Maturity Ratings in Boys (continued)

Stage 4

Pubic Hair: Coarse and curly hair, as in the adult; area covered greater than in stage 3 but not as great as in the adult and not yet including the thighs

Genitalia

- **Penis:** Further enlarged in length and breadth, with development of the glans

- **Testes and Scrotum:** Further enlarged; scrotal skin darkened

Stage 5

Pubic Hair: Hair adult quantity and quality, spread to the medial surfaces of the thighs but not up over the abdomen

Genitalia

- **Penis:** Adult in size and shape

- **Testes and Scrotum:** Adult in size and shape

Photos reprinted from *Pediatric Endocrinology and Growth* 2nd ed., Wales & Wit, 2003, with permission from Elsevier.

Table 18-7	Sex Maturity Ratings in Girls: Pubic Hair
Stage 1	Preadolescent—no pubic hair except for the fine body hair (vellus hair) similar to that on the abdomen
Stage 2 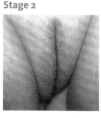	Sparse growth of long, slightly pigmented, downy hair, straight or only slightly curled, chiefly along the labia
Stage 3 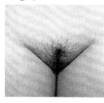	Darker, coarser, curlier hair, spreading sparsely over the pubic symphysis
Stage 4 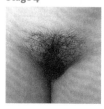	Coarse and curly hair as in adults; area covered greater than in stage 3 but not as great as in the adult and not yet including the thighs
Stage 5 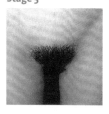	Hair adult in quantity and quality, spread on the medial surfaces of the thighs but not up over the abdomen

Photos reprinted, with permission from the American Academy of Pediatrics, *Assessment of Sexual Maturity Stages in Girls*, 1995.

Table 18-8 Physical Signs of Sexual Abuse

Physical Signs That May Indicate Sexual Abuse in Children*

1. Marked and immediate dilatation of the anus in knee–chest position, with no constipation, stool in the vault, or neurologic disorders
2. Hymenal notch or cleft that extends >50% of the inferior hymenal rim (confirmed in knee–chest position)
3. Condyloma acuminata in a child older than 3 years
4. Bruising, abrasions, lacerations, or bite marks of labia or perihymenal tissue
5. Herpes of the anogenital area beyond the neonatal period
6. Purulent or malodorous vaginal discharge in a young girl (all discharges should be cultured and viewed under a microscope for evidence of a sexually transmitted infection)

Physical Signs That Strongly Suggest Sexual Abuse in Children*

1. Lacerations, ecchymoses, and newly healed scars of the hymen or the posterior fourchette
2. No hymenal tissue from 3 to 9 o'clock (confirmed in various positions)
3. Healed hymenal transections, especially between 3 and 9 o'clock (complete cleft)
4. Perianal lacerations extending to external sphincter

A sexual abuse expert must evaluate a child with concerning physical signs for a complete history and sexual abuse examination.

---

*Any physical sign must be evaluated in light of the entire history, other parts of the physical examination, and laboratory data.

CHAPTER 19

The Pregnant Woman

The Health History

Common Concerns

- Initial prenatal history
  - Confirmation of pregnancy
  - Symptoms of pregnancy
  - Concerns about and attitudes toward the pregnancy
  - Current health and past medical history
  - Past obstetric history
  - Risk factors for maternal and fetal health
  - Family history
  - Plans for breast-feeding
- Determining gestational age and expected date of delivery

Focus the *initial prenatal visit* on confirming the pregnancy, assessing the health status of the mother and any risks for complications, and counseling to ensure a healthy pregnancy. Ask about the following topics:

- *Confirmation of pregnancy.* Has the patient had a confirmatory urine pregnancy test, and when? When was her last menstrual period (LMP)? Has an ultrasound been done to establish dates? Explain that serum pregnancy tests are rarely required to confirm pregnancy.

- *Symptoms of pregnancy.* absence of menses, breast fullness or tenderness, nausea or vomiting, fatigue, and urinary frequency. Explain that serum or urine testing for beta human chorionic gonadotropin (HCG) offers the best confirmation of pregnancy.

- *Maternal concerns and attitudes.* Review the mother's feelings about the pregnancy and whether she plans to continue to term. Ask about any fears and about support from the father.

- *Current health and past medical history.* Does the patient have any acute or chronic medical concerns, past or present? Pay particular attention to issues that affect pregnancy, such as abdominal surgeries, hypertension, diabetes, cardiac conditions including any that were surgically corrected in childhood, asthma, hypercoagulability states involving lupus or anticardiolipin antibodies, mental health disorders including postpartum depression, HIV, sexually transmitted infections, abnormal Pap smears, and exposure to diethylstilbestrol (DES) in utero.

- *Past obstetric history.* Ask about prior pregnancies and outcomes. Has she had any complications during past pregnancies, including labor and delivery? Has she had a premature or growth-retarded infant, or a baby large for gestational age? Has there been a prior fetal demise?

- *Risk factors for maternal and fetal health.* Does the patient use tobacco, alcohol, or illicit drugs? Does she take any medications, over-the-counter drugs, or herbal prescriptions? Does she have any toxic exposures at work, home, or otherwise? Is her nutritional intake adequate, or is she at risk for problems stemming from obesity? Does she have an adequate social support network and income sources? Are there unusual sources of stress at home or work? Is there any history of physical abuse or domestic violence?

- *Family history* of chronic illnesses or genetically transmitted diseases: sickle cell anemia, cystic fibrosis, muscular dystrophy, and others.

- *Plans for breast-feeding. Education and encouragement during pregnancy are recommended.*

Gestational age and *expected date of delivery.*

- *Gestational age.* Count the number of weeks and days from the first day of the LMP. Counting this *menstrual age* from the LMP–although biologically distinct from the date of conception, it is the standard means of calculating fetal age, yielding an average pregnancy length of 40 weeks. Rarely, the actual date of conception is known (as with in vitro fertilization.) In these cases, use a *conception age,* which is 2 weeks less than the menstrual age. However, this number should never be used to make clinical judgements that rely on the menstrual age for standards of care.

- *Expected date of delivery (EDD).* The expected date of delivery is 40 weeks from the first date of the LMP. Using *Naegele's rule,* the EDD can be estimated by taking the LMP, adding 7 days, subtracting 3 months and adding 1 year.

- *Tools for calculations.* Pregnancy wheels and online calculators are commonly used to expedite these calculations, but they should be checked for accuracy.

- *Limitations on pregnancy dating.* Patient recall of the LMP is highly variable. The LMP can also be biased by hormonal contraceptives or lengthly menstrual cycles. Check LMP dating against physical exam markers such as fundal height, clarifying discrepancies against ultrasound evaluation.

Subsequent Prenatal Visits. Obstetric visits traditionally follow a set schedule: monthly until 30 gestational weeks, then biweekly until 36 weeks, then weekly until delivery. Update and document the history at every visit, especially fetal movement, contractions, leakage of fluids and vaginal bleeding. At every visit, assess: vital signs (especially blood pressure and weight), fundal height, verification of FHR, and fetal position and activity.

Health Promotion and Counseling: Evidence and Recommendations

Important Topics for Health Promotion and Counseling

- Nutrition
- Weight gain
- Exercise
- Substance abuse
- Domestic violence
- Prenatal laboratory screenings
- Immunizations

Nutrition and Weight Gain. Evaluate nutritional status during the first prenatal visit, including: diet history; measurement of height, weight, and body mass index (BMI); and a hematocrit. Prescribe needed vitamin and mineral supplements. Develop a nutrition plan appropriate to cultural preferences, typically three balanced meals each day, including 300 additional kcal plus prenatal supplements. Caution against excess amounts of vitamin A, which can become toxic; fish with mercury exposure such as sharks, swordfish, or even canned tuna; unpasteurized dairy products; and undercooked meats.

Weigh the woman at each visit, with the results plotted on a graph, using the updated recommendations below.

Recommendations for Total and Rate of Weight Gain During Pregnancy, by Prepregnancy BMI, 2009

Prepregnancy BMI	BMI*	Total Weight Gain (lbs)	Rates of Weight Gain[†] 2nd and 3rd Trimester (lbs/wk)
Underweight	<18.5	28–40	1 (1–1.3)
Normal weight	18.5–24.9	25–35	1 (0.8–1)
Overweight	25–29.9	15–25	0.6 (0.5–0.7)
Obese (includes all classes)	≥30	11–20	0.5 (0.4–0.6)

*To calculate BMI, go to www.nhlbisupport.com/bmi.
[†]Calculations assume a 0.5–2 kg (1.1–4.4 lbs) weight gain in the first trimester (based on Siega-Riz et al., 1994; Abrams et al., 1995; Carmichael et al., 1997)

Source: Rasmussen KM, Yaktine AL (eds) and Institute of Medicine. Committee to Reexamine IOM Pregnancy Weight Guidelines. Weight gain during pregnancy: re-examing the guidelines. Washington, DC: National Academics Press, 2009. (Available at http://www.iom.edu/Reports/2009/Weight-Gain-During-Pregnancy-Reexamining-the-Guidelines.aspx.) Accessed February 26, 2011.

Exercise. Recommend 30 minutes of moderate exercise or more on most days of the week unless contraindications exist. Women initiating exercise during pregnancy should consider programs developed specifically for pregnant women. Immersion in hot water should be avoided. After the first trimester, women should avoid exercise in the supine position, which can compress the inferior vena cava, resulting in dizziness and decreased placental blood flow. In the third trimester, advise against exercises that may cause loss of balance. Contact sports or activities that risk abdominal trauma are unwise in all trimesters. Pregnant woman should avoid overheating, dehydration, and any exertion that causes notable fatigue or discomfort.

Substances of Abuse. Promote abstinence as the immediate goal during pregnancy. Pursue universal screening in a neutral manner for:

- *Tobacco.* Tobacco use accounts for a third of all low-birth-weight babies and many poor pregnancy outcomes, including placental abruption and preterm labor. Cessation is the goal, but any decrease in usage is favorable.

- *Alcohol.* Fetal alcohol syndrome is the leading cause of preventable mental retardation in the United States. Abstinence is widely recommended throughout pregnancy.

- *Illicit drugs including narcotics.* Women with addictions should be referred for treatment immediately and counseled and screened for hepatitis C and HIV.

- *Prescription drugs.* Ask about commonly abused prescription drugs, including narcotics, stimulants, benzodiazepines.

Domestic Violence. Pregnancy is a time when risk of intimate partner violence increases. Up to one in five women experience some form of abuse during pregnancy. Pursue universal screening of all pregnant women without regard to socioeconomic status. Ask, "Since you've been pregnant, have you been slapped or otherwise physically hurt by anyone?" Nonverbal clues include frequent changes in appointments at the last minute, unusual behavior during visits, partners that refuse to leave the patient alone, and bruises or other injuries. When abuse becomes apparent, ask the patient how you might best help her. Respect limits she places on sharing information. Maintain an updated list of shelters, counseling centers, hotline numbers and other trusted local referrals. Plan future appointments at accelerated intervals. Complete a thorough physical exam as much as she permits and document all injuries on a body diagram.

> **National Domestic Violence Hotline**
>
> - Web site: www.thehotline.org
> - 1-800-799-SAFE (7233)
> - TTY for hearing impaired: 1-800-787-3224

Prenatal Laboratory Screenings. Initially include blood type and Rh, antibody screen, complete blood count—especially hematocrit and platelet count, rubella titer, syphilis test, hepatitis B surface antigen, HIV, STI screen for gonorrhea and chlamydia and urinalysis with culture. Timed screenings include an oral glucose tolerance test for gestational diabetes around 24 weeks, and a vaginal swab for group B *streptococcus* between 35 to 37 weeks' gestation. Pursue additional tests related to the mother's risk factors, such as screening for aneuploidy, screening for Tay-Sachs or other genetic diseases, amniocentesis, or checking for infectious diseases such as hepatitis C.

Immunizations. As indicated, give tetanus and influenza vaccinations in the second or third trimester. The following vaccines are safe during pregnancy: pneumococcal, meningococcal, and hepatitis B. The following vaccines are NOT safe during pregnancy: measles/mumps/rubella, polio, varicella. However, all women should have rubella titers drawn during pregnancy and be immunized after birth if nonimmune. Rho (D) immunoglobulin, or RhoGAM, should be given to all Rh-negative women at 28 weeks' gestation and again within 3 days of delivery to prevent sensitization to an Rh-positive infant.

Techniques of Examination

Preparing for the Examination

Show respect for the woman's comfort and privacy, as well as for her individual needs and sensitivities. Ask her to wear her gown with the opening in front to ease the examination of both breasts and the pregnant abdomen.

Positioning
- The semisitting position with the knees bent (see p. 366) affords the most comfort and protects abdominal organs and vessels from the weight of the gravid uterus.
- Avoid prolonged periods of lying on the back. Make your abdominal palpation efficient and accurate.
- The pelvic examination also should be relatively quick.

Equipment
- *Gynecologic speculum and lubrication:* Because of vaginal wall relaxation during pregnancy, a larger-than-usual speculum may be needed.
- *Sampling materials:* The cervical brush may cause bleeding, so the Ayre wooden spatula or "broom" sampling device is preferred during pregnancy. Additional swabs may be needed to screen for sexually transmitted infections, group B strep, and wet mount preparations.
- *Tape measure:* Use a plastic or paper tape measure to assess the size of the uterus after 20 gestational weeks.
- *Doppler fetal heart rate monitor and gel:* Apply a "Doppler" or "Doptone" to the gravid belly to assess fetal heart rate after 10 weeks of gestation.

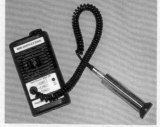

EXAMINATION TECHNIQUES

POSSIBLE FINDINGS

HEIGHT, WEIGHT, AND VITAL SIGNS

Observe the general health, emotional state, nutritional status, and coordination as the pregnant woman comes into the room.

Measure the height and weight. Calculate BMI. First-trimester weight loss should not exceed 5% of prepartum weight.

Weight loss of more than 5% in excessive vomiting, or *hyperemesis*

Measure the blood pressure at every visit. In midpregnancy, it may be lower than in the nonpregnant state.

Gestational hypertension: if systolic blood pressure (SBP) ≥140 mm Hg and diastolic blood pressure (DBP) ≥90 mm Hg, first occurring after week 20 and *without proteinuria*

Chronic hypertension: if SBP ≥140 mm Hg and DBP ≥90 mm Hg prior to pregnancy, before week 20, and after 12 weeks postpartum

Preeclampsia: if SBP ≥140 mm Hg and DBP ≥90 mm Hg after week 20 and *with proteinuria*

HEAD AND NECK

- *Face.* Check for the mask of pregnancy, *chloasma*, or irregular brownish patches around the forehead and cheeks, across the bridge of the nose, or along the jaw.

  Facial edema after 20 weeks in gestational hypertension

- *Hair*

  Hair loss should not be attributed to pregnancy.

- *Eyes.* Note the conjunctival color.

  Anemia of pregnancy may cause conjunctival pallor.

- *Nose*, including nasal congestion

  Nosebleeds are more common during pregnancy. Erosion of nasal septum if use of intranasal cocaine.

- *Mouth*

  Gingival enlargement common

- *Thyroid gland.* Inspect and palpate. Modest symmetric enlargement is common.

  Significant enlargement is abnormal and should be investigated.

| EXAMINATION TECHNIQUES | POSSIBLE FINDINGS |

THORAX AND LUNGS

Inspect the thorax for contours. Observe the pattern of breathing. Auscultate the lungs.

Respiratory alkalosis in later trimesters. Elevated respiratory rate in infection, pulmonary embolism, *peripartum cardiomyopathy*.

HEART

Palpate the apical impulse.

Impulse may be higher than normal in the fourth intercostal space because of transverse and leftward rotation of the heart from the higher diaphragm.

Auscultate the heart. A venous hum and systolic or continuous mammary souffle (see p. 165) are common.

Murmurs may signal anemia; new diastolic murmurs should be investigated. If signs of heart failure, consider *peripartum cardiomyopathy*.

BREASTS

Inspect the breasts and nipples for symmetry and color.

The venous pattern may be marked, the nipples and areolae are dark, and Montgomery's glands are prominent.

Palpate for masses.

During pregnancy, breasts are tender and nodular; focal tenderness in *mastitis*. Investigate any new discrete masses.

Compress each nipple between your index finger and thumb.

This may express colostrum from the nipples; investigate if abnormal bloody or purulent discharge.

ABDOMEN

Place the pregnant woman in a semisitting position with her knees flexed.

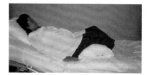

EXAMINATION TECHNIQUES

- Inspect any scars or striae, the shape and contour of the abdomen, and the fundal height.
- Assess the shape and contour to estimate pregnancy size.

POSSIBLE FINDINGS

Purplish striae and linea nigra are normal.

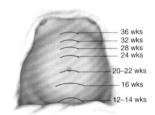

EXPECTED HEIGHT OF UTERINE FUNDUS OF PREGNANCY

- Palpate for:
  - *Organs and masses*
  - *Fetal movements,* usually detected after 24 weeks

  - *Uterine contractility*

Ultrasound confirmation of fetal health and movement may be needed.

Irregular contractions after 12 weeks or after palpation during the third trimester

Prior to 37 weeks, regular uterine contractions or bleeding are abnormal, suggesting *preterm labor.*

- If woman is >20 weeks pregnant, *measure fundal height* with a tape measure from the top of the symphysis pubis to the top of the uterine fundus. After 20 weeks, measurement in centimeters should roughly equal the weeks of gestation.

If fundal height is more than 4 cm higher than expected, consider multiple gestation, a large fetus, extra amniotic fluid, or uterine leiomyoma. If more than 4 cm lower, consider low level of amniotic fluid, missed abortion, transverse lie, growth retardation, or fetal anomaly.

- *Auscultate the fetal heart tones,* noting rate (FHR), location, and rhythm. A Doptone detects the FHR after 10 weeks. The FHR is audible with a fetoscope after 18 weeks.

Lack of an audible FHR may indicate pregnancy of fewer weeks than expected, fetal demise, or false pregnancy.

EXAMINATION TECHNIQUES

- *Location.* From 10 to 18 weeks, the FHR is in the midline of the lower abdomen; later depends on fetal position. Use modified *Leopold's maneuvers* to palpate the fetal head and back and identify where to listen.

- *Rate.* The *rate* usually is 120 to 160 beats per minute. After 32 to 34 weeks, the FHR should increase with fetal movement.

- *Rhythm.* In the third trimester, expect a variance of 10 to 15 beats per minute (BPM) over 1 to 2 minutes.

POSSIBLE FINDINGS

An FHR that drops noticeably near term with fetal movement could indicate poor placental circulation.

Lack of beat-to-beat variability late in pregnancy warrants investigation with an FHR monitor.

GENITALIA, ANUS, AND RECTUM

Inspect the *external genitalia*.

Parous relaxation of the introitus, labial varicosities, enlargement of the labia and clitoris, scars from an *episiotomy* or perineal lacerations

Palpate *Bartholin's* and *Skene's glands*. Check for a *cystocele* or *rectocele*.

Bartholin's cyst

Examine the *internal genitalia*.

Speculum Examination

- Inspect the *cervix* for color, shape, and healed lacerations.

  Purplish color of pregnancy; lacerations from prior deliveries

- Perform a *Pap smear*, if indicated.

  Specimens may be needed for diagnosis of vaginal or cervical infection

- Inspect the *vaginal walls*.

  Bluish or violet color, deep rugae, leukorrhea in normal pregnancy; vaginal irritation, itching, and discharge in infection

EXAMINATION TECHNIQUES

Bimanual Examination

Insert two lubricated fingers into introitus, palmar side down, with slight pressure downward on the perineum. Slide fingers into the posterior vaginal vault. Maintaining downward pressure, gently turn fingers palmar side up.

- Assess cervical os and degree of effacement. Place your finger gently in the os, and then sweep it around the *surface of the cervix*.

  POSSIBLE FINDINGS: Closed external os if nulliparous; os open to size of fingertip if multiparous

- Estimate the *length of the cervix*. Palpate the lateral surface from the cervical tip to the lateral fornix.

  Prior to 34 to 36 weeks, cervix should retain normal length of ≥3 cm.

- Palpate the *uterus* for size, shape, consistency, and position.

  Hegar's sign, or early softening of the isthmus; pear-shaped uterus up to 8 weeks, then globular

- Estimate *uterine size*. With your internal fingers placed at either side of cervix, palmar surfaces upward, gently lift the uterus toward the abdominal hand. Capture the fundal portion of the uterus between your two hands and gently estimate size.

  An irregularly shaped uterus suggests uterine myomata or a *bicornuate uterus,* two distinct uterine cavities separated by a septum.

- Palpate the *left and right adnexa*.

  Early in pregnancy, it is important to rule out tubal (*ectopic*) pregnancy.

- Evaluate pelvic floor strength as you withdraw the examining fingers.

- Inspect the anus. Rectal and rectovaginal examinations are usually not indicated.

  Hemorrhoids may engorge later in pregnancy.

| EXAMINATION TECHNIQUES | POSSIBLE FINDINGS |

EXTREMITIES

Inspect the legs for *varicose veins*.

Palpate the hands and legs for *edema*.

Watch for swelling of *preeclampsia* or deep venous thrombosis.

Check knee and ankle deep tendon reflexes.

Hyperreflexia may signal *preeclampsia*.

SPECIAL TECHNIQUES

LEOPOLD'S MANEUVERS

To identify:
- The upper and lower fetal poles, namely, the proximal and distal fetal parts
- The maternal side where the fetal back is located
- The descent of the presenting part into the maternal pelvis
- The extent of flexion of the fetal head
- Estimated fetal weight and size

Common deviations include *breech presentation* (fetal buttocks present at the outlet of the maternal pelvis) and absence of the presenting part well down into the maternal pelvis at term.

FIRST MANEUVER
(Upper Fetal Pole)

Stand at the woman's side, facing her head. Keep the fingers of both examining hands together. Palpate gently with the fingertips to determine what part of the fetus is in the upper pole of the uterine fundus.

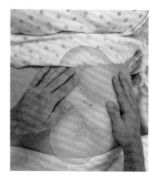

| EXAMINATION TECHNIQUES | POSSIBLE FINDINGS |

SECOND MANEUVER
(Sides of the Maternal Abdomen)

Place one hand on each side of the woman's abdomen, aiming to capture the body of the fetus between them. Use one hand to steady the uterus and the other to palpate the fetus. Look for the back on one side and the extremities on the other.

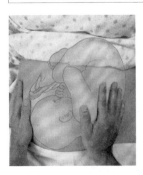

THIRD MANEUVER
(Lower Fetal Pole and Descent into Pelvis)

Face the woman's feet. Palpate the area just above the symphysis pubis. Note whether the hands diverge with downward pressure or stay together to learn if the presenting part of the fetus, head or buttocks, is descending into the pelvic inlet.

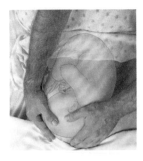

FOURTH MANEUVER
(Flexion of the fetal head)

This maneuver assesses the flexion or extension of the fetal head, presuming that the fetal head is the presenting part in the pelvis. Still facing the woman's feet, with your hands positioned on either side of the gravid uterus as in the third maneuver, identify the fetal front and back sides. Using one hand at a time, slide your fingers down each side of the fetal body until you reach the "cephalic prominence," that is, where the fetal brow or occiput juts out.

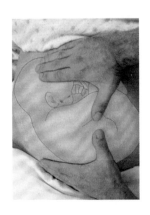

EXAMINATION TECHNIQUES

Recording Your Findings

Recording the Physical Examination—The Pregnant Woman

"32-year-old G3,P1102 at 18 weeks' gestation as determined by LMP presents to establish prenatal care. Patient endorses fetal movement; denies contractions, vaginal bleeding, and leakage of fluids. On external exam, low transverse cesarean scar is evident; fundus is palpable just below umbilicus. On internal exam, cervix is open to fingertip at the external os but closed at the internal os; cervix is 3 cm long; uterus enlarged to size consistent with 18-week gestation. Speculum exam shows leucorrhea with positive Chadwick's sign. FHT by Doppler are between 140 and 145 BPM." *Describes healthy woman at 18 weeks' gestation*.

CHAPTER

20

The Older Adult

Older adults now number more than 39 million in the United States, growing to 88 million by 2050. Life span at birth is currently 84 years for women and 82 years for men. The "demographic imperative" is to maximize not only life span but also "health span" for older adults so that seniors maintain full function for as long as possible, enjoying rich and active lives in their homes and communities.

- Assessing the older adult entails a focus on healthy or "successful" aging; understanding and mobilizing family, social, and community supports; skills directed to functional assessment, "the sixth vital sign"; and promoting the older adult's long-term health and safety.

- The aging population displays marked heterogeneity. Investigators distinguish "usual" aging, with its complex of diseases and impairments, from optimal aging. Optimal aging occurs in those people who escape debilitating disease entirely and maintain healthy lives late into their 80s and 90s. Studies of centenarians show that genes account for approximately 20% of the probability of living to 100, with healthy lifestyles accounting for approximately 20% to 30%.

The Health History

APPROACH TO THE PATIENT

As you talk with older adults, convey respect, patience, and cultural awareness. Be sure to address patients by their last name.

Adjusting the Office Environment. Make sure the office is neither too cool nor too warm. Face the patient directly, sitting at eye level. A well-lit room allows the older adult to see your facial expressions and gestures.

More than 50% of older adults have hearing deficits. Free the room of distractions or noise. Consider using a "pocket talker," a microphone that amplifies your voice and connects to an earpiece inserted by the patient. Chairs with higher seating and a wide stool with a handrail leading up to the examining table help patients with quadriceps weakness.

Shaping the Content and Pace of the Visit.   Older people often reminisce. Listen to this process of life review to gain important insights and help patients as they work through painful feelings or recapture joys and accomplishments.

Balance the need to assess complex problems with the patient's endurance and possible fatigue. Consider dividing the initial assessment into two visits.

Eliciting Symptoms in the Older Adult.   Older patients may overestimate healthiness even when increasing disease and disability are apparent. To reduce the risk of late recognition and delayed intervention, adopt more directed questions or *health screening tools.* Consult with family members and caretakers.

Acute illnesses present differently in older adults than in younger age groups. Be sensitive to changes in presentation of myocardial infarction and thyroid disease. Older patients with infections are less likely to have fever.

Recognize the symptom clusters typical of different *geriatric syndromes,* notable interacting clusters of symptoms, for example, falls, dizziness, depression, urinary incontinence, and functional impairment. Searching for the usual "unifying diagnosis" may pertain to fewer than 50% of older adults.

Cognitive impairment may affect the patient's history. Even elders with mild cognitive impairment, however, can provide sufficient history to reveal concurrent disorders. Use simple sentences with prompts to trigger necessary information. If impairments are more severe, confirm symptoms with family members or caregivers.

Addressing Cultural Dimensions of Aging.   By 2050, the older adult population will increase by 230%, and the minority older adult population by 510%. Cultural differences affect the epidemiology of illness and mental health, acculturation, the specific concerns of the elderly, the potential for misdiagnosis, and disparities in health outcomes. Review the components of self-awareness needed for cultural responsiveness, discussed in Chapter 3 (pp. 40–41). Ask about spiritual advisors and native healers. Cultural values particularly affect decisions about the end of life. Elders, family, and even an extended community group may make these decisions with or for the older patient.

COMMON CONCERNS

- Activities of daily living
- Instrumental activities of daily living
- Medications
- Smoking and alcohol
- Acute and persistent pain
- Nutrition
- Frailty
- Advance directives and palliative care

Place symptoms in the context of your overall *functional assessment*, always focusing on helping the older adult to maintain optimal well-being and level of function.

Activities of Daily Living. Daily activities provide an important baseline for the future. You might say "Tell me about your typical day" or "Tell me about your day yesterday." Then move to a greater level of detail: "You got up at 8 AM? How is it getting out of bed?"

Activities of Daily Living and Instrumental Activities of Daily Living

Physical Activities of Daily Living (ADLs)	Instrumental Activities of Daily Living (IADLs)
Bathing	Using the telephone
Dressing	Shopping
Toileting	Preparing food
Transferring	Housekeeping
Continence	Laundry
Feeding	Transportation
	Taking medicine
	Managing money

Medications. Adults older than 65 take approximately 30% of all prescriptions. Roughly 30% take more than eight prescribed drugs each day! Take a thorough medication history, including name, dose, frequency, and indication for each drug. Explore all components of polypharmacy, including concurrent use of multiple drugs, underuse, inappropriate use, and nonadherence. Ask about use of over-the-counter medications, vitamin and nutrition supplements, and mood-altering drugs. Medications are the most common modifiable risk factor associated with falls.

Smoking and Alcohol. At each visit, advise elderly smokers to quit. An estimated 2% to 20% of older adults have alcohol-related problems. This percentage is expected to rise as the population ages in coming decades. Despite the prevalence of alcohol problems among the elderly, rates of detection and treatment are low. Use the CAGE questions to uncover problem drinking (see p. 46), which contributes to drug interactions and worsens comorbid illnesses.

Acute and Persistent Pain. Pain and associated complaints account for 80% of clinician visits, usually for musculoskeletal complaints like back and joint pain. Older patients are less likely to report pain, leading to undue suffering, depression, social isolation, physical disability, and loss of function.

Inquire about pain each time you meet with the older patient. Ask specifically, "Are you having any pain right now? How about over the past week?" Unidimensional scales such as the Visual Analog Scale, graphic pictures, and the Verbal 0–10 Scale have all been validated and are easiest to use.

Characteristics of Acute and Persistent Pain

Acute Pain	Persistent Pain
Distinct onset	Lasts more than 3 months
Obvious pathology	Often associated with psychological or functional impairment
Short duration	Can fluctuate in character and intensity over time
Common causes: postsurgical, trauma, headache	Common causes: arthritis, cancer, claudication, leg cramps, neuropathy, radiculopathy

Source: Reuben DB, Herr KA, Pacala JT, et al. Geriatrics at Your Fingertips: 2004, 6th ed. Malden, MA: Blackwell Publishing, for the American Geriatrics Society, 2004:149.

Nutrition. Taking a diet history and using the Rapid Screen for Dietary Intake and the Nutrition Screening Checklist (p. 62) are especially important in older adults.

Frailty. The prevalence of this multifactorial syndrome related to declines in physiologic reserves, muscle mass, energy and exercise capacity is 4% to 22%. Pursue related interventions.

Advance Directives and Palliative Care. Initiate these discussions *before* serious illness develops. Advance care planning involves providing information, invoking the patient's preferences, identifying proxy decision makers, and conveying empathy and support. Use clear, simple language. Ask about preferences relating to written "Do Not Resuscitate" orders specifying life support measures "if the heart or lungs were to stop or give out." Seek a written health care proxy or durable power of attorney for health care, "someone who can make decisions reflecting your wishes in case of confusion or emergency." Include these discussions in office settings rather than the uncertain and stressful environment of emergency or acute care.

The goal of *palliative care* is "to relieve suffering and improve the quality of life for patients with advanced illnesses and their families through specific knowledge and skills, including communication with patients and family members; management of pain and other symptoms; psychosocial, spiritual, and bereavement support; and coordination of an array of medical and social services."

Health Promotion and Counseling: Evidence and Recommendations

Important Topics for Health Promotion and Counseling in the Older Adult

- When to screen
- Cancer screening
- Depression, dementia, and cognitive impairment
- Elder mistreatment and abuse

When to Screen. As the life span for older adults extends into the 80s, new issues for screening emerge. In general, base screening decisions on each older person's particular circumstances, rather than on age alone. Consider life expectancy, time interval until benefit from screening accrues, and patient preference. The American Geriatrics Society recommends that if life expectancy is short, give priority to treating conditions that will benefit the patient in the time that remains.

- Screen for age-related changes in *vision* and *hearing*. These are included in the 10-Minute Geriatric Screener (pp. 380–381).

- Recommend regular aerobic *exercise,* resistance training to increase strength, and balance exercise like tai chi.

- *Immunizations.* Include the pneumococcal vaccine once after age 65, annual influenza vaccinations, Td boosters every 10 years, and the *herpes zoster* vaccine.

- Promote *household safety.* Correct poor lighting, chairs at awkward heights, slippery or irregular surfaces, and environmental hazards.

Cancer Screening. Cancer screening can be controversial because of limited evidence about adults older than age 70 to 80. The U.S. Preventive Services Task Force (USPSTF) guidelines are summarized below:

- *Breast cancer* (2009): *Mammography* every 2 years between ages 50 and 74; insufficient evidence thereafter.

- *Cervical cancer* (2003): Routine screening up to age 65 if low risk.

- *Colorectal cancer* (2008): Colonoscopy every 10 years, beginning at age 50; This examination is difficult for many older patients, sigmoidoscopy every 5 years with high-sensitivity fecal occult blood tests (FOBTs) every 3 years, or FOBTs every year ages 50 to 75.

- *Prostate cancer* (2008): Insufficient evidence to declare recommendation.

- *Skin cancer* (2006), lung cancer (2004): Insufficient evidence. American Geriatrics Society recommends checking for skin and oral cancers in high-risk patients.

Depression, Dementia, and Cognitive Impairment. Depression affects 10% of older men and 18% of older women. Use the two screening questions in Chapter 5 p. 68.

Dementia is "an acquired syndrome of decline in memory and at least one other cognitive domain such as language, visuospatial, or executive function sufficient to interfere with social or occupational functioning." It affects 13% of Americans over age 65. Prominent features include:

- Normal alertness but short-term memory deficits and subtle language errors.

- Visuospatial perceptual difficulties and loss of orientation to place.

- Changes in executive function, or ability to perform sequential tasks.

- In later stages, impaired judgment, aphasia, apraxia and loss of ADLs.

Most dementias represent Alzheimer's disease (50% to 85%) or vascular multi-infarct dementia (10% to 20%). Dementia often has a slow, insidious onset. The early stages of *mild cognitive impairment* may be detected only on neurocognitive testing. Watch for family complaints of new or unusual behaviors. Investigate contributing factors such as medications, depression, metabolic abnormalities, or other medical and psychiatric conditions.

Elder Mistreatment and Abuse. Screen older patients for possible *elder mistreatment*, which includes abuse, neglect, exploitation, and abandonment. Prevalence is approximately 1% to 10% of the older population; however, many more cases may remain undetected.

Techniques of Examination

Assessment of the older adult departs from the traditional format of the history and physical examination. Enhanced interviewing, emphasis on daily function and key topics related to elder health, and functional assessment are especially important.

ASSESSING FUNCTIONAL STATUS: THE "SIXTH VITAL SIGN"

Assessing Functional Ability. Functional status is the ability to perform tasks and fulfill social roles associated with daily living across a wide range of complexity. Several performance-based assessment instruments are available. The screening tool below is brief, has high inter-rater agreement, and can be used easily by office staff. It covers the three important domains of geriatric assessment: physical, cognitive, and psychosocial function. It addresses key sensory modalities and urinary incontinence, an often unreported problem that greatly affects social interactions and self-esteem in the elderly. One mnemonic that helps students assess incontinence is DIAPERS: **D**elirium, **I**nfection, **A**trophic urethritis/vaginitis, **P**harmaceuticals, **E**xcess urine output (e.g., due to heart failure, hyperglycemia), **R**estricted mobility, **S**tool impaction.

10-Minute Geriatric Screener

Problem and Screening Measure	Positive Screen
Vision: Two Parts: Ask: "Do you have difficulty driving, or watching television, or reading, or doing any of your daily activities because of your eyesight? If yes, then: Test each eye with Snellen chart while patient wears corrective lenses (if applicable).	Yes to question and inability to read >20/40 on Snellen chart
Hearing: Use audioscope set at 40 dB. Test hearing using 1,000 and 2,000 Hz.	Inability to hear 1,000 or 2,000 Hz in both ears or either of these frequencies in one ear
Leg mobility: Time the patient after instructing: "Rise from the chair. Walk 20 feet briskly, turn, walk back to the chair, and sit down."	Unable to complete task in 15 seconds
Urinary incontinence: Two Parts: Ask: "In the last year, have you ever lost your urine and gotten wet?" If yes, then ask: "Have you lost urine on at least 6 separate dates?"	Yes to both questions
Nutrition/weight loss: Two parts: Ask: "Have you lost 10 lbs over the past 6 months without trying to do so?" Weigh the patient.	Yes to the question or weight <100 lbs

(continued)

10-Minute Geriatric Screener (continued)

Problem and Screening Measure	Positive Screen
Memory: Three-item recall	Unable to remember all three items after 1 minute
Depression: Ask: "Do you often feel sad or depressed?"	Yes to the question
Physical disability: Six questions: "Are you able to...: ▸ "Do strenuous activities like fast walking or bicycling?" ▸ "Do heavy work around the house like washing windows, walls, or floors?" ▸ "Go shopping for groceries or clothes?" ▸ "Get to places out of walking distance?" ▸ "Bathe, either a sponge bath, tub bath, or shower?" ▸ "Dress, like putting on a shirt, buttoning and zipping, or putting on shoes?"	No to any of the questions

Source: More AA, Siu AL. Screening for common problems in ambulatory elderly: clinical confirmation of a screening instrument. Am J Med 1996;100:438–440.

Further Assessment for Preventing Falls. Each year approximately 35% to 40% of healthy community-dwelling older adults experience falls. Incidence rates in nursing homes and hospitals are almost three times higher, with related injuries in approximately 25%.

The American Geriatrics Society (AGS) recommends risk factor assessment for falls during routine primary care visits, with more intensive assessment in *high-risk groups*—those with first or recurrent falls, nursing home residents, and those prone to fall-related injuries. Assess how the fall occurred, seeking details from any witnesses, and identify risk factors, medical comorbidities, functional status, and environmental risks. Couple your assessment with interventions for prevention, including gait and balance training and exercise to strengthen muscles, vitamin D supplementation, reduction of home hazards, discontinuation of psychotropic medication, and multifactorial assessment with targeted interventions. The AGS recommendations are provided on the next page.

Prevention of Falls in Older Persons Living in the Community

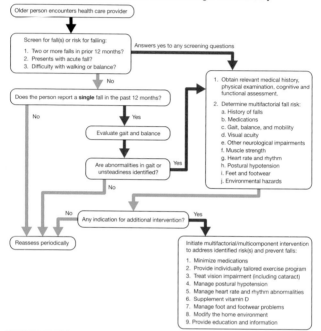

Source: Panel on Prevention of Falls in Older Persons, American Geriatrics Society and British Geriatrics Society. Summary of the Updated American Geriatrics Society/British Geriatrics Society. Clinical Practice guideline for prevention of falls in older persons, 2010. J Am Geriatr Soc 59:148–157, 2011. Also at http://www.americangeriatrics.org/files/documents/health_care_pros/JAGS.Falls.Guidelines.pdf. Accessed January 24, 2011. See also U.S. Preventive Services Task Force. Interventions to Prevent Falls in Older Adults, Topic Page. December 2010. At http://www.uspreventiveservicestaskforce.org/uspstf/uspsfalls.htm. Accessed January 24, 2011.

EXAMINATION TECHNIQUES	POSSIBLE FINDINGS

PHYSICAL EXAMINATION OF THE OLDER ADULT

Vital Signs. Measure blood pressure, checking for increased systolic blood pressure (SBP) and widened pulse pressure (PP), defined as SBP minus diastolic blood pressure (DBP).

Isolated systolic hypertension (SBP ≥140) after age 50 triples the risk of coronary heart disease in men. PP ≥60 is a risk factor for cardiovascular and renal disease and stroke.

EXAMINATION TECHNIQUES	POSSIBLE FINDINGS

Review the JNC 7 categories of hypertension to guide early detection and treatment.

Assess the patient for *orthostatic hypotension*, defined as a drop in SBP of ≥20 mm Hg or DBP of ≥10 mm Hg or HR increase of ≥20 BPM, within 3 minutes of standing. Measure in two positions: supine after the patient rests for up to 10 minutes, then within 2 to 3 minutes after standing up.

Orthostatic hypotension occurs in 10% to 20% of older adults and in up to 30% of frail nursing home residents, especially when they first arise in the morning. Watch for lightheadedness, weakness, unsteadiness, visual blurring, and, in 20% to 30% of patients, syncope.

Assess for medications, autonomic disorders, diabetes, prolonged bedrest, blood loss, and cardiovascular disorders.

Measure heart rate, respiratory rate, and temperature. The apical heart rate may yield more information about arrhythmias in older patients. Use thermometers accurate for lower temperatures.

Respiratory rate ≥25 breaths per minute indicates lower respiratory infection or possible CHF or COPD.

Hypothermia is more common in elderly patients.

Weight and height are especially important and needed for calculation of the body mass index (p. 53). Weight should be measured at every visit. Obtain oxygen saturation using a pulse oximeter.

Low weight is a key indicator of poor nutrition.

Undernutrition in depression, alcoholism, cognitive impairment, malignancy, chronic organ failure (cardiac, renal, pulmonary), medication use, social isolation, and poverty

Skin. Note physiologic changes of aging, such as thinning, loss of elastic tissue and turgor, and wrinkling.

Dry, flaky, rough, and often itchy

Check the extensor surface of the hands and forearms.

White depigmented patches (*pseudoscars*); well-demarcated, vividly purple macules or patches that may fade after several weeks (*actinic purpura*)

Look for changes from sun exposure. There may be *actinic lentigines*, or "liver spots," and *actinic keratoses,* superficial flattened papules covered by a dry scale (p. 94).

Distinguish such lesions from a *basal cell carcinoma* and *squamous cell carcinoma* (p. 95). Dark, raised, asymmetric lesion with irregular borders is suspicious for *melanoma*

| EXAMINATION TECHNIQUES | POSSIBLE FINDINGS |

Inspect for the benign *comedones*, or blackheads, on the cheeks or around the eyes; *cherry angiomas* (p. 93); and *seborrheic keratoses*, (p. 94).

Inspect for painful vesicular lesions in a dermatomal distribution.

Herpes zoster from reactivation of latent varicella-zoster virus in the dorsal root ganglia

In older bedbound patients, especially when emaciated or neurologically impaired, inspect for damage or ulceration.

Pressure sores if obliteration of arteriolar and capillary blood flow to the skin or shear forces with movement across sheets or lifting upright incorrectly

HEENT. Inspect the eyelids, the bony orbit, and the eye.

Senile ptosis arising from weakening of the levator palpebrae, relaxation of the skin, and increased weight of the upper eyelid

Ectropion or *entropion* of lower lids (p. 116)

Yellowing of the sclera and *arcus senilis*, a benign whitish ring around the limbus

Test visual acuity, using a pocket Snellen chart or wall-mounted chart.

More than 40 million Americans have refractive errors—*presbyopia*.

Examine the lenses and fundi.

Cataracts, glaucoma, and macular degeneration all increase with aging.

Inspect each lens for opacities.

Cataracts are the world's leading cause of blindness.

Assess the cup-to-disc ratio, usually ≤1:2.

Increased cup-to-disc ratio suggests open-angle *glaucoma* and possible loss of peripheral and central vision, and blindness. Prevalence is three to four times higher in African Americans.

Inspect the fundi for colloid bodies causing alterations in pigmentation called *drusen*. These may be hard and sharply defined, or soft and confluent with altered pigmentation.

Macular degeneration causes poor central vision and blindness: types include *dry atrophic* (more common but less severe) and *wet exudative* (or neovascular).

Chapter 20 | The Older Adult

EXAMINATION TECHNIQUES	POSSIBLE FINDINGS
Test hearing by the whispered voice (see p. 108) or audioscope. Inspect ear canals for cerumen.	Removing cerumen often quickly improves hearing.
Examine the oral cavity for odor, appearance of the gingival mucosa, any caries, mobility of the teeth, and quantity of saliva.	*Malodor* in poor oral hygiene, periodontitis, or caries *Gingivitis* if periodontal disease
Inspect for lesions on mucosal surfaces. Ask patient to remove dentures so you can check gums for denture sores.	Dental plaque and cavitation if caries. Increased tooth mobility; risk of tooth aspiration Decreased salivation from medications, radiation, Sjögren's syndrome, or dehydration *Oral tumors,* usually on lateral borders of tongue and floor of mouth
Thorax and Lungs. Note subtle signs of changes in pulmonary function.	Increased anteroposterior diameter, purse-lipped breathing, and dyspnea with talking or minimal exertion in *chronic obstructive pulmonary disease*
Cardiovascular System. Review blood pressure and heart rate.	Isolated systolic hypertension and a widened pulse pressure are cardiac risk factors. Search for *left ventricular hypertrophy (LVH)*.
Inspect the jugular venous pulsation (JVP), palpating the carotid upstrokes, and listen for any overlying carotid bruits.	A *tortuous atherosclerotic aorta* can raise pressure in the left jugular veins by impairing drainage into right atrium. Carotid bruits in possible *carotid stenosis*.
Assess the point of maximal impulse (PMI), and then heart sounds.	Sustained PMI is found in LVH; diffuse PMI is found within heart failure (see p. 155). In older adults, S_3 in dilatation of the left ventricle from heart failure or cardiomyopathy; S_4 in hypertension

EXAMINATION TECHNIQUES	POSSIBLE FINDINGS
Listen for cardiac murmurs in all areas (see p. 157). Describe timing, shape, location of maximal intensity, radiation, intensity, pitch, and quality of each murmur.	A systolic crescendo–decrescendo murmur in the second right interspace in *aortic sclerosis* or *aortic stenosis*. Both carry increased risk of cardiovascular disease and death. A harsh holosystolic murmur at the apex suggests *mitral regurgitation,* also common in the elderly.
For systolic murmurs over the clavicle, check for delay between the brachial and radial pulses.	Delay during simultaneous palpation (but not compression) of brachial and radial pulses in *aortic stenosis.*

Breasts and Axillae. Palpate the breasts carefully for lumps or masses.

Possible breast cancer

Abdomen

Listen for bruits over the aorta, renal arteries, and femoral arteries.	*Bruits* in atherosclerotic vascular disease
Inspect the upper abdomen; palpate to the left of the midline for aortic pulsations.	Widened aorta and pulsatile mass may be found in *abdominal aortic aneurysm.*

Female Genitalia and Pelvic Examination. Take special care to explain the steps of the examination and allow time for careful positioning. For the woman with arthritis or spinal deformities who cannot flex her hips or knees, an assistant can gently raise and support the legs, or help the woman into the left lateral position.

Inspect the vulva for changes related to menopause; identify any labial masses. Bluish swellings may be varicosities.	Benign masses include condylomata, fibromas, leiomyomas, and sebaceous cysts. Bulging of the anterior vaginal wall below the urethra in urethrocele
Inspect the urethra for *caruncles,* or prolapse of fleshy erythematous mucosal tissue at the urethral meatus.	Clitoral enlargement in *androgen-producing tumors* or use of androgen creams

EXAMINATION TECHNIQUES	POSSIBLE FINDINGS
Speculum Examination. Inspect vaginal walls, which may be atrophic, and cervix.	Estrogen-stimulated cervical mucus with ferning in use of hormone replacement therapy, *endometrial hyperplasia*, and *estrogen-producing tumors*
Obtain endocervical cells for the Pap smear. Use a blind swab if the atrophic vagina is too small.	
Removing speculum, ask patient to bear down.	Uterine prolapse, cystocele, urethrocele, or rectocele.
Perform the bimanual examination.	See Table 14-6, Positions of the Uterus, and Uterine Myomas, p. 239.
	Mobility of cervix restricted if inflammation, malignancy, or surgical adhesion
	Palpable ovaries in *ovarian cancer*.
Perform the rectovaginal examination if indicated.	Enlarged, fixed, or irregular uterus if adhesions or malignancy. Rectal masses in *colon cancer*.
Male Genitalia and Prostate. Examine the penis; retract foreskin if present. Examine the scrotum, testes, and epididymis.	Smegma, penile cancer, and scrotal hydroceles
Do a rectal examination.	Rectal masses in *colon cancer*. *Prostate hyperplasia* if enlargement; *prostate cancer* if nodules or masses.
Peripheral Vascular System. Auscultate the abdomen for aortic, renal, femoral artery bruits.	Bruits over these vessels in *atherosclerotic disease*.
Palpate pulses.	Diminished or absent pulses in *arterial occlusion*. Confirm with an office ankle–brachial index (see pp. 209–210).

EXAMINATION TECHNIQUES	POSSIBLE FINDINGS
Musculoskeletal System. Screen general range of motion and gait. Conduct *timed "get up and go"* test.	Review examination techniques for individual joints in Chapter 16, Musculoskelatal System. See Table 20-1, Timed Get Up and Go Test, p. 390.
If joint deformity, deficits in mobility, or pain with movement, conduct a more thorough examination.	Degenerative joint changes in *osteoarthritis;* joint inflammation in *rheumatoid* or *gouty arthritis.* See Tables 16-1 to 16-4, pp. 277–282.
Nervous System. Refer to results of 10-Minute Geriatric Screener, pp. 380–381. Pursue further examination if any deficits. Focus especially on memory and affect.	Learn to distinguish delirium from depression and dementia. See Table 20-2, Delirium and Dementia, pp. 391–392 and Table 20-3, Screening for Dementia: The Mini-Cog, p. 393.
Assess gait and balance, particularly standing balance; timed 8-foot walk; stride characteristics like width, pace, and length of stride; and careful turning.	Abnormalities of gait and balance, especially widening of base, slowing and lengthening of stride, and difficulty turning, are correlated with risk of falls.
Although neurologic abnormalities are common in older adults, their prevalence without identifiable disease increases with age, ranging from 30% to 50%.	Physiologic changes of aging: unequal pupil size, decreased arm swing and spontaneous movements, increased leg rigidity and abnormal gait, presence of the snout and grasp reflexes, and decreased toe vibratory sense.
Assess any tremor, rigidity, bradykinesia, micrographia, shuffling gait, and difficulty turning in bed, opening jars, and rising from a chair.	Seen in Parkinson's disease. Tremor is slow frequency and at rest, with a "pill-rolling" quality, aggravated by stress and inhibited during sleep or movement. *Essential tremor* is often bilateral, symmetric, with positive family history, and diminished by alcohol

EXAMINATION TECHNIQUES

Recording Your Findings

As you read through this physical examination, you will notice some atypical findings. Test yourself to see if you can interpret these findings in the context of all you have learned about the examination of the older adult.

Recording the Physical Examination—The Older Adult

> Mr. J is an older adult who appears healthy but underweight, with good muscle bulk. He is alert and interactive, with good recall of his life history. He is accompanied by his son.
>
> **Vital Signs:** Ht (without shoes) 160 cm (5′). Wt (dressed) 65 kg (143 lb). BMI 28. BP 145/88 right arm, supine; 154/94 left arm, supine. Heart rate (HR) 98 and regular. Respiratory rate (RR) 18. Temperature (oral) 98.6°F.
>
> **10-Minute Geriatric Screener:** (see pp. 380–381)
>
> **Vision:** Patient reports difficulty reading. Visual acuity 20/60 on Snellen chart.
>
> Needs further evaluation for glasses and possibly hearing aid.
>
> **Hearing:** Cannot hear whispered voice in either ear. Cannot hear 1,000 or 2,000 Hz with audioscope in either ear.
>
> **Leg Mobility:** Can walk 20 feet briskly, turn, walk back to chair, and sit down in 14 seconds.
>
> **Urinary Incontinence:** Has lost urine and gotten wet on 20 separate days.
>
> Needs further evaluation for incontinence, including "DIAPER" assessment (see p. 380), prostate examination, and postvoid residual, which is normally ≤50 mL (requires bladder catheterization).
>
> **Nutrition:** Has lost 15 lbs over the past 6 months without trying.
>
> Needs nutritional screen (see p. 62).
>
> **Memory:** Can remember three items after 1 minute.
>
> **Depression:** Does not often feel sad or depressed.
>
> **Physical Disability:** Can walk fast but cannot ride a bicycle. Can do moderate but not heavy work around the house. Can go shopping for groceries or clothes. Can get to places out of walking distance. Can bathe each day without difficulty. Can dress, including buttoning and zipping, and can put on shoes.
>
> Consider exercise regimen with strength training.
>
> **Physical Examination:** Record the vital signs and weight. Carefully describe your findings for each relevant segment of the peripheral examination, using terminology found in the "Recording Your Findings" sections of the prior chapters.

Aids to Interpretation

Table 20-1 **Timed Get Up and Go Test**

Performed with patient wearing regular footwear, using usual walking aid if needed, and sitting back in a chair with arm rest.

On the word, "Go," the patient is asked to do the following:
1. Stand up from the arm chair
2. Walk 3 meters (in a line)
3. Turn
4. Walk back to chair
5. Sit down

Time the second effort.

Observe patient for postural stability, steppage, stride length, and sway.

Scoring:
- **Normal:** completes task in <10 seconds
- **Abnormal:** completes task in >20 seconds

Low scores correlate with good functional independence; high scores correlate with poor functional independence and higher risk of falls.

Reproduced from: Get-up and Go Test. In: Mathias S, Nayak USL, Isaacs B. "Balance in elderly patient" The "Get Up and Go" Test. Arch Phys Med Rehabil 1986;67:387–389; Podsiadlo D, Richardson S. The Timed "Up and Go": A test of basic functional mobility for frail elderly persons. J Am Geriatr Soc 1991;39:142–148.

Table 20-2 Delirium and Dementia

	Delirium	Dementia
Clinical Features		
Onset	Acute	Insidious
Course	Fluctuating, with lucid intervals; worse at night	Slowly progressive
Duration	Hours to weeks	Months to years
Sleep/Wake Cycle	Always disrupted	Sleep fragmented
General Medical Illness or Drug Toxicity	Either or both present	Often absent, especially in Alzheimer's disease
Mental Status		
Level of Consciousness	Disturbed. Person less clearly aware of the environment and less able to focus, sustain, or shift attention	Usually normal until late in the course of the illness
Behavior	Activity often abnormally decreased (somnolence) or increased (agitation, hypervigilance)	Normal to slow; may become inappropriate
Speech	May be hesitant, slow or rapid, incoherent	Difficulty in finding words, aphasia
Mood	Fluctuating, labile, from fearful or irritable to normal or depressed	Often flat, depressed
Thought Processes	Disorganized, may be incoherent	Impoverished. Speech gives little information

(continued)

Table 20-2 Delirium and Dementia (continued)

	Delirium	Dementia
Thought Content	Delusions common, often transient	Delusions may occur
Perceptions	Illusions, hallucinations, most often visual	Hallucinations may occur.
Judgment	Impaired, often to a varying degree	Increasingly impaired over the course of the illness
Orientation	Usually disoriented, especially for time. A known place may seem unfamiliar.	Fairly well maintained, but becomes impaired in the later stages of illness
Attention	Fluctuates. Person easily distracted, unable to concentrate on selected tasks	Usually unaffected until late in the illness
Memory	Immediate and recent memory impaired	Recent memory and new learning especially impaired
Examples of Cause	Delirium tremens (due to withdrawal from alcohol) Uremia Acute hepatic failure Acute cerebral vasculitis Atropine poisoning	*Reversible:* Vitamin B_{12} deficiency, thyroid disorders *Irreversible:* Alzheimer's disease, vascular dementia (from multiple infarcts), dementia due to head trauma

Table 20-3 — Screening for Dementia: The Mini-Cog

Administration

The test is administered as follows:

1. Instruct the patient to listen carefully to and remember 3 unrelated words and then to repeat the words.
2. Instruct the patient to draw the face of a clock, either on a blank sheet of paper or on a sheet with the clock circle already drawn on the page. After the patient puts the numbers on the clock face, ask him or her to draw the hands of the clock to read a specific time.
3. Ask the patient to repeat the 3 previously stated words.

Scoring

Give 1 point for each recalled word after the clock drawing test (CDC) distractor.

Patients recalling none of the three words are classified as demented (Score = 0).

Patients recalling all three words are classified as nondemented (Score = 3).

Patients with intermediate word recall of 1–2 words are classified based on the CDT (Abnormal = demented; Normal = nondemented).

Note: The CDT is considered normal if all numbers are present in the correct sequence and position, and the hands readably display the requested time.

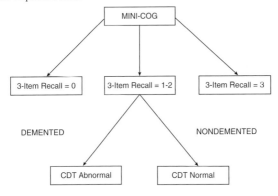

From Borson S, Scanlan J, Brush M, et al. The Mini-Cog: a cognitive 'vital signs' measure for dementia screening in multi-lingual elderly. Int J Geriatr Psychiatry 2000;15(11): 1021–1027. Copyright John Wiley & Sons Limited. Reproduced with permission.

Index

Page numbers followed by "b" indicate boxed material; those followed by "t" indicate end-of-chapter tables.

A

ABCDE screening, 83, 96t
Abdomen, 179–193
   in children, 336, 342
   concerning symptoms, 179–184
   examination of, 12, 186–193
   fullness of, 181
   health history, 179–184
   health promotion and counseling, 184–186
   in older adults, 386
   pain or tenderness, 179–182, 197t
   during pregnancy, 366–368
   recording findings, 193b
Abdominal aortic aneurysm, 190, 199, 201, 203, 386
Abdominal fullness, 181
Abdominal reflexes, 302, 313t
Abscess
   of brain, 99
   lung, 142t
   peritonsillar, 109, 342
Abstract thinking, 74
Abuse
   of alcohol, 71, 184–185
   of drugs, 46, 71, 363
   intimate partner, 47, 47b, 363, 363b
   of older adults, 379
   during pregnancy, 363, 363b
   sexual, in children, 343, 357t
Acoustic nerve, 291b, 293
Acquired immunodeficiency syndrome (AIDS). *See also* HIV infection
   Kaposi's sarcoma, 95t
Acromioclavicular arthritis, 282t
Actinic keratoses, 94t, 383
Actinic lentigines, 383
Actinic purpura, 383
Activities of daily living (ADLs), 375, 375b
Acute stress disorder, 81t
Adam's bend test, 345
Adnexa (ovaries), 228, 232, 369, 387
Adolescents
   examination of, 344–346
   hypertension in, 330b, 350t
   recommended preventative care for, 349t
   sexual maturity ratings in, 353t–356t
Advance directive, 377
Adventitious breath sounds, 132, 133b, 135
Agoraphobia, 80t
Airway, upper *vs.* lower, 335b
Alcohol abuse, 71, 184–185
Alcohol use
   CAGE questionnaire for, 46, 184
   interviewing about, 46
   in older adults, 376
   during pregnancy, 363
Allen test, 205
Allergic rhinitis, 101
Allergies, 3, 101, 325
Alopecia areata, 97t
Alzheimer's disease, 379
Amblyopia, 339
Amenorrhea, 226
Anal reflex, 303
Analgesic rebound headache, 112t
Anatomic snuffbox, 263
Androgen-producing tumors, 386
Angina pectoris, 137t, 147
Angioedema, 122t
Angioma
   cherry, 93t, 384
   spider, 93t
Angular cheilitis, 122t
Ankle jerks, 302
Ankle reflex, 302

395

Ankle–brachial index, 209t–210t
Ankles
  examination of, 274–275, 297
  ulcers of, 208t
Anorexia, 182
Anorexia nervosa, 61t, 226
Anterior cruciate ligament, 273, 284t
Anterior drawer sign, 273
Anteverted uterus, 239t
Anticipatory guidance, 325–326
Anus, during pregnancy, 369
Anxiety disorders, 80t–81t
Aorta
  abdominal aortic aneurysm, 190, 199, 201, 203, 386
  coarctation of the, 335
  dissecting aneurysm, 137t, 147
  examination of, 190
  tortuous atherosclerotic, 385
Aortic insufficiency, 154, 155b, 202
Aortic regurgitation, 156–158
Aortic sclerosis, 386
Aortic stenosis, 154, 156–157, 159, 351t, 386
Apgar score, 326, 327b
Aphasia, assessment for, 72b
Aphthous ulcer, 124t
Apical impulse
  assessment of, 56, 155–156
  in children, 335
  in older adults, 385
  during pregnancy, 366
Apnea, 334
Appearance, assessment of, 72
Appendicitis, 180, 181, 197t
  assessment for, 192–193
Arcus senilis, 384
Argyll Robertson pupil, 104
Arms
  examination of, 202–203
  flaccid, 306
Arousal, 212
Arousal system, 286
Arrhythmias, 57, 161t–164t, 330
Arterial insufficiency, 206, 207t–208t
Arterial occlusion, 202, 204, 387
Arteriosclerosis obliterans, 204
Arthralgia, 255
Arthritis
  acromioclavicular, 282t
  acute septic, 255
  in ankles and feet, 274–275
  degenerative (osteoarthritis), 255, 262, 281t, 388
  gonococcal, 254, 263
  gouty, 388
  of hip, 269
  knee, 270–271, 283t
  patterns of pain in, 281t
  rheumatoid, 254–55, 262–263, 281t, 388
Articular structures, 251
Asbestosis, 140t
Ascites, assessment of, 191–192
Assessment, 15–23
  clinical reasoning in, 15–16
  comprehensive vs. focused, 1, 9, 31
  organizing data, 23–24
  recording, 27b–29b
  test selection for, 25b–27b
  tips for, 24b
Asterixis, 304
Asthma, 139t, 142t, 146t
Ataxia, 288
Ataxic breathing, 65t
Atelectasis, 132
Atherosclerotic disease, 387
Athetosis, 314t
Atrial fibrillation, 57, 154
Atrial septal defect, 335
Attention
  assessment of, 73, 392t
  defined, 69b
Attention deficit disorder, 338
Auricle, examination of, 107
Auscultation
  of abdomen, 187, 187b
  of chest, 132, 132b, 135
  of fetal heart, 367–368
  of heart, 156–158, 158b
  of infant heart, 335
Axillae
  examination of, 11, 172
  in older adults, 386
Axillary temperature, 57

B

Babinski response, 303
Back
  examination of, 11
  stiffness of, 278t
Back pain, low, 254, 256, 277t–278t
Bacterial vaginitis, 235t
Baker's cyst, 271, 284t
Balance, 388, 390t
Balanitis, 214
Balloon sign, 272

Index

Ballotte, patella, 272
Barlow test, 337
Barrel chest, 144t
Bartholin's gland, 225, 368
Basal cell carcinoma, 95t, 383
Basal ganglia, 285
Basal ganglia disorder, 313t
Behavior
　assessment of, 72
　in delirium and dementia, 391t
　in older adults, 390t
Bell's palsy, 293, 312t
Benign prostatic hyperplasia (BPH), 242, 246t–247t, 248t–249t, 387
Biceps reflex, 301
Bicipital tendinitis, 282t
Biliary obstruction, 183b
Bimanual examination, 232, 369, 387
Biot's breathing, 65t
Birth history, 324
Bitemporal hemianopsia, 115t
Bladder, disorders of, 183–184, 196t–197t
Bleeding
　gastrointestinal, 242
　from nose, 102
　postmenopausal, 226
　sputum and, 141t–143t
　subarachnoid, 99–100, 113t, 287
　uterine, 226
　vitreous, 100
Blood, in stool, 182
Blood pressure
　assessment of, 54–56, 153–154
　in children, 330, 339
　classifications for, 56b, 150b
　cuff size, 54b
　high. *See* Hypertension
　low, 154, 383
　measuring, 55b
　in older adults, 382–383, 385
　during pregnancy, 365
　tips for accurate, 55b
Blood pressure cuff, sizing, 54b
Body mass index (BMI), 52–54
　calculation of, 53b
　chart for, 54b
　in children, 338
　excessively low, 61t
　for obesity, 52
　during pregnancy, 362b
Bone density, criteria for, 257b
Bouchard's nodes, 264
Bowel sounds, 187b
Bowlegged, 328

Brachial pulse, 202
Brachioradialis reflex, 302
Brain
　abscess of, 99
　tumors of, 99–100, 113t
Brainstem, 285
Breast self-examination (BSE), 169, 173b–174b
Breastfeeding, 360
Breasts, 167–175
　in adolescents, 345, 353t
　anatomy of, 169
　cancer of, 167–169, 168b, 175t–177t, 378
　concerning symptoms, 167–169
　cysts of, 168b, 171
　discharge from, 172
　examination of, 11, 169–172
　health history, 167–169
　in infants, 336
　male, 172
　masses of, 167, 168b
　in older adults, 386
　during pregnancy, 366
　recording findings, 174b
　in review of systems, 5
　sexual maturity ratings for, 353t
Breath odor, 52
Breath sounds, 132, 132b, 135
　adventitious, 132, 133b, 135
Breathing
　abnormal, 65t
　assessment of, 57, 129
　in children, 330
　in comatose patient, 319t
　effort of, 57
　normal, 57, 65t
　in older adults, 383
　shortness of breath, 128, 147
Breech presentation, 370
Brief psychotic disorder, 82t
Bronchial breath sounds, 132b
Bronchiectasis, 142t
Bronchiolitis, 330
Bronchitis, chronic, 139t, 142t, 146t
Bronchophony, 133, 133b
Bronchovesicular breath sounds, 132b
Brudzinski's sign, 303
Bruits
　abdominal, 187b, 386
　carotid, 154
Bulge sign, 271
Bulimia nervosa, 61t

Bulla, 89t
Burrow, 90t
Bursa, 251
Bursitis, 255
  in hip, 268
  in knee, 270–271, 283t
  olecranon, 262
  in shoulder, 259, 282t

C

CAGE questionnaire, 46, 184
Calcium
  food sources of, 63t
  recommended dietary intake for, 258b
Calf swelling, 200
Cancer
  breast, 167–169, 168b, 175t–177t, 378
  cervical, 228, 237t, 378
  colorectal, 182, 185b–186b, 194t, 242, 378, 387
  lip, 122t
  ovarian, 228, 387
  penis, 218t
  prostate, 242, 249t, 378, 387
  rectal, 249t
  screening in older adults, 378
  skin, 95t, 378, 383
  testicular, 221t
  tongue, 124t
  vulvar, 234t
Candidiasis
  in infants, 333
  oral, 124t, 333
  tongue, 123t
  vaginitis, 235t
Canker sore, 124t
Capacity, altered, 42
Carcinoma
  basal cell, 95t, 383
  cervical, 237t
  of lip, 122t
  of penis, 218t
  squamous cell, 95t, 383
  of tongue, 124t
  of vulva, 234t
Cardiac examination, 155–159
  auscultation, 156–159
  heart sounds, 156
  in infants, 335
  inspection and palpation, 155–156
  murmurs, 157–159, 158b
  during pregnancy, 366
  sequence for, 155b
Cardiac syncope, 288
Cardinal directions of gaze, 104–105
Cardiomyopathy, 155
  hypertrophic, 159
  peripartum, 366
Cardiovascular disease
  major risk factors for, 149b
  screening for, 148–153
Cardiovascular system, 147–160
  cardiac examination, 155–159
  concerning symptoms, 147
  examination of, 12, 153–159
  health history, 147
  health promotion and counseling, 148–153
  in older adults, 385–386
  during pregnancy, 366
  recording findings, 160b
  in review of systems, 5
Carotid bruits, 154
Carotid pulse, 154
Carotid stenosis, 385
Carpal tunnel syndrome, 262, 265–266, 296
Cartilaginous joints, 252b
Caruncles, 386
Cataracts, 100, 102, 384
Cauda equina, 286
Cauda equine syndrome, 254
Cellulitis, 200, 203
Central nervous system, 285–286
  disorders of, 313t
Cerebellar disorders, 297, 313t
Cerebellum, 286
Cerebrovascular accident (CVA), 103
Cervical myelopathy, 280t
Cervical radiculopathy, 279t, 296
Cervicitis, 237t
Cervix
  abnormalities of, 237t
  cancer of, 228, 237t, 378
  examination of, 231
  during pregnancy, 369
  shapes of Os, 236t
Chalazion, 117t
Chancre
  female genitalia, 234t
  lip, 122t
  male genitalia, 214, 220t
Cheilitis, angular, 122t
Cherry angioma, 93t, 384
Chest. *See* Thorax (chest)
Chest pain, 127, 137t–138t, 147

Index

Chest wall pain, 138t
Cheyne-Stokes breathing, 65t
Chief complaint, 1b, 3, 323
Childhood illnesses, 3–4
Children. *See also* Adolescents
  development of, 323b, 324–325
  examination of, 338–344
  health history, 323–326
  health promotion and counseling, 325–326
  heart murmurs in, 335, 342, 351t–352t
  hypertension in, 330b, 339, 350t
  infants, 329–337
  interviewing, 338b
  newborns, 326–328
  recommended preventative care for, 349t
  recording findings, 346b–347b
  sexual abuse in, 343, 357t
  sexual maturity ratings in, 353t–356t
Chills, 49
Chloasma, 365
Choanal atresia, 333
Cholecystitis, 193
Chondromalacia, 270
Chorea, 314t
Chronic obstructive pulmonary disease (COPD), 135, 139t, 146t, 385
Chronic pain, defined, 59
Cirrhosis, 182, 183b
Clavicle fracture, 336
Clinical breast examination (CBE), 169
Clinical reasoning, 15–16. *See also* Assessment
Clinician
  behavior and appearance, 35
  self-reflection of, 39
Clitoris, 230
Clubbing, 98t
Cluster headache, 99, 111t
Coarctation of the aorta, 335
Cognitive function
  assessment of, 73
  higher, 70b, 74
Cognitive impairment, 290b
  mild, 379
  in older adults, 378–379
Cogwheel rigidity, 316t
Collaborative partnerships, 41
Colles' fracture, 263
Colonoscopy, 243
Colorectal cancer, 182, 185b–186b, 194t, 242, 243, 378, 387

Coma, 305
  Glasgow Coma Scale, 320t
  structural, 319t
  toxic-metabolic, 319t
Comatose patient
  assessment of, 304–306
  pupils in, 305–306, 319t, 321t
Comedones, 384
Communication
  nonverbal, 33
  respectful, 40–41
Comprehensive health history. *See* Health history
Concussion, headache due to, 114t
Conductive hearing loss, 101, 121t, 293
Condylar joints, 253b
Condyloma acuminatum, 233t
Condyloma latum, 234t
Condylomata acuminata, 219t
Congestive heart failure, 335. *See also* Heart failure
Consciousness, level of, 305b
  assessment of, 51, 72
  in comatose patient, 319t
  defined, 69b
  in delirium and dementia, 391t
  loss of, 288
Constipation, 182
Constructional ability, assessment of, 74
Coordination, 297–298, 313t
Corneal light reflex, 339
Corneal reflexes, 104, 293
Corticospinal lesion, 298
Costovertebral angle, 190
Cough, 141t–143t
Crackles, 133b
Cranial nerves, 286
  assessment of, 292–294
  examination of, 13
  functions of, 291b
Cranial neuralgias, 113t
Crohn's disease, 182, 195t, 242, 244
Crossed straight-leg raise, 277
Croup, 334b
Crust, skin, 91t
Cryptorchidism, 215, 221t
Cultural competence, defined, 40
Cultural considerations
  health disparities in pain management, 59–60
  in older adults, 374–375
  patient with language barrier, 43, 43b
  working with interpreter, 43b

Cultural humility, 40–41
Culture, defined, 40
Cutaneous stimulation reflexes, 302–3
Cyanosis, 86t
Cyclothymic episode, 79t
Cystocele, 230, 238t, 368
Cystourethrocele, 230, 238t
Cysts, 88t
  Baker's, 271
  breast, 168b, 171
  congenital, 333
  epidermoid, 233t
  periauricular, 333
  pilar, 103
  pilonidal, 244
  thyroglossal duct, 333
Cytomegalovirus, 182

D

Dacryocystitis, 117t
Data
  identifying, 323
  organizing, 23–24
  subjective *vs.* objective, 2b
Death, interviewing about issues related to, 47
Decerebrate rigidity, 306
Decorticate rigidity, 306
Deep tendon reflexes, 301, 313t
Deep venous thrombosis, 204
Degenerative joint disease, 255, 262, 281t, 388
Delirium, 290b, 391t–392t
Delusional disorder, 82t
Dementia, 290b
  in older adults, 378–379
  screening for, 393t
  vs. delirium, 391t–392t
Dental caries, 341
Dependent edema, 147
Depression, 290b
  health promotion and counseling for, 70–71
  low back pain and, 256
  in older adults, 378–379
de Quervain's tenosynovitis, 263, 265, 296
Dermatomes, 317t–318t
Development, child, 323b, 324–325
Developmental delay/abnormality, 329, 338, 344

Diabetes
  in cardiovascular disease, 149b
  screening for, 150b–151b
Diabetes insipidus, 184
Diabetes mellitus, 184
Diabetic retinopathy, 119t
Diarrhea, 182, 194t–196t
Diet
  health promotion and counseling for, 50–51, 256
  in older adults, 376
  during pregnancy, 361
  recommendations for hypertension, 64t
  screening checklist, 62t
  sources of nutrients, 63t
Diethylstilbestrol (DES), 237t
Diffuse esophageal spasm, 138t
Digital rectal examination, 242–243
Diphtheria, 125t
Diplopia, 101, 288
Discharge
  breast, 172
  penile, 213
  vaginal, 226, 235t, 343
Discriminative sensations, 300
Disease, defined, 36
Disease/illness model, defined, 36
Dissecting aortic aneurysm, 137t, 147
Distal weakness, 288
Distress, signs of, 51
Diverticulitis, 181, 197t
Dizziness, 287
Do Not Resuscitate (DNR), 47, 377
Doll's eye movements, 306
Domestic violence, 47, 47b, 363, 363b
Doppler method, blood pressure, 330
Dorsalis pedis pulse, 204
Down's syndrome, 331
Drawer sign
  anterior, 273
  posterior, 274
Dress, patient, 52, 72
Drug abuse, 46, 71, 363
Drug use
  allergies and, 3
  diarrhea related to, 194t
  health history, 3, 46
  in older adults, 375–376
  during pregnancy, 363
  prescription abuse, 46
  urinary incontinence related to, 197t
Drusen, 384
Dullness, percussion notes, 131b, 135
Dupuytren's contracture, 262, 264

Index

Durable medical power of attorney, 42
Dying patient, 47
Dysarthria, 288
Dyskinesia, oral-facial, 315t
Dyslipidemia
 in cardiovascular disease, 149b
 classification of, 151
 in metabolic syndrome, 152b
 screening for, 151, 152b
 treatment of, 152b
Dysmenorrhea, 226
Dyspareunia, 227
Dyspepsia, 181
Dysphagia, 182
Dyspnea, 139t–140t, 147
Dysrhythmias, 57, 161t–164t, 330
Dysthymic disorder, 79t
Dystonia, 315t
Dysuria, 183

E

Ear canal, 107
Earache, 101
Eardrum, 107–108, 120t
Ears
 in children, 340
 examination of, 11, 107
 health history of, 101
 in infants, 332, 333b
 in older adults, 385
 pain in, 101
 recording findings, 110b
 in review of systems, 5
Eating disorders, 61t, 226
Ecchymosis, 94t
Echoing, 33
Ectopic pregnancy, 181, 369
Ectropion, 116t
Edema, 147
 dependent, 147
 pitting, 204
 during pregnancy, 370
Effusion
 of knee, 271–272
 pleural, 131, 146t
Egophony, 133, 133b
Ejaculation, 212
Elbow, 262, 296
Elder mistreatment, 379
Elderly patients. *See* Older adults
Empathetic response, 32

Empowerment, patient, 34, 34b
Endocervical broom, 231
Endocervical polyp, 237t
Endocrine system, 6
Endometrial hyperplasia, 387
Endometriosis, 226
Enteroviral infections, 333
Entropion, 116t
Environment for examination, 9, 35, 373–374
Epidermoid cyst, 233t
Epididymis, 215, 222t
Epididymitis, 222t
Episcleritis, 117t
Episiotomy, 368
Epistaxis, 102
Epitrochlear lymph nodes, 11, 203
Epstein's pearls, 333
Erectile dysfunction, 212
Erosion, skin, 92t
Esophageal spasm, diffuse, 138t
Esophagitis, reflex, 138t
Estrogen-producing tumors, 387
Ethics, professionalism and, 48, 48b
Excoriation, 92t
Exercise
 health promotion and counseling for, 51, 256
 during pregnancy, 362
Exophthalmos, 116t
Expected date of delivery (EDD), 360–361
Expressions, facial, 52, 72
Extinction, sensation, 301
Extra-articular structures, 251
Extraocular muscles, 101
Extremities, lower. *See also specific structures*
 examination of, 12, 370
Eyelid
 abnormalities of, 116t–117t
 in older adults, 384
 retraction, 116t
Eyes
 abnormalities of, 116t–117t
 in children, 339–340
 in comatose patient, 305–306
 disorders of, 112t
 examination of, 11, 103–104
 health history of, 100–101
 in infants, 332, 332b
 in older adults, 384
 during pregnancy, 365
 recording findings, 110b
 in review of systems, 5

F

Face
  expressions of, 52, 72
  of infants, 331, 332b
  paralysis of, 103, 312t
  during pregnancy, 365
Facial nerve, 291b, 293
Failure to thrive, 329
Fainting, 288
Fall prevention, 258, 381–382
Fallot, tetralogy of, 351t–352t
Family history, 2b, 4, 149b, 153, 360
Family planning, 229
Fasciculations, 314t
Fatigue, 49
Fecal occult blood test (FOBT), 243
Feeding history, 324
Feet
  swelling of, 200
  ulcers of, 208t
Female genital examination, 225–232
  anatomical considerations, 225
  concerning symptoms, 225–227
  examination techniques, 13–14, 229–232, 229b
  health history, 225–227
  health promotion and counseling, 227–229
  recording findings, 233b
  sexually transmitted infections (STIs) in, 227–228, 231
Female genitalia
  in adolescents, 345
  in children, 343
  examination of, 13–14
  in infants, 336
  in older adults, 386–387
  during pregnancy, 368–369
  in review of systems, 6
  sexual maturity ratings for, 356t
Femoral hernia, 216, 223t, 232
Femoral pulse, 204
Fetal alcohol syndrome, 331, 363
Fetal heart rate (FHR), 367–368
Fever, 49, 57
Fibroadenoma, of breast, 168b, 171
Fibromyalgia, 255, 279t
Fibrous joints, 252b
Fingernails, 85, 98t
Fingers, 264, 296
Fissure, 92t
Fissured tongue, 123t
Flaccid paralysis, 306
Flaccidity, 316t

Flail chest, 144t
Flat percussion note, 131b
Flu shots, 128
Folate, food sources of, 63t
Fontanelles, 331
Forced expiratory time, 135
Forgetfulness, 290b
Fracture
  clavicle, 259, 336
  Colles', 263
  osteoporosis and, 257b
  scaphoid, 263
Frailty, 377
Functional assessment, 375
Functional status, 379–380
Fundal height, 367
Funnel chest, 144t

G

Gait
  assessment of, 52, 267–268, 297–298
  in older adults, 388, 390t
Gastroesophageal reflux disease (GERD), 181
Gastrointestinal reflux, 143t
Gastrointestinal system
  bleeding, 242
  chest pain and, 138t
  pain related to, 180–183
  in review of systems, 5
  symptoms related to, 182–183
Gaze, cardinal directions of, 104–105
Gegenhalten, 316t
General survey
  in infants, 329–330
  in physical examination, 10, 51–52
  recording findings, 60
  in review of systems, 5
Generalized anxiety disorder, 81t
Genital herpes, 219t, 234t
Genital warts, 219t, 233t
Genitalia
  ambiguous, 336
  examination of, 13–14
  female, 225. *See also* Female genital examination
  male, 211. *See also* Male genital examination
  in review of systems, 6
Geographic tongue, 123t
Geriatric competencies, minimum, 391t–393t

Geriatric Screener, 10-Minute, 378, 380b–381b
Geriatric syndromes, 374
Gestational age, 327b, 328b, 348t, 360–361
Gestational hypertension, 365b
"Get Up and Go" test, 388, 390t
Giant cell arteritis, 114t
Gingivitis, 385
Glasgow Coma Scale, 320t
Glaucoma
  acute, 101, 112t
  health promotion and counseling for, 102–103
  open-angle, 100, 384
Glaucomatous cupping, 118t
Glossopharyngeal nerve, 291b, 294
Goiter, 102, 110, 126t
Gonococcal arthritis, 254, 263
Gout, 255, 388
Gray matter, 285
Great arteries, transposition of the, 335, 352t
Grip strength, hand, 265
Growth, of child, 324
Guarding, abdominal, 188
Gums, 109

H

Hair
  examination of, 85
  loss of, 97t, 199
  pubic, 354t–356t
Hairy leukoplakia, 123t
Hairy tongue, 123t
Hand
  arterial supply to, 205
  flaccid, 306
  grip strength of, 265
Head, 99–102
  circumference of, 329
  examination of, 11, 103–111
  health history, 99–102
  health promotion and counseling, 102–103
  in infants, 331
  in older adults, 384–385
  during pregnancy, 365
  recording findings, 110b
  in review of systems, 5
Headache, 99, 287
  cluster, 99, 111t
  migraine, 100, 111t
  primary, 111t
  red flags for, 100b
  secondary, 112t–114t
  tension, 99, 111t
Health care proxy, 42, 47
Health disparities
  in cardiovascular screening and risk factors, 149
  in diabetes screening and diagnosis, 151
  in pain management, 59–60
  in osteoporosis risk factors, 256–257
  in risk of prostate cancer, 242–243
Health history, 2–7, 2b
  in children, 323–326
  components of, 1b–2b
  comprehensive vs. focused, 1, 9, 31
  concerning symptoms, 49–50
  interview and, 31–48
  in older adults, 373–377
  prenatal, 359–361
Health Insurance Portability and Accountability Act (HIPAA), 42
Health maintenance, 4
Health promotion and counseling, 227–229
  abdominal aortic aneurysm, 201
  alcohol abuse, 71, 184–185
  cardiovascular disease screening, 148–153
  cervical cancer screening, 228
  in children, 325–326
  colorectal cancer, 185b–186b
  colorectal cancer screening, 243
  depression, 70–71
  diet, 50–51, 62t, 63t, 256
  exercise, 51, 256
  fall prevention, 258
  family planning, 229
  flu shots, 128
  hearing loss, 103
  hepatitis prevention, 185
  low back pain, 256
  for menopause, 229
  nutrition, 50–51, 62t, 63t, 256
  in older adults, 377–379, 391t
  optimal weight, 50–51
  oral health, 103
  osteoporosis, 256–257, 257b–258b
  ovarian cancer screening, 228
  peripheral neuropathy, 290
  peripheral vascular disease, 200–201
  pneumococcal vaccine, 128
  during pregnancy, 361–364

Health promotion and counseling (*continued*)
  prostate cancer screening, 242–243
  renal artery disease, 201
  sexually transmitted infections (STIs) prevention, 213–214, 228
  skin cancer screening, 83
  smoking cessation, 128b
  stroke prevention, 289–290
  substance abuse, 71
  suicide risk, 71
  testicular self-examination, 214
  vision loss, 102–103
Health supervision visits, 325
Hearing
  assessment of, 108, 121t
  in infants, 333b
  in older adults, 385
Hearing loss, 293
  conductive, 101, 121t
  health promotion and counseling, 103
  sensorineural, 101, 121t
Heart. *See also* Cardiovascular system
  examination of. *See* Cardiac examination
  in infants, 335
  in older adults, 385–386
  during pregnancy, 366
Heart failure
  congestive, 335
  left ventricular, 139t, 143t, 146t, 147, 155, 159
Heart murmurs
  assessment of, 156–158
  causes of, 165t
  in children, 335, 342, 351t–352t
  grading of, 158b
  in older adults, 386
  during pregnancy, 366
  systolic murmur identification, 159
Heart rate
  assessment of, 56–57, 153
  fetal, 367–368
  in older adults, 383
Heart rhythm, 57, 161t–164t, 330
Heart sounds
  assessment of, 156, 161t–164t
  in infants, 335
Heartburn, 181
Heberden's nodes, 264
HEENT (head, ears, eyes, nose, and throat), 99–102
  examination of, 11, 103–110
  health history, 99–102

health promotion and counseling, 102–103
in older adults, 384–385
recording findings, 110b
in review of systems, 5
Height
  assessment of, 52
  in infants, 329
  in older adults, 383
Hematoma, subdural, 329
Hemianopsia, 103, 115t
Hemoptysis, 141t–143t
Hemorrhage
  subarachnoid, 99–100, 113t, 287
  vitreous, 100
Hemorrhagic telangiectasia, hereditary, 122t
Hemorrhoids, 249t, 369
Hepatitis, 181, 182
  alcoholic, 179, 183b
  prevention of, 185
  types of, 183b, 185
Hepatomegaly, 188–189, 342
Hereditary hemorrhagic telangiectasia, 122t
Hernia
  in children, 328, 336, 343
  in female, 232
  femoral, 216, 223t, 232
  indirect *vs.* direct, 216, 223t
  inguinal, 216, 232, 336, 343
  scrotal, 218t
  umbilical, 328
Herpes simplex
  female genital, 234t
  in infants, 333
  lip, 122t
  male genital, 219t
Herpes zoster, 384
Higher cognitive functions, defined, 70b
Hinge joints, 253b
Hip dysplasia, congenital, 337
Hips, examination of, 267–268, 296–297
History. *See* Health history
HIV infection
  female genital examination, 228
  male genital examination, 213–214
Hoarseness, 102
Homonymous hemianopsia, 115t
Hormone replacement therapy (HRT), 229
Housemaid's knee, 270, 283t

Index

Human immunodeficiency virus (HIV). *See* HIV infection
Human papillomavirus (HPV), 219t, 242
Hydrocele, 215, 218t, 336
Hydrocephalus, 103, 329
Hymen, imperforate, 230
Hyperglycemia, 100
Hyperopia, 100
Hyperpnea, 65t
Hyperpyrexia, defined, 57
Hyperresonance, 131, 131b
Hypertension
  in cardiovascular disease, 149b
  in children, 330b, 339, 350t
  classification of, 56b, 150b
  dietary recommendations for, 64t
  gestational, 365b
  isolated systolic, 56, 382
  during pregnancy, 365, 365b
  pulmonary, 335
  screening for, 150
Hyperthyroidism, 102, 103
Hypertonia, 316t
Hypoglossal nerve, 291b, 294
Hypomanic episode, 79t
Hypoplastic left heart, 335
Hypospadias, 214, 218t
Hypotension, orthostatic, 154, 383
Hypothalamus, 285
Hypothermia
  causes of, 57
  defined, 57
Hypothesis, generating, 38–39
Hypothyroidism, 102
Hypotonia, 316t, 337
Hypovolemia, 154

I

Illicit drug abuse, 71, 363
Illness, defined, 36
Immunizations, 4, 325
  in older adults, 378
  during pregnancy, 364
Imperforate hymen, 230
Impulse, point of maximal, 56, 155–156, 335, 366, 385
Incontinence, urinary, types of, 184, 196t–197t
Infantile automatisms, 337
Infants
  assessment of, 329–337
  head circumference, 329
  hypertension in, 330b
  maturity classification for, 348t
  recommended preventative care for, 349t
Infection
  diarrhea related to, 194t
  sexually transmitted. *See* Sexually transmitted infections (STIs)
Inflammatory bowel disease (IBD), 194t, 195t
Inguinal hernia, 216, 232, 336, 343
Inguinal lymph nodes, 203
Insight, patient, 69b, 73
Intention tremor, 314t
Intercourse, pain with, 227
Intermittent claudication, 199, 207t
Interpreter, working with, 43b
Interviewing, 31–48
  children, 338b
  comprehensive *vs.* focused, 1, 9, 31
  cultural humility in, 40–41
  ethics and professionalism, 48, 48b
  format of, 31
  patient with hearing loss, 44
  patient with vision loss, 44
  patient's perspective in, 37, 37b
  preparation for, 34–35
  sensitive topics, 45–47
  sequence for, 35–39
  specific situations, 41–45
  techniques for, 32–34
Intimate partner abuse, 47, 47b
Intracranial pressure, increased, 331
Introitus, 230
Involuntary movements, 295, 313t, 314t–315t
Iron, food sources of, 63t
Irritable bowel syndrome, 182
Ischiogluteal bursa, 268
Isolated systolic hypertension, 56, 382

J

Jaundice, 86t, 182
Joint pain, 281t
  assessment of, 254–255, 254b
  monoarticular, 254
  polyarticular, 254
Joints. *See also* specific joint
  concerning symptoms, 253–255
  examination of, 258–275, 258b
  recording findings, 276b
  stiffness, 255
  types of, 252b–253b

Judgment, patient, 70b, 73, 392t
Jugular veins, 154
Jugular venous pressure, 154
Jugular venous pulsations, 154, 385

K

Kaposi's sarcoma, 95t
Keloid, 91t
Keratoses
   actinic, 94t
   seborrheic, 94t
Kernig's sign, 303
Kidneys, examination of, 190
Klinefelter's syndrome, 221t
Knee
   anatomical considerations, 269
   examination of, 269–274, 297
   painful, 283t–284t
Knee reflex, 302
Koplik's spots, 125t
Korotkoff sounds, 159
Kussmaul breathing, 65t
Kyphoscoliosis, thoracic, 145t

L

Labia, 230
Labor, preterm, 367
Labyrinthitis, 101
Lachman test, 273
Language, 70b, 72
Language barrier, 43, 43b
Laryngitis, 141t
Laryngotracheobronchitis, 334b
Last period start (LMP), 226
Lateral collateral ligament, 273, 284t
Lateral meniscus, 272, 283t
Lead-pipe rigidity, 316t
Left ventricular heart failure, 139t, 143t, 146t, 147, 155, 159
Left ventricular hypertrophy, 155, 385
Legs
   coldness, numbness, pallor on, 199
   examination of, 203–204
   flaccid, 306
   hair loss on, 199
   length measurement, 276
   peripheral vascular disease and, 199–200, 203–204, 207t–210t
   swelling of, 200
Leopold's maneuvers, 368, 370–371
Lesions
   brainstem, 101
   corticospinal, 298
   skin, 51, 87t–94t
   upper motor neuron, 301
Lethargy, 305
Leukocoria, 332
Leukonychia, 98t
Leukoplakia, hairy, 123t
Level of consciousness, 305b, 319t, 391t
Lhermitte's sign, 280t
Libido, 212
Lichenification, 91t
Lifestyle, in cardiovascular disease, 153, 153b
Ligaments, 251
   knee, 273–274, 284t
Light reflex, 106b
Lighting, 9
Likelihood ratio, 26b–27b
Lips, 109, 122t
Listening, active, 32
Literacy, low, 44
Liver
   enlarged, 188–189, 342
   examination of, 188–189
   normal, 188
   risk factors for disease, 183b
Lumbar spinal stenosis, 277t
Lumbosacral radiculopathy, 304
Lungs
   abscess of, 143t
   anterior, 12
   cancer of, 140t, 143t
   concerning symptoms, 127–128
   disorders of, 137t–140t, 146t
   examination of, 129–135
   health history, 127–128
   health promotion and counseling, 128
   in infants, 334, 334b–335b
   in older adults, 385
   posterior, 11
   during pregnancy, 366
   recording findings, 136b
Lymph nodes
   axillae, 172
   cervical, 109
   epitrochlear, 203
   in infants, 333
   inguinal, 203
Lymphadenopathy, 203, 333

M

Macular degeneration, 100, 102, 384
Macule, 87t
Major depressive episode, 78t–79t
Malabsorption syndrome, 195t
Male genital examination, 211–217
  anatomical considerations, 211
  concerning symptoms, 211–213
  examination techniques, 13, 214–217
  health history, 211–213
  recording findings, 217b
  sexually transmitted infections (STIs) in, 213–214, 219t–220t
  testicular self-examination, 214
Male genitalia
  in adolescents, 345
  in children, 343
  examination of, 13
  in infants, 336
  in older adults, 387
  in review of systems, 6
  sexual maturity ratings for, 354t–355t
Malignant melanoma, 96t
Malocclusion, 342
Malodor, 385
Mammography, 168
Manic episode, 78t–79t
Masseter muscles, 259, 293
Maximal impulse, point of, 56, 155–156, 335, 366, 385
McBurney's point, 192
McMurray test, 272
Medial collateral ligament, 273, 284t
Medial meniscus, 272, 283t
Melanoma, 96t, 383
Melena, 182
Memory
  defined, 69b
  in delirium and dementia, 394t
  recent, 74
  remote, 73
Ménière's disease, 101
Meningeal signs, 303
Meningitis, 99, 113t, 303, 331
Meniscus of knee, 272, 283t
Menopause, 226, 229
Menstrual history, 225
Mental health history, 45–46
Mental health screening, red flags for, 68b
Mental status, 67–82
  in children, 338
  concerning symptoms, 69
  disorders of, 76t–82t
  examination of, 13, 71–75, 71b
  health history, 69–70
  health promotion and counseling, 70–71
  in infants, 329
  recording findings, 75b
  red flags for mental health screening, 68b
  unexplained symptoms and, 67, 67b–68b
Metabolic syndrome, 152, 152b
Methicillin-resistant *Staphylococcus aureus* (MRSA) precautions, 14
Microcephaly, 331
Migraine headache, 100, 111t
Mini-Cog exam, 290b, 393t
Mini-Mental State Examination (MMSE), 74, 75b
Mitgehen, 316t
Mitral regurgitation, 156–157, 386
Mitral stenosis, 139t, 143t, 147, 155b, 156–157
Mitral valve prolapse, 159
Mixed episode, 79t
Mood
  assessment of, 73, 391t
  defined, 70b
  disorders of, 78t–79t
Motor system (motor activity)
  assessment of, 13, 52, 72, 294–98
  disorders of, 313t
Mouth
  abnormalities of, 122t–124t
  assessment of, 109
  cancers of, 122t, 124t
  candidiasis of, 124t, 333
  in children, 341–342
  health history of, 102
  in infants, 333
  in older adults, 385
  during pregnancy, 365
Movements, involuntary, 295, 313t, 314t–315t
MRSA precautions, 14
Multiple sclerosis, 296
Murmurs. *See* Heart murmurs
Murphy's sign, 193
Muscle bulk, 295, 313t
Muscle strength
  assessment of, 295–297, 295b
  in motor system disorders, 313t
Muscle tone, 313t
  assessment of, 295
  disorders of, 316t

Musculoskeletal system, 251–276
  abnormalities of, 277t–281t
  in children, 344
  concerning symptoms, 253–255
  examination of, 11–12, 258–275, 258b
  health history, 253–255
  health promotion and counseling, 256–258
  in infants, 336–337
  joint assessment, 251, 252b–253b
  in older adults, 388
  recording findings, 276b
  in review of systems, 6
Myalgia, 255
Myasthenia gravis, 288, 295
Mycoplasma, 141t
Myelopathy, cervical, 280t
Myocardial infarction, 137t, 147, 180
Myoma, of uterus, 239t
Myopathy, 288, 295
Myopia, 100
Myxedema, 103

N

Naegele's rule, 360–361
Nails
  abnormalities of, 98t
  examination of, 85
Nasal congestion, 101
Nausea, 181
Near reaction, pupillary, 104
Neck
  examination of, 11, 109–110
  health history, 102
  in infants, 333
  pain in, 254, 279t–280t
  during pregnancy, 365
  in review of systems, 5
Negative predictive value, 26b
Nerves
  cranial, 13, 286, 291b, 292–294
  peripheral, 286–287
  spinal, 287
Nervous system, 285–307
  central, 285–286
  in children, 344
  concerning symptoms, 287–289
  examination of, 12–13
  health promotion and counseling, 289–290
  in older adults, 388
  peripheral, 286–387

  recording findings, 307b
  in review of systems, 6
Neuralgias, cranial, 113t
Neurologic screening, in newborns, 328
Neuropathic ulcers, 208t
Neuropathy, peripheral, 290
Nevi, ABCDE screening for, 83, 96t
Newborns
  Apgar score, 326, 327b
  assessment of, 326–328
  birth weight, 327b
  classification of, 327b–328b, 348t
  head circumference, 329
  hypertension in, 330b
Night sweats, 49
Nipple
  discharge of, 172
  inspection of, 170
  Paget's disease of, 170, 177t
  retraction or deviation, 170, 176t
Nocturia, 184
Nose
  assessment of, 108
  bleeding from, 365
  examination of, 11
  health history of, 101–102
  in infants, 333
  in older adults, 384–385
  during pregnancy, 365
  recording findings, 110b
  in review of systems, 5
Numbness, 199
Nursing bottle caries, 341
Nutrients, sources of, 63t
Nutrition
  health promotion and counseling for, 50–51, 256
  in older adults, 376
  during pregnancy, 361
  screening checklist, 62t
  sources of nutrients, 63t
Nystagmus, 332

O

Obesity
  body mass index (BMI) for, 52
  in cardiovascular disease, 149b
  during pregnancy, 362b
Objective data, 2b
Obsessive-compulsive disorder, 81t
Obstetric history, 360
Obstructive pulmonary disease, 147

Obtundation, 305
Obturator sign, 192
Occlusion, arterial, 202, 204, 387
Oculocephalic reflex, 306
Oculomotor nerve, 291b, 292
Odor, body and breath, 52
Odynophagia, 182
OLD CARTS mnemonics, 38
Older adults, 373–389
  abuse of, 379
  cancer screening in, 378
  concerning symptoms, 375–377
  cultural considerations, 374–375
  delirium and dementia, 391t–392t
  examination of, 379–388
  fall prevention in, 381–382
  health history, 373–389, 373–377
  health promotion and counseling, 377–379
  Mini-Cog exam, 393t
  recording findings, 389b
Olfactory nerve, 291b, 292
Onycholysis, 98t
Open-angle glaucoma, 100, 384
Ophthalmoscope, 105b
OPQRST mnemonics, 38
Optic disc
  abnormalities of, 118t
  examination of, 105–106, 106b–107b
Optic nerve, 291b, 292
Optic neuritis, 101
Oral health, health promotion and counseling, 103
Oral mucosa, 109
Oral temperature, 57–58
Oral-facial dyskinesias, 315t
Orchitis, 221t
Orgasm, 212
Orientation
  assessment of, 73, 392t
  defined, 69b
Orthopnea, 147
Orthostatic hypotension, 154, 383
Ortolani test, 337
Osteoarthritis, 255, 262, 281t, 388
Osteopenia, 257b
Osteoporosis, 256–257, 257b–258b
Otitis externa, 101, 340
Otitis media, 101, 120t, 340–341
Ovaries
  cancer of, 228, 387
  examination of, 232, 369
Ovulation, 229

P

Paget's disease, of nipple, 170, 177t
Pain
  abdominal, 179–182, 197t
  acute, 376, 376b
  in arms and legs, 199
  assessment of, 59–60
  chest, 127, 137t–138t, 147
  chronic, 59
  in health history, 50
  joint, 254–255, 254b, 281t
  knee, 283t–284t
  low back, 254, 256, 277t–278t
  neck, 254, 279t–280t
  in older adults, 376
  persistent, 376, 376b
  sensation of, 299
  shoulder, 282t
Pain management, 60
  health disparities in, 59–60
Palliative care, 377
Pallor, 199
Palpitations, 147
Panic attack, 80t
Panic disorder, 80t
Pap smear, 230–231, 368, 387
Papilledema, 118t
Papule, 87t
Paradoxical pulse, 159
Paralysis
  of face, 312t
  flaccid, 306
Paratonia, 316t
Parietal pain, 180
Parkinsonism, 313t
Paronychia, 98t
Paroxysmal nocturnal dyspnea (PND), 147
Paroxysmal supraventricular tachycardia, 330, 335
Partnering with patient, 33–34
Partnerships, collaborative, 41
Patch, skin, 87t
Patellofemoral compartment, 270
Patellofemoral disorder, 270, 283t
Patient
  with altered capacity, 42
  angry or disruptive, 42–43
  comfort of, 9
  confusing, 41
  crying, 42
  dying, 47
  empowerment of, 34, 34b
  with impaired hearing, 44

Patient (*continued*)
  with impaired vision, 44
  with language barrier, 43, 43b
  with limited intelligence, 44
  with low literacy, 44
  with personal problems, 44
  perspective, 37, 37b
  positioning of, 8b, 10
  seductive, 44–45
  silent, 41
  talkative, 42
Peau d'orange, 170, 177t
Pectus carinatum (pigeon chest), 145t
Pectus excavatum (funnel chest), 144t
Pediatrics. *See* Children
Pelvic examination, 229–232, 229b
  in older adults, 386–387
  during pregnancy, 368–369
Pelvic floor, 238t, 369
Pelvic inflammatory disease (PID), 181, 226, 232
Pelvic muscles, 232
Penis
  abnormalities of, 218t
  cancer of, 218t
  in children and adolescents, 354t–355t
  discharge from, 213
  examination of, 214
Perceptions, patient, 69b, 73, 392t
Percussion, chest, 131, 131b, 135
Perforation, eardrum, 120t
Pericardial friction, 156
Pericarditis, 137t, 159
Peripheral nerves, 286–287
Peripheral nervous system, 286–287, 313t
Peripheral neuropathy, 290
Peripheral vascular disease, 200–201
Peripheral vascular system, 199–206
  concerning symptoms, 199–200
  disorders of, 199–201, 207t–208t
  examination of, 12, 202–206
  health history, 199–200
  health promotion and counseling, 200–201
  in older adults, 387
  recording findings, 206b
  in review of systems, 6
Peritonsillar abscess, 109, 342
Personal history, 2b, 4
Personal hygiene, 52, 72
Pes anserine bursitis, 271, 283t
Petechia, 93t
Peutz-Jeghers syndrome, 122t

Phalen's sign, 266
Pharyngitis, 125t
  streptococcal, 102, 341
Pharynx
  abnormalities of, 125t
  in children, 341
  examination of, 11, 102, 109
  in infants, 333
  in older adults, 384–385
Phimosis, 214
Phobias, types of, 80t
Physical activity, 51, 256
Physical examination, 7–14
  approach to, 7
  in children, 338–344
  general survey in, 51–52
  health history in, 49–50
  health promotion and counseling in, 50–51
  of older adults, 379–388
  pain in, 59–60
  patient positioning for, 8b, 10
  during pregnancy, 364–371, 364b
  preparation for, 7b
  recording findings, 60
  sequence for, 8b, 10
  standard and universal precautions in, 14
  vital signs, 54–58
Physical status
  in children, 338
  in infants, 329
Pigeon chest, 145t
Pilar cyst, 103
Pilonidal cyst, 244
Pinguecula, 117t
Plantar reflex, 303, 313t
Plaque, skin, 88t
Pleural effusion, 131, 146t
Pleural pain, 138t
Pleurisy, 180, 197t
Pneumatic otoscope, 340
Pneumococcal vaccine, 128
Pneumonia, 140t–141t, 330, 334b
Pneumothorax, 140t, 146t
Point localization, 301
Point of maximal impulse, 385
  assessment of, 56, 155–156
  in children, 335
  in older adults, 385
  during pregnancy, 366
Polydactyly, 336
Polymyalgia rheumatica, 255
Polyneuropathy, 288, 295

Polyps
  endocervical, 237t
  of rectum, 249t
Polyuria, 184
Popliteal cyst, 271, 284t
Popliteal pulse, 204
Position sensation, 299–300
Positive predictive value, 26b
Postconcussion headache, 114t
Posterior cruciate ligament, 274
Posterior drawer sign, 274
Posterior tibial pulse, 204
Postictal state, 289
Postmenopausal bleeding, 226
Postnasal drip, 141t
Posttraumatic stress disorder, 81t
Postural hypotension, 154, 383
Postural tremor, 314t
Posture, assessment of, 52, 72
Potassium, food sources of, 64t
Precocious puberty, 343
Predictive value, 25b–26b
  negative, 26b
  positive, 26b
Preeclampsia, 365b, 370
Pregnancy
  amenorrhea due to, 226
  concerning symptoms, 359–361
  ectopic, 181, 369
  examination during, 364–371, 364b
  family planning and, 229
  health promotion and counseling, 361–364
  hypertension during, 365b
  prenatal laboratory screenings, 363–364
  recording findings, 372b
  symptoms of, 226
Premature ejaculation, 212
Prenatal visit
  initial, 359–360
  subsequent, 361
Prepatellar bursitis, 270, 283t
Presbyopia, 100, 384
Prescription drug use. *See* Drug use
Present illness, 2b, 3, 3b, 323
Pressure sores, 384
Presyncope, 287
Prevention
  primary, 148
  secondary, 148
Primary prevention, 148
Primitive reflexes, 337
Problem list, 30b
Proctitis, 244

Professionalism, and ethics, 48, 48b
Pronator drift, 298
Prostate
  benign prostatic hyperplasia, 242, 246t–247t, 248t–249t
  cancer of, 242–243, 249t, 378, 387
  concerning symptoms, 241–242
  examination of, 244–245
  in older adults, 387
  recording findings, 245
Prostate-specific antigen (PSA), 242–243
Prostatitis, 183–184, 249t
Proximal weakness, 288
Pseudoscars, 383
Psoas sign, 192
Psoriasis, 88t, 103
Psychiatric disorders. *See* Mental status
Psychotic disorders, 82t
Pterygoid muscles, 259
Ptosis, 116t
  senile, 384
Puberty
  delayed, 230
  precocious, 343
Pubic hair, 354t–356t
Pulmonary embolism, 140t, 143t
Pulmonary fibrosis, 140t
Pulmonary function, assessment of, 135
Pulmonary tuberculosis, 142t
Pulmonary valve atresia, 335
Pulmonary valve stenosis, 156, 335
Pulse
  apical, 56, 155
  brachial, 202
  carotid, 154
  in children, 330
  dorsalis pedis, 204
  femoral, 204
  grading of, 202b
  in older adults, 386
  paradoxical, 159
  popliteal, 204
  posterior tibial, 204
  pulsus alternans, 159
  radial, 56, 202
Pulse pressure, 382
Pulsus alternans, 159
Pupils
  Argyll Robertson, 104
  in comatose patient, 305–306, 319t, 321t
  examination of, 104
  near reaction, 104

Purpura, 93t
Pustule, 89t
Pyelonephritis, 183
Pyloric stenosis, 336
Pyrexia, defined, 57

Q

Questioning
  guided, 32–33, 32b
  open-ended, 36, 39

R

Radial pulse, 56, 202
Radiculopathy
  cervical, 279t, 296
  lumbosacral, 304
Rales, 133b
Range of motion (ROM)
  ankle, 275
  elbow, 262
  hip, 268–269
  measuring, 276
  shoulder, 260
  spine, 267
  wrist and hands, 262, 264
Rapport, 35
Raynaud's disease, 200, 202
Reasoning, clinical, 15–16
Reassurance, 33
Rebound tenderness, 188
Record, patient
  checklist for, 27b–29b
  organizing, 27b–30b
Rectal examination, 13–14
  in female, 245
  in male, 244–245
  in older adults, 387
  during pregnancy, 369
Rectal thermometer, 58
Rectocele, 230, 238t, 368
Rectovaginal examination, 232, 387
Rectum
  abnormalities of, 249t
  cancer of, 249t
  concerning symptoms, 241–242
  examination of, 244–245
  health history, 241–242
  recording findings, 245
Red reflex, 105
Referred pain, 180, 278t
Reflex esophagitis, 138t

Reflexes
  assessment of, 13, 301–303
  corneal light, 339
  cutaneous stimulation, 302–303
  grading of, 301b
  in infants, 337
  in motor system disorders, 313t
  during pregnancy, 370
  primitive, 337
Reliability, 25b
Renal artery disease, 201
Resonant percussion note, 131b
Respiratory infection, upper, 334
Respiratory rate
  abnormal, 65t
  assessment of, 57, 129
  in children, 330
  in comatose patient, 319t
  normal, 57, 65t
  in older adults, 383
Respiratory rhythm
  abnormal, 65t
  assessment of, 57, 129
Respiratory system, 127–136
  anterior thorax, 12, 134–135
  concerning symptoms, 127–128
  disorders of, 137t–140t, 144t–146t
  examination of, 129–135
  health history, 127–128
  health promotion and counseling, 128
  posterior thorax, 11, 130–134
  recording findings, 136b
  in review of systems, 5
Reticular activating system, 286
Retina, examination of, 106b–107b
Retinal detachment, 100–101
Retinoblastoma, 332
Retinopathy, diabetic, 119t
Retroflexed uterus, 239t
Retroverted uterus, 239t
Review of systems, 2b, 4–7
Rheumatic fever, 254
Rheumatoid arthritis, 254–255, 262–263, 281t, 388
Rhinitis, 101
Rhinorrhea, 101
Rhonchi, 133b
Right ventricular enlargement, 156
Rigidity, 316t
Ringworm, 97t
Rinne test, 108, 121t, 293
Romberg test, 298

Rotator cuff, 259–260
  tear, 260–261
  tendinitis, 282t
Rovsing's sign, 192

S

Sacroiliitis, 254
Safety, 378
Salpingitis, 197t
Sarcoidosis, 140t
Sarcoma, Kaposi's, 95t
Scabies, 90t
Scale, skin, 90t
Scaphoid fracture, 263
Scapula, winging of, 304
Scar, 91t
Schizoaffective disorder, 82t
Schizophrenia, 82t
Schizophreniform disorder, 82t
Sciatica, 277t
Scoliometer, 345
Scoliosis, assessment of, 345
Screening
  for breast cancer, 168–169
  for cardiovascular disease, 148–153
  for cervical cancer, 228
  in children, 325
  for colorectal cancer, 243
  for diabetes, 150b–151b
  for dyslipidemia, 151, 152b
  for hypertension, 150
  in older adults, 377–378
  for ovarian cancer, 228
  prenatal laboratory, 363–364
  for prostate cancer, 242–243
  for skin cancer, 83, 96t
Scrotum
  abnormalities of, 218t
  edema of, 218t
  examination of, 215
  in hernia, 218t
Seborrheic keratoses, 94t, 384
Secondary prevention, 148
Seizure, 289
Self-awareness, 40
Self-care capacity, in older adults, 390t
Self-examination
  breast, 169, 173b–174b
  testicular, 214, 216b–217b
Senile ptosis, 384
Sensitivity, statistical, 25b–26b
Sensorineural hearing loss, 101, 121t, 293

Sensory system, assessment of, 13, 298–301
Serous effusion, 120t
Sexual abuse, in children, 343, 357t
Sexual history, 45
Sexual maturity ratings, in adolescents, 353t–356t
Sexually transmitted infections (STIs)
  counseling for, 213–214, 228, 243
  in females, 227–228, 231
  in males, 213–214, 219t–220t
Short stature, 329
Shortness of breath, 128, 147
Shoulder
  examination of, 259–261
  painful, 282t
Signing breathing, 65t
Sinuses
  assessment of, 11, 108
  health history of, 101–102
  in review of systems, 5
Sinusitis, 112t
Skene's gland, 225, 368
Skin, 83–98
  cancer of, 83, 94t–96t, 378
  color of, 51, 86t
  concerning symptoms, 83
  examination of, 10, 84–85
  health promotion and counseling for, 83
  in infants, 331
  lesions of, 51, 87t–94t
  nevi, 83, 96t
  in older adults, 383–384
  recording findings, 85
  in review of systems, 5
  tags, 336
Skin cancer
  ABCDE screening for, 83, 96t
  in older adults, 378
  types of, 95t–96t
Skin lesions
  assessment of, 51
  primary, 87t–90t
  secondary, 90t–92t
  vascular and purpuric, 93t–94t
Smoking
  in cardiovascular disease, 153
  in older adults, 376
  during pregnancy, 362–363
  readiness for cessation, 128b
Sneezing, 101
Social development, 324
Social history, 2b, 4
Social phobia, 80t

Sodium, food sources of, 64t
Somatoform disorders, 76t–78t
Spasticity, 316t
Specificity, statistical, 25b–26b
Speculum examination, 230–231, 368
Speech
 aphasia, 72b
 assessment of, 72
 in delirium and dementia, 391t
 development of, 324
Spermatic cord, 215, 222t
Spermatocele, 222t
Spheroidal joints, 253b
Spider angioma, 93t
Spider vein, 93t
Spinal accessory nerve, 291b, 294
Spinal cord, 286
Spinal nerve, 287
Spinal stenosis, 199
 lumbar, 277t
Spine, examination of, 266–267
Spleen, examination of, 189
Splenomegaly, 189
Spontaneous pneumothorax, 140t
Sprains, 255, 274–275, 284t
Squamous cell carcinoma, 95t, 383
Stance, assessment of, 298
Standard precautions, 14
Steatorrhea, 182
Stereognosis, 300
Sternomastoid muscles, 294
Stiffness
 back, 278t
 joint, 255
Stool, 182–183
Strabismus, 332, 339
Straight leg rise, 304
Strep throat, 102
Stress disorder, acute, 81t
Stridor, 129, 334b
Stroke
 face paralysis in, 312t
 prevention of, 289–290
 types of, 308t–309t
 vascular territories of, 310t–311t
Structural coma, 319t
Stupor, 305
Sty, 117t
Subacromial bursitis, 282t
Subarachnoid hemorrhage, 99–100, 113t, 287
Subdeltoid bursitis, 282t
Subdural hematoma, 329
Subjective data, 2b

Substance abuse, 46, 71, 363
Subtalar joint, 275
Suicide risk, 71
Summarization, 34
Supernumerary teeth, 333
Supinator reflex, 302
Sutures, cranial, 331
Swallowing, 182
Swelling
 of feet, 200
 of infant head, 331
 joint, 255
 of legs, 200
Symptoms
 seven attributes of, 3b, 38b
 unexplained and mental status, 67, 67b–68b
Syncope, 288
Syndactyly, 336
Synovial joints, 252b–253b
Syphilis
 female genital, 234t
 lip, 122t
 male genital, 220t
 primary, 220t, 234t
 secondary, 234t
 tongue, 124t
Systemic lupus erythematosus (SLE), 255
Systems review, 2b, 4–7
Systolic hypertension, isolated, 56, 382
Systolic murmur, 159

T

Tachycardia, paroxysmal supraventricular, 330
Tachypnea, 65t
Tactile fremitus, 130
Talocalcaneal joint, 275
Tangential lighting, 9
Tavistock principles, 48b
Teeth, 109
 in children, 341–342
 supernumerary, 333
Telangiectasia, hereditary hemorrhagic, 122t
Temperature, body, assessment of, 57–58
Temperature sensation, 299
Temporal muscles, 259, 293
Temporomandibular joint, examination of, 259

Index

Tendonitis, 255
  of shoulder, 282t
Tendons, 251
10-Minute Geriatric Screener, 378, 380b–381b
Tenosynovitis, 264
Tension headache, 99, 111t
Terry's nails, 98t
Testes
  abnormalities of, 221t
  cancer of, 221t
  examination of, 215
  sexual maturity ratings, 354t–355t
  small, 221t
  undescended, 336
Testicular self-examination, 214, 216b–217b
Tetralogy of Fallot, 351t–352t
Thalamus, 285
Thermometers, 58
Thorax (chest), 127–136
  anterior, 12, 134–135
  concerning symptoms, 127–128
  deformities of, 144t–145t
  disorders of, 137t–140t, 144t–146t
  examination of, 129–135
  health history, 127–128
  health promotion and counseling, 128
  in infants, 334, 334b–335b
  in older adults, 385
  posterior, 11, 130–134
  during pregnancy, 366
  recording findings, 136b
Thought content
  assessment of, 73, 392t
  defined, 69b
Thought processes
  assessment of, 73, 391t
  defined, 69b
Throat
  abnormalities of, 125t
  in children, 333, 341–342
  examination of, 11, 102, 109
  health history, 102
  in older adults, 384–385
  recording findings, 110b
  in review of systems, 5
  sore, 102, 125t
Thromboangiitis obliterans, 202
Thrombophlebitis, 203
Thrush, 333
Thumbs, examination of, 264–265

Thyroid gland
  abnormalities of, 126t
  examination of, 110
  in health history, 102
  during pregnancy, 365
TIA (transient ischemic attack), 288, 289
Tibia, torsion of the, 337
Tibial pulse, posterior, 204
Tibiofemoral joint, 270
Tibiotalar joint, 275
Tics, 315t
Tinea capitis, 97t
Tinnitus, 101
Tinsel's sign, 265
Tobacco use. *See* Smoking
Tongue
  abnormalities of, 123t–124t
  assessment of, 109
  in children, 333, 341
Tonsillitis, 109
Tonsils, 109, 342
Torsion of spermatic cord, 222t
Torsion of the tibia, 337
Torticollis, 279t
Tortuous atherosclerotic aorta, 385
Total anomalous pulmonary venous return, 335
Touch sensation, 299
Toxic-metabolic coma, 319t
Tracheal breath sounds, 132b
Tracheobronchitis, 138t, 141t
Transient ischemic attack (TIA), 288, 289
Transmitted voice sounds, 133, 133b
Transposition of the great arteries, 335, 352t
Transverse tarsal joint, 275
Trapezius muscles, 294
Traumatic flail chest, 144t
Tremors, 314t
  essential, 388
  in older adults, 388
Triceps reflex, 301
Trichomonas vaginitis, 235t
Trichotillomania, 97t
Tricuspid regurgitation, 154
Trigeminal nerve, 291b, 292–293
Trigeminal neuralgia, 113t
Trigger finger, 264
Trochanteric bursa, 268
Tuberculosis, pulmonary, 142t
Tug test, 107

Tumors
　andogen-producing, 386
　of brain, 99–100, 113t
　estrogen-producing, 387
　skin, 94t–95t
　of testis, 321t
Turgor, skin, 84, 331
Two-point discrimination, 300
Tympanic membrane temperature, 58
Tympanic percussion note, 131b
Tympanosclerosis, 120t

U

Ulcerative colitis, 195t
Ulcers
　aphthous, 124t
　arterial insufficiency, 208t
　of feet and ankles, 208t
　neuropathic, 208t
　of skin, 92t, 384
　venous insufficiency, 208t
Umbilical cord, 328
Umbilical hernia, 328
Universal precautions, 14
Upper motor neuron lesion, 301
Urethral caruncle, 230
Urethral orifice, 230
Urethritis, 183–184, 213, 230
Urinary frequency, 183
Urinary incontinence, types of, 184, 196t–197t
Urinary system
　concerning symptoms, 179b
　examination of, 183–184
　in review of systems, 6
Urinary urgency, 183
Urination, 183–184
Urine, 183
Uterus
　bicornuate, 369
　examination of, 232
　myoma of, 239t
　positions of, 239t
　during pregnancy, 367, 369
　prolapsed, 238t

V

Vagina
　adenosis of, 237t
　discharge from, 226, 235t, 343
　examination of, 231–232
Vaginitis, 235t, 343

Vaginosis, 235t
Vagus nerve, 291b, 294
Validation, 33
Validity, test, 25b
Valsalva maneuver, 159
Values, defined, 40
Varicocele, 215, 222t
Varicose veins, 204, 370
Vasovagal (vasodepressor) syncope, 288
Veins
　jugular, 154
　spider, 93t
　varicose, 124t, 204, 370
Venereal warts, 219t, 233t
Venous insufficiency, 207t–208t
Venous stasis ulcers, 200
Ventricular heart failure, left, 139t, 143t, 146t, 147, 155, 159
Ventricular hypertrophy
　left, 155, 385
　right, 156
Ventricular septal defect, 352t
Vertigo, 101, 287
Vesicle, 89t
Vesicular breath sounds, 132b
Vibration sensation, 299–300
Visceral pain, 179
Vision
　in children, 339, 340b
　disorders of, 102–103, 112t, 115t
　headaches and, 112t
　health promotion and counseling for, 102–103
　in infants, 332, 332b
　interviewing patient with impairment, 44
　in older adults, 384
Visual field defects, 115t
Vital signs
　assessment of, 10, 54–58
　blood pressure, 54–56
　in children, 330, 339
　functional status, 379–380
　heart rate and rhythm, 56–57
　in older adults, 382–383
　during pregnancy, 365
　recording findings, 60
　respiratory rate and rhythm, 57
　temperature, 57–58
Vitamin D
　food sources of, 63t
　recommended dietary intake for, 258b
Vitreous floaters, 101

Vitreous hemorrhage, 100
Vocabulary, assessment of, 74
Voice sounds, transmitted, 133, 133b
Vomiting, 181
Vulva, 233t–234t
Vulvovaginitis, 183

W

Warts, genital, 219t, 233t
Weakness, 49, 288
Weaver's bottom, 268
Weber test, 108, 121t, 293
Weight
    assessment of, 52–53
    body mass index (BMI) and, 52–54
    changes in, 50
    in children, 338
    health history, 50
    in infants, 329
    in older adults, 383
    optimal, 50–51
    during pregnancy, 361, 362b
Wheal, 88t
Wheezes, 129, 133b
Whiplash, 279t
Whispered pectoriloquy, 133, 133b
White matter, 285
Winging of scapula, 304
Wrist, 262, 264, 296

X

Xanthelasma, 117t